Psychiatry

Psychiatry

Sixth Edition

Andrew Sims and David Owens
Academic Unit of Psychiatry, University of Leeds

Baillière Tindall
London · Philadelphia · Sydney · Tokyo · Toronto

Baillière Tindall 24–28 Oval Road
W. B. Saunders London NW1 7DX

The Curtis Center
Independence Square West
Philadelphia, PA 19106–3399, USA

55 Horner Avenue
Toronto, Ontario, M8Z 4X6, Canada

Harcourt Brace Jovanovich Group
(Australia) Pty Ltd
30–52 Smidmore Street
Marrickville
NSW 2204, Australia

Harcourt Brace Jovanovich Japan Inc
Ichibancho Central Building,
22–1 Ichibancho
Chiyoda-ku, Tokyo 102, Japan

First published 1964
Fifth edition 1983
Sixth edition 1993

A catalogue record for this book is available from the British Library

ISBN 0–7020–1586–5

Typeset by Mathematical Composition Setters Ltd, Salisbury, Wiltshire
Printed and bound in Great Britain at The Bath Press, Avon

Contents

Preface

A civilized society, it has been said, can reasonably be judged by the quality of care given to its most disadvantaged members, the mentally ill. This being so, learning about the characteristics of the mentally ill, how to treat them most effectively, and how services are provided is clearly of great importance for every medical student; it is they for whom *Psychiatry* is written.

Much has changed since the last edition of this book: *Psychiatry, Concise Medical Textbooks*, 5th edition. This is reflected in comprehensive changes to its substance. All areas of psychiatry have developed over the last few years – biological, psychological and social, both in the understanding of factors which cause disorder and in methods of treatment. The terms used in psychiatric classification have also shown extensive alteration; this book is now based upon the 10th edition of the International Classification of Diseases. The practical arrangements for the delivery of mental health care is much changed, as is the ideology of carers and the expectations of those receiving treatment.

Amongst the medical profession a sophisticated level of mental health care and knowledge is now expected, not only from psychiatrists but from other hospital and public health doctors and especially from general practitioners. This has been matched by the increased prominence given to psychiatry in the undergraduate curriculum.

These developments have necessitated the changes in this new edition. Whilst maintaining the basis of descriptive psychopathology established in the past by Professor E.W. Anderson and Professor Sir William Trethowan, this has had to be somewhat abbreviated in order to accommodate much new material. As the specialty of psychiatry has developed, so any consideration that this book might be appropriate for the postgraduate trainee has now been abandoned: it is wholly directed at the medical undergraduate.

Sir William Trethowan, author, either alone or in collaboration, of the last three editions has now retired. His contribution to previous editions, as to the whole of British psychiatry, has been enormous. David Owens has joined me as author of this edition. He brings a much-needed new perspective, especially on the social aspects of psychiatry. Even between the writing of this book and its publication there have been further changes in psychiatric knowledge and practice; we expect that the subject will go on developing so that future patients will be helped even more effectively.

We are grateful to Gillies Owens (Senior Lecturer and Network Leader, Special Education Needs) and Catherine Gascoigne (Team Leader, Extended Education), both of Northumberland College of Arts and Technology, for their help with the chapter on Learning disability. For typing the many drafts of the manuscript, we also owe thanks to Monika Stephenson and Jackie Waller – both of the University of Leeds.

Andrew Sims
Leeds, 1992

1

Introduction

Mental disorders, their consequences and their treatment are given more attention and prominence in society now than in the past. There are at least four major reasons for this, and these do not include the popular but false myth that mental illness is due to the 'stress of modern life'. First, illness has always been very common, but with the eradication or successful treatment of many of the serious physical illnesses of younger life, mental illness accounts for a higher proportion of residual disability. Second, the public have become more sophisticated and make more demands for health; not only for the arrest of major disease processes, but also for a better quality of life in all areas of physical and mental functioning. Third, there has been a proliferation of both pharmacological and psychotherapeutic treatments in psychiatry. As many of these have proved effective, the expectations of the public have been further increased. Fourth, psychiatric patients with long-term disability are now more conspicuous as the old mental hospitals have either closed or decreased their numbers so that there are more patients with residual symptoms in the community.

There is no evidence that mental illness in general is more common now than in the past, or more common in developed countries than in under-developed; the evidence points to mental illnesses being of similar frequency in different parts of the world and at different times with some local differences for specific conditions.

There is a trend towards improvement of mental health in western societies, with lower rates for mental handicap and the organic conditions of childhood due to preventable diseases, less frequent occurrence of long-term effects of untreated psychosis in early adult life, and because of better obstetric care and more effective treatment of chronic infection, lowered incidence of psychiatric sequelae.

Health and illness

No simple definition of mental disorder or psychiatric illness will be universally satisfactory. In fact, the term 'mental illness' is so wide ranging as to be misleading, as it includes both conditions such as Huntington's chorea that kill prematurely after disabling for years, and the minor emotional disorders commonly seen in primary care. It is not possible to propose a single health-care strategy that includes all mental illnesses, but the following are always needed: compassion and skill from the health-care professionals, carefully conducted psychiatric research, and the provision by the authorities of adequate (and that usually means increased) resources for treatment.

To be able to decide what is *disorder* of mental equilibrium, we need to know what is *in order* or normal. However, the term 'normal' is used in many different ways and is best reserved in medicine as a statistical concept, something that is close to the mean.

A narrow definition states that mental disorder is organic disease of the brain, either structural or chemical; this is not the situation, however, with the majority of mental illnesses. Most doctors in the field of psychiatry work with an operational definition which is ultimately tautologous – that mental disorder describes the condition experienced by the people they are asked to see. It works well enough in a benevolent society where the individual with symptoms finds the appropriate helping professional, but when the state decrees who is mentally ill this distinction breaks down.

Another approach regards illness as carrying biological disadvantage by either increased mortality or decreased fecundity; that is, a reduced number of offspring. Carried into the mental disorders, one can see how this fits the major psychiatric illnesses of manic-depressive psychosis, in which there is greatly increased risk of suicide, or schizophrenia, the sufferers from which, especially males, are much less likely to procreate. However, this concept is more difficult to apply for some other mental illnesses.

The World Health Organization's definition of health, 'a state of complete physical, mental and social well-being and not merely the absence of disease or infirmity', is too comprehensive to be practical as a criterion for determining mental illness. Many people who make no complaint and would not be amenable to psychiatric treatment are far from fulfilling these criteria of health.

Illness behaviour is a sociological concept, and it implies that different people will perceive, evaluate and act upon their symptoms in different ways. Having experienced symptoms and reckoned that these amount to illness, an individual may then regard himself as ill (assume the *sick role*) and act in a way which he believes to be appropriate for that illness. Most often illness behaviour occurs with genuine disease, but sometimes the symptoms and behaviour occur when there is no underlying organic condition to account for it; any concept of mental illness needs to account for such *somatization*.

The nature of mental disorder

When mental disorder is suspected there will be disturbance of the way the person feels, especially about himself, or behaves (including, of course, verbal behaviour), or both. In practice, just diagnosing 'mental disorder' is quite inadequate, and one must look for the distinctive patterns of individual mental illnesses. There are, of course, mixed and atypical cases, and one disorder may occasionally change into another. However, *diagnosis* is just as important in psychiatry as in the rest of medicine, and there cannot be appropriate treatment without accurate diagnosis; diagnosis in psychiatry does not imply, however, a single word but a brief account of the important elements of the case, sometimes called a 'diagnostic formulation' (see Chapter 3).

Mental illness is virtually always multifactorial in nature. Even where a single causative agent can be isolated – for example, alcohol misuse – by the time the patient presents for treatment there are multiple psychological and social components in the total disorder and distress, as well as the contribution of the specific chemical and its direct biological consequences. In the assessment of all mental illness, then, biological, psychological and social factors will always need to be taken into account. We hope that the importance of these different influences in mental illnesses will be obvious throughout this book. Mental illness, even within the same diagnostic category, may present with different manifestations and different degrees of severity. This means that the patient, the patient's relatives and the doctor may all have a different impression of the patient and may be misled by symptoms. For this reason recognition of mental illness varies enormously; for example, amongst different general practitioners, a ninefold difference in identification rates of mental illness has been shown. The descriptions of illness that follow are mostly placed within diagnostic categories. However, it must be borne in mind that these categories are not totally discrete, nor immutable, and more than one condition may coexist or follow each other in the same patient. Traditionally, four major groups

Table 1.1 *Major diagnostic groups of psychiatric disorders*

1 Learning disability
2 Organic states
3 Psychoses
4 Neuroses and personality disorders

of conditions have been recognized in psychiatry, and someone coming new to the study of the subject may find it helpful, with the diagnosis of any individual patient, to consider in which of these main groups does the predominant diagnosis lie (Table 1.1)

In learning disability, there will be evidence of intellectual disability or learning difficulty established within the first 18 months of life and this will have affected the subsequent life course. Organic states are identifiable when a disease of the brain or generalized illness affecting the brain has resulted in a disordered mental state. In psychoses, the major examples of which are manic-depressive psychosis and schizophrenia, there is a disturbance in the patient's judgement of reality and this results in symptoms and disturbances in behaviour and daily living. With neuroses, personality disorders and related conditions, the difference from normal behaviour and experience is quantitative rather than qualitative. These conditions, which include anxiety states and much of the depressive disorder encountered in primary care, occur in about one-sixth of the population within any year.

History of psychiatry

Descriptions of mentally ill people and the effect they had on those around them go back to earliest times. From an ancient Egyptian papyrus comes the expression 'Kneeling of the mind' as an eloquent description of depression. Similarly, a mad person was described as 'the man who is between the hands of the gods'. Mental illness is a much neglected factor in human history. Too little attention has been given to the way psychiatric symptoms may

have influenced the behaviour and decisions of prominent people, and how notions about mental illness and, for instance, witchcraft, may have affected the actions of the populace. What we know of the mental state of King Henry VIII of England would support the presumed diagnosis of neurosyphilis; how much did this mould the far-reaching decisions he made? We know that the recurrent psychotic illness of George III had a marked influence upon psychiatry and the way the mentally ill were treated subsequently. How much did the misidentification of mentally ill old women in New England in the late seventeenth century as being 'demon-possessed' affect not only their own lives but the quality of life of the whole community?

It would be inappropriate for this book to do more than point out some of the historical themes. The institution became central for the practice of humane management in the nineteenth century. Originally, the intention was to protect the mentally ill who were exposed both to danger and exploitation by providing *asylum*, a safe place away from the big city; there were also overtones of custodial containment so that the rest of society would not see them. Mental health law and social attitudes to the mentally ill have always been influential and have often lagged behind the innovations of the reformers. A recurring dilemma is the conflict between freedom for the individual and restraint for his own and others' protection. Treatment from earliest times has oscillated from the organic, biological, pharmacological to the previously magical, and now more psychosocial type of management. Good practice has usually been typified by both approaches. For a more detailed look at the development of psychiatry in Britain from the middle of the nineteenth century, readers are referred to Berrios and Freeman (1991).

The significance of mental disorder

For the individual sufferer mental illness completely dominates every aspect of life. Feelings about oneself, capacity for activity and all areas of social relationships are affected, including the family, marriage, sexual activity, work, recreation, management of finances, relationship with the law, public life and so on. There are usually two main components in psychiatric complaint; dissatisfaction about how the individual feels concerning themselves, and impairment of the capacity for equal and mutually rewarding relationships.

The study of abnormal states of mind is known as psychopathology; that is, the systematic study of abnormal experience and behaviour. *Descriptive psychopathology* describes and categorizes the abnormal experiences as recounted by the patient and observed in his behaviour. The psychiatrist attempts to observe and understand the psychic events, so that the observer can, as far as possible, know for himself what the patient's experience must feel like. *Explanatory psychopathology* goes a step further but does so on tricky ground; it attempts to explain the symptoms or behaviour on the basis of preconceived theoretical formulations; for example, psychoanalysis. *Experimental psychopathology* explores the relationships between abnormal phenomena by inducing a change in one and observing associated changes in others; for example, what happens to a schizophrenic patient's experience of hearing voices when 'white noise' is played into the ear in which voices are normally heard? This enables hypotheses to be formulated and tested in further experiments. This is clearly the way to proceed in understanding both of the above two types of psychopathology. We are, however, at a very early stage in this process in psychiatry.

The mentally ill have suffered in almost all societies, not only from the distressing symptoms inside their own minds and the personal consequences of their own disturbed behaviour, but also from the marked stigma that has been attached to mental illness. Rejection, ostracism, derision, concealment and active persecution have sometimes been the lot of the mentally ill, and their families have suffered shame, humiliation and financial loss because of their sick member. The mentally ill have often been punished for psychotic behaviour or the consequences of phobic ideas, and they have almost always been misunderstood. It is probable that the stigma attached to mental illness has been one of the major factors holding back the development of psychiatry as a specialty. Mental health charities giving research grants receive less money in donations than animal charities. Resources going into mental health as a percentage of all hospital spending in the United Kingdom decreased in the thirty years since 1960. Recruitment to psychiatry amongst medical graduates was in the past inhibited not only by misgivings of the potential candidate's family, but also by ridicule from senior members of the medical profession; thankfully, this has now much reduced. The mentally ill themselves have been subjected to all sorts of indignities and disadvantages. We now have much better care and treatment for the mentally ill and the prognosis for most mental illnesses has improved, yet some stigma remains.

Psychiatric care in different settings

In the last thirty years there has been a quiet, but comprehensive revolution in the care of the mentally ill, the setting in which it takes place, and the range of treatments available. In the past a sufferer from a serious mental illness, such as schizophrenia, was likely to be admitted to hospital during the acute onset of the first episode of the illness and might then remain in mental hospital for decades, if not for the rest of his life. A sufferer from a minor psychiatric disorder such as neurotic illness was likely to receive no treatment at all. The range and diversity of treatment settings has increased enormously, as have the strategies and methods of treating different psychiatric conditions. This is exemplified by changes in the mental hospital population (see Figures 1.1 and 1.2).

Figures 1.1 and 1.2 demonstrate what has happened to inpatient numbers in psychiatric hospitals over a century. During the nineteenth century following the County Asylums Act (1808), mental hospitals or county lunatic asylums, as they were then known, were built and progressively increased in size. The numbers continued to increase, with only small diminution during the two world wars, until

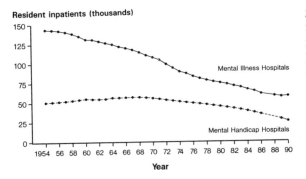

Resident inpatients (thousands)

Figure 1.1 Inpatients resident in mental illness hospitals, England and Wales (1954–90)

greater diversity in the types of hospital accommodation and other settings available for treatment. The price of greater freedom for patients, however, has been an increase in the number of those who are psychiatrically ill and incarcerated in prison or alternatively homeless and uncared for.

Psychiatric inpatient units may be found both in mental hospitals, now considerably reduced in size, and in district general hospitals. The development of psychiatric units in district general hospitals has followed the recognition that psychiatry needs to be drawn closer to the rest of medicine and needs to share many of the facilities found in the hospital. The mental hospitals themselves have changed enormously, with much of the original hospital land, including farms and other small industries, sold off for building land or motorways. Within the hospital buildings, many wards have been emptied or replaced with other functions and the number of patients on each ward has been vastly reduced. Most of the wards in a mental hospital in the 1990s will be receiving acute

reaching a peak in the mid-1950s. There were then several major changes occurring at about the same time and reversing the previous trend. These were the introduction of neuroleptic drugs in the mid-1950s; a new Mental Health Act altering the legal status of patients; improvement in attitude towards the mentally ill following pioneering work in some mental hospitals; and changes in expectations of both patients and their relatives. There is now much

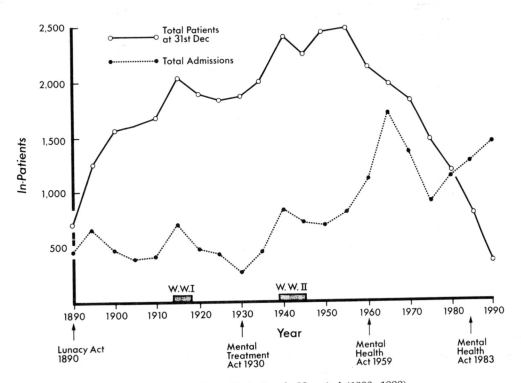

Figure 1.2 Patients resident on 31 December, High Royds Hospital (1890–1990)

admissions, and a third of patients are aged over 65.

With the move into the community and the knocking down, often actually, of the walls of the mental hospital, has come increasing recognition of a need to deal appropriately, for their own safety and for the safety of others, with those patients who are behaviourally disturbed, potentially violent and who exhibit 'challenging' behaviour. A range of facilities are now usually available, with part of some psychiatric hospitals offering a greater level of security, a higher level of staffing and concentrating only upon such patients in an intensive care unit. There are also Regional Secure Units treating the mentally ill who have come into contact with the law and are potentially disturbed or violent. Special Hospitals take, in the main, patients who have exhibited a high level of dangerousness.

There has been a great increase over the last twenty years in the numbers and diversity of placements in Day Hospitals and Day Centres. It has been recognized that rehabilitation can be carried out more effectively in many instances if the patient is living at home at night and at the weekends and is receiving treatment directed towards his reintegration into society during the day. There are also conditions, particularly the neurotic disorders, for which admission as an inpatient to hospital may reinforce symptoms that can better be removed using a model of relearning rather than of passive submission to treatment.

Outpatient care has also increased in importance and diversified. There is now a wider range of conditions that may appropriately be treated in the outpatient department, and the methods of treatment available and the mental health disciplines giving such treatment have also increased. The scale of this increase is shown in Figure 1.3.

One of the most marked changes in the delivery of mental health care has been the emphasis placed recently upon care in the community. This has involved a range of services and treatment being provided in the patient's own home, and also mental health assessment and treatment being carried out in smaller centres and units within the local community.

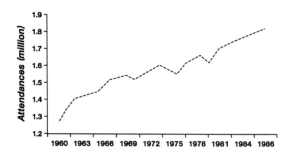

Figure 1.3 Mental illness outpatient attendances, England and Wales (1960–86)

Increasingly, many psychiatrists work for some of their time in general practice health centres, either seeing new patients or previous patients for follow-up interviews or discussing problem situations and cases with the general practitioners and associated health centre staff. Child psychiatry has, for many years, been carried out at least in part in child and family centres and this has necessitated close working relationships with other professional staff. The various changes in the care of patients in different settings has necessitated changes in the practice of psychiatry, particularly a much greater emphasis on multidisciplinary working. Psychiatrists now regularly work with community psychiatric nurses, social workers, occupational therapists and clinical psychologists and often also with physiotherapists, dietitians and other healthcare workers. It is imperative that psychiatrists have a good working relationship with the general practitioners in the geographical area they both serve, and it is important for them together to work out which part of the total care for their patients they will each provide.

Education in psychiatry

Education in the evaluation and treatment of mental disorders now starts at the medical undergraduate stage. Practising doctors in all specialties will have some contact with mental illness and the symptoms and changes in behaviour it causes. It is now recognized that the behavioural sciences, including psychology, sociology and social anthropology, are important in pre-clinical training. These, with the neurosciences, form the essential basic scientific background for the subsequent acquisition of psychiatric theory. Some relevant knowledge of philosophy and medical ethics is also important.

Subsequent psychiatric knowledge and understanding are based upon psychopathology and epidemiology. Psychopathology is described and defined in Chapter 2. Epidemiology – that is, how illnesses are distributed in populations – is of crucial importance in understanding the natural history, prognosis and treatment of different psychiatric conditions in different societies and groups.

Learning about psychiatric diagnosis and treatment can only take place effectively in a clinical situation. Ideally, this will involve hospital and community settings, and the student should be encouraged to see and help in the treatment of patients under the supervision of a senior and experienced psychiatrist who is enthusiastic about, and prepared to give time to, teaching. The learning of interviewing skills, always an essential part of undergraduate psychiatry, is valuable also for other areas of medicine, and the examination of mental state and full history-taking have wider application than just psychiatry.

The attitudes of the doctor are supremely important in helping patients with mental illness. It is an uncomfortable fact for the psychiatrist, and also for the medical undergraduate learning psychiatry, that we have to look at ourselves and our attitudes before we can be of any use to our patients. In psychiatric treatment the aim may be relief of symptoms, decrease in the risk of suicide, enabling the person to function more effectively or helping the patient to accept themselves as they are. Treatment may, on occasions, be long-term and the results of treatment and the degree of change possible may be frustratingly slight. Dealing with psychiatric patients, especially with those who are suffering from neurotic disorders, is personally challenging to the student and to the doctor, perhaps because their own doubts and neurotic fears may tend to re-emerge. For these reasons part of education in psychiatry is to look at one's own attitudes, personal philosophy and means of emotional support. Psychiatry is probably the most interesting and challenging specialty for the doctor, whether it is practised alongside another area of medicine or as a psychiatrist; that is the opinion of the authors!

Further reading

Berrios, G.E. and Freeman, H. (1991) *150 Years of British Psychiatry 1841–1991*, London: Gaskell.

Clare, A.W. (1976) *Psychiatry in Dissent: Controversial Issues in Thought and Practice*, London: Tavistock.

Gelder, M., Gath, D. and Mayou, R. (1989) *Oxford Textbook of Psychiatry*, 2nd edn, Oxford: Oxford University Press.

Kendell, R.E. and Zealley, A.K. (1988) *Companion to Psychiatric Studies*, 4th edn, Edinburgh: Churchill Livingstone.

Wing, J.K. (1978) *Reasoning about Madness*, Oxford: Oxford University Press.

2

Psychopathology

The twin bases of psychiatric knowledge are epidemiology – that is, the distribution of diseases or syndromes in defined populations – and psychopathology. *Psychopathology* is the systematic study of abnormal experience, cognition (the use of knowledge, hence intellectual processes) and behaviour. Examination of the mental state is therefore the equivalent of the detailed physical examination in general medicine.

Diagnosis, in medicine, categorizes problems in order to solve or ameliorate them using appropriate techniques and skills. The diagnosis indicates what this individual patient holds in common with some others, and thus suggests that a successful treatment plan used for somebody else with the same diagnosis may well lead to benefit in this case also. A detailed history and a careful examination are the essentials for making a diagnosis in general medicine; so it is in psychiatry, the examination concentrating upon the mental state. The symptoms and signs of mental illness are elicited, and the skilful use of descriptive psychopathology adds precision to this. To say that a patient is miserable is informative, but tells you little about how he may be helped. To describe him as suffering from a depressive episode as part of a manic-depressive illness suggests to the psychiatrist ways in which this man's suffering may be relieved.

Every medical student knows that *symptoms* are the complaints which the patient makes and *signs* are the indicators of illness that the doctor finds on examination. This is still a valid distinction for psychiatry, but both symptoms and signs may be revealed in the conversation of the patient. Symptoms are the complaints; for example, 'I feel miserable'. The signs are the way the patient's speech indicate abnormalities of psychological functioning with or without the patient being aware that this abnormality exists. For instance, when a patient says that he is able to increase the power of the sun by taking all his clothes off, his statement is a sign indicating the presence of delusion. Both symptoms and signs are important in psychiatry, for making the diagnosis and also for establishing the relationship between patient and therapist.

The abnormal experiences of the patient can be accounted for in a number of different ways. The chief difference is between those methods that seek to *explain* the abnormal behaviour in terms of underlying theoretical constructs, and *descriptive psychopathology*, which avoids underlying theoretical explanations of cause (Figure 2.1). Descriptive psychopathology describes and categorizes the abnormal experiences as recounted by the patient and observed in his behaviour. Observation of *behaviour* needs to be both meticulous and informed; for instance, both noticing the stereotyped behaviour of a schizophrenic patient and knowing its significance.

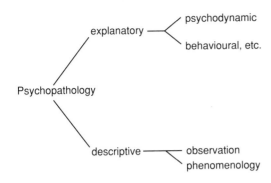

Figure 2.1 Psychopathology

Phenomenology, in psychiatry, is the observation and categorization of abnormal psychic events, the internal experiences of the patient, in order to understand them so that the observer can, as far as possible, know for himself what the patient's experience must feel like. It is not possible for me to observe my patient's hallucination, nor is it possible for him to recognize that what he is hearing is auditory hallucination. What I can do is try to understand what he is describing using the human characteristics I hold in common with him: that is, the ability to perceive, a common language and shared capacity for emotional experience. From him is required a detailed description of his internal experience.

Listening and observing are crucial for understanding, and great care must be taken in asking precise questions. *Empathy* is the ability to feel oneself into the situation of the other person, and the method of empathy implies asking appropriate, persistent and insightful questions so that the patient is able to describe exactly what he is experiencing, and the doctor is able to understand this description and use his capacity for empathy to recreate this experience in his own mind. Finally, the doctor describes this experience back to the patient in such a clear way that the patient recognizes it as being his own internal experience. This is the essential starting place for the skilled use of empathy as a tool in psychopathology.

An important distinction for psychopathology was made by the German psychiatrist Jaspers, between *understanding* and *explanation*. Explanation is the usual business of science, using external senses and observation to make causal connections by following a chain of events. Understanding, in Jaspers' sense, involves empathy in that we are able to understand the patient's subjective experience by using our own capacity as human beings.

When my patient, involved as a policeman in a major disaster, informs me that he feels homicidal anger towards his superiors, explanation involves listing the causes for his emotion; understanding involves my putting myself into his position, his background and feelings at the time, and trying to empathize with his current state of frustration, misery, alienation and impotent rage.

It is important also to make the distinction between *form and content*. The form of the psychic experience is the description of its structure in psychopathological terms; for example, an hallucination. Content is the colouring of the experience or the description of it which the patient actually gives. My patient tells me that he has a message that he is 'to root out the Angel of Death'. When I discuss this with him further he says that he is hearing a voice from outside his head which is deep and masculine, and seems to come from above and behind him, and this voice is giving him orders. The form is of an auditory hallucination; the content is that this voice is a message, and what the message actually says. The form is of diagnostic value; hallucinations occur in certain psychiatric conditions and are highly unlikely in others. The content is determined by the individual's background experience and his predominant interests; it has social and cultural determinants.

Organic change and psychopathology

In Chapter 7, on organic states, are described methods of examining the cognitive state which assess whether there is organic impairment of mental function. Generalized disorder of the brain regularly produces particular mental abnormalities irrespective of the precise nature of the brain disease. Of course, localized disturbance of the brain will also produce specific symptoms typical for that neuro-anatomical site or function. Psychopathology is concerned with observing the behaviour and describing the subjective state of patients, and with aggregating symptoms that commonly occur to indicate syndromes or disorders. Much progress is still to be made in relating these symptoms to particular neuropathological or neurochemical disturbance. Amongst organic disturbances some symptoms are regularly found, and these symptoms can be somewhat similar to the disturbances that may occur in conditions that are not organically mediated; part of the usefulness of precise psycho-pathology is to make the distinction between these different types of symptoms. A patient after severe head injury may suffer from memory loss; a recently arrested offender may say that he cannot remember what he has done or where he has been. It is a not unreasonable task for the psychopathologist to make the dis-tinction between these two different accounts of disturbed memory.

Consciousness is a state of awareness of the self and the environment; it implies an inner aware-ness of experience, the capacity to react to objects intentionally, and a knowledge of a conscious self. To be unconscious is to have no subjective experience, and this can take three quite different forms, as demonstrated in Figure 2.2. A person can be in full normal conscious-ness, or they can be in an intermediate state of partial consciousness, or they can be wholly unconscious because they are (1) in coma, or (2) in deep sleep, or (3) totally unaware of the object of attention. In each of these the term 'unconscious' is legitimately used, but the organic state of the brain is totally different for these three situations. The word 'conscious' only becomes meaningful when one takes into account the object of which the person is conscious, what he is aware of; this is the only way this function can be tested.

Consciousness can be assessed quantitatively on a continuum from full alertness and aware-ness in normal consciousness to coma. In *clouding of consciousness*, a lesser stage of impair-ment, there is difficulty with thinking, attention, perception, memory and usually drowsiness

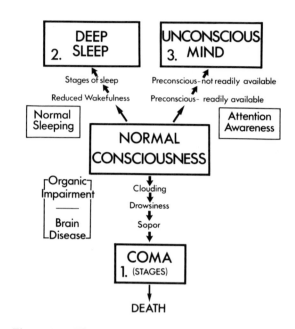

Figure 2.2 Three meanings of unconsciousness

but sometimes excitability. In *drowsiness*, the patient is slow in action and in speech, sluggish in intent and sleepy in subjective experience. Without stimulation the patient will drift into 'sleep'. In *sopor*, the next deepening stage, the patient is mostly unconscious, but strong stimuli will momentarily return him to responsiveness. In *coma*, the patient is no longer rousable but deeply unconscious. Coma itself has a succession of increasing stages culminating in *brain death*.

Some of the terminology used about qualitative changes of consciousness is much complicated by the way different authors use the same word with subtly different meanings. It is recom-mended that the word '*delirium*' is used to describe an acute organic impairment of the brain in which there is severe disturbance of consciousness and also abnormality of percep-tion and mood. The patient is preoccupied with the experience and so there is lack of attention to the outside world; illusions and hallucina-tions frequently occur; delusions may also occur. There is a disturbance of mood which may vary from stark terror to frivolous buf-foonery. *Delirium tremens*, especially associated with withdrawal of alcohol, is one form of this condition and shows the characteristic features (see Chapter 7).

The term *'confusion of thinking'* is very misleading, even confusing! It should be used simply to describe subjective disturbance of the thinking process and not as a term pathognomonic of organic psychosyndromes. It may occur in organic states or functional psychoses, and is also associated with powerful emotion in neurotic disorders: 'I feel confused in my thinking.'

Attention is the active or passive focusing of consciousness upon an experience. *Concentration* is the deliberate maintaining of this focus of consciousness upon an experience or on the task in hand. *Orientation* is an awareness of one's setting in time and place, and of one's personal identity. Attention describes an observation of another person's state from outside, whilst *awareness* is that person's own description of the same state. These functions are particularly disturbed by organic disease of the brain, but also occur in other psychiatric conditions even with life crises.

Attention may be decreased in normal people in sleep, fatigue and boredom. It may be altered in psychogenic states, such as in hysterical dissociation or in organic states with lowering of consciousness; for example, after head injury or in an acute toxic state with alcohol. *Narrowing* of attention occurs with depressive illness. *Loss of attention* occurs in the hyperkinetic syndrome of childhood.

Orientation, then, is the capacity of a person to know what is real in his current setting in time, space and person. Impaired orientation is usually indicative of either an acute or chronic organic state. It indicates loss of *intellectual grasp*, in that the perceptual cues on which an individual makes judgements are misinterpreted. Characteristically, *disorientation* may fluctuate during the day and is worse in the evening and at night. Disorientation for time occurs at an early stage in the illness, with space disturbed at a later stage, and for person usually only in a very advanced organic state.

Evaluating *memory disorder* is useful, as it shows that different functions of memory may be disturbed in different types of condition:

- *Registration* is the capacity to add new information to the memory store – disturbance is exemplified by a person with alcohol intoxication having no memory for their activities during consciousness the previous evening, even when they are reminded of what they did;

- *Retention* is the ability to store knowledge which can subsequently be returned to consciousness – retention can be divided into immediate, recent and remote memory – impairment of recent memory is characteristic of early dementia of any type;

- *Retrieval* is the capacity to return stored material from memory – impairment is particularly characteristic of the memory disorder of amnesic syndrome (Korsakov Syndrome; Chapter 8);

- *Recall* is the return of stored remembered information into consciousness at a chosen moment – failure of recall is characteristic of psychogenic memory disturbance (for example, an inability to remember an eponymous disease during a medical viva examination!);

- *Recognition* is the feeling of familiarity which accompanies the return of stored material to consciousness.

- *Confabulation* is a falsification of memory occurring in clear consciousness in association with organically derived amnesia. It is particularly frequent early in the course of Korsakov Syndrome following chronic alcohol abuse. A confabulating patient, thirty years after the end of World War II, claimed that she had been down to the Food Office the day before to collect her ration book. Suggestibility is prominent in confabulation, with the patient including the interviewer's suggested material into answers and questions. Actual experiences are often remembered but taken out of their chronological order; for instance, a 65-year-old woman who said that her baby was crying all the previous night.

- *Perseveration* is a response that was appropriate to a first stimulus being given inappropriately to a second, different stimulus. This may be shown verbally or in motor activity. It is often demonstrated quite by accident during the history and mental state examination. For example, when a patient was asked where he was born, he said 'Accrington'. Shortly afterwards, when asked where he was working, he repeated 'Accrington' inappropriately and mistakenly.

Disorder of the sense of *time* may also occur in both organic psychiatric conditions and in psychogenic states. The three functions of importance are an ability to separate events into past, present and future, the capacity to estimate duration of time, and the ability to put events in sequence. These are necessary for intellectual processes to be carried out. Obviously, disorder of time sense is intimately connected with disturbance of consciousness, attention and memory.

Pathology of perception

For psychiatric diagnosis the most significant abnormality of perception is undoubtedly *hallucination*. However, the importance of detailed psychopathology in this area lies in the ability it gives the clinician to decide what is and what is not hallucination.

Abnormalities of perception are usually described in terms of sensory distortions and false perceptions. *Sensory distortions* include alterations in the intensity and quality of perception. For instance, heightened intensity of auditory perception is called *hyperacusis*. The patient does not hear better than usual, but he complains that sounds are uncomfortably loud. It is found in depressive illness, associated with migraine, and particularly with toxic states such as the 'hangover' following alcohol excess. The quality of perception may also be altered in abnormal mental states; for example, changes in colour may be described by subjects taking mescaline or LSD, changes in shape by patients with parietal lobe lesions.

In *false perception*, which includes illusion, hallucination and pseudohallucination, objects are perceived without an appropriate stimulus. In illusion, the object is misinterpreted through fantasy; the frightened child believes the curtains blowing are an armed intruder.

Hallucination is a false perception without an external causative object. It is not a distortion of a real perception but something new, and it may occur simultaneously with and alongside real perception. It has no external stimulus, but the subjective experience is identical to normal perception; so what the doctor as an observer calls hallucination, the patient as sufferer experiences as an entirely normal sensory experience: subjectively it is indistinguishable from normal perception. The sensory experience that is considered to be hallucination by others is not corroborated by a sensation in any other sensory modality and so the individual has to account for this in their explanation of their own experience. Thus a patient hearing an hallucinatory voice, but seeing no one in the room, may explain it by saying, 'There must be an electronic device', or, perhaps, 'It is spirits that are causing the sound'.

Hallucinations can take place at the same time as normal sensory stimuli, and more than one hallucination may be experienced at the same time, or in rapid succession. Attention will not remove the hallucination. Although hallucination may occur in any of the sensory modalities, *auditory hallucinations* are the commonest and they have the greatest diagnostic significance. 'Hearing voices' is particularly characteristic of schizophrenia. It is especially so when the voices are in the third person and they say the patient's own thoughts out aloud, or they give a running commentary on the patient's actions, or they argue or discuss vigorously with each other. Hearing voices, usually of single words or second person imperatives, may also occur with chronic alcoholic hallucinosis, or with affective psychoses. The patient does not necessarily describe them as 'voices', but may talk of them as 'messages' or in some other way.

Visual hallucinations are particularly characteristic of organic states. These may be a result of abnormalities of the visual pathways or occipital lobes in which it may be difficult or impossible to distinguish hallucination from sensory distortion. Visual hallucinations commonly occur in acute organic disturbance such as delirium tremens, in the post-concussional state, in epileptic twilight states and in various metabolic disturbances such as hepatic failure.

They may also occur in toxic states from glue- or petrol-sniffing or with drugs such as lysergic acid diethylamide (LSD).

Hallucinations of *bodily sensation* occur and may be superficial, kinaesthetic or visceral. *Superficial* hallucinations may be abnormal perceptions of heat or cold (thermic), or touch (haptic) or of fluid (hygric) on the skin. *Kinaesthetic hallucinations* are false perceptions of the muscle or joint sense. The patient may describe his limbs as being bent or twisted, or his muscles squeezed. *Visceral* hallucinations are false perceptions of the organs; for example, pain or heaviness or stretching. These hallucinations of bodily sensation occur in schizophrenic illness and may be described in bizarre terms with the characteristic experience of passivity; that is, the individual believes his bodily sensation to be influenced by forces outside himself: 'I can feel my brain being stretched in sheets down my spinal column.'

Olfactory hallucinations – that is, of smell – and *gustatory* hallucinations – of taste – may occur in schizophrenia, associated with epilepsy or in other organic states. It is important to make the distinction between olfactory hallucination in which the patient has a false perception of smell, from delusion of smell in which the patient may believe he or she smells without having any associated perception.

It is important to know of the existence of *pseudohallucination*, in which the perception is experienced as located in subjective space, and hence perceived with the 'inner eye' (or ear). It usually has an 'as if' quality and the experience is figurative, not concrete or real; so the person with such an experience would not expect others around him to share his experience. He knows that it depends upon his previous life history and background for its own existence. Characteristic of pseudohallucination is the experience occurring after bereavement, in which a normal, healthy widow has a full and vivid experience of the lost spouse's presence, visually or auditorally, but knows at the same time that this is pictorial and in inner space: 'I heard his laugh in the next room.'

False beliefs

These include *primary* and *secondary delusions, over-valued ideas* and *sensitive ideas of reference*. A delusion is a false, unshakeable idea or belief which is out of keeping with the patient's educational, cultural and social background; it is held with extraordinary conviction and subjective certainty. As far as the subjective belief of the person holding the delusion is concerned, delusion is indistinguishable from any other idea that he may hold, and quite different from fantasy. Delusions are therefore not *imaginary beliefs*. Delusion has been regarded as a fundamental feature of the legal definition of insanity or mental illness (see page 226).

An *over-valued idea* is an acceptable, comprehensible idea pursued by the individual beyond the bounds of reason. It is usually associated with abnormal personality. *Morbid jealousy* is quite frequently manifested as an over-valued idea. A man wonders if his wife is being unfaithful to him. He takes time off work and hires a car that she will not recognize to follow her when she goes into town. He checks her underwear, he arrives home unexpectedly in the middle of the day, he asks their young children whether there have been any visitors. In fact, he goes to totally unreasonable lengths to check on his wife's behaviour. This man has an abnormality of personality of paranoid type. In psychiatry the word 'paranoid' means *self-referent* and is not limited to persecutory; thus a patient who believes that everybody around him secretly believes he is the king is still suffering from paranoid – that is, self-referent – delusions.

Sensitive ideas of reference ascribe the situation in which a person consistently believes that other people are against him, belittling him, making derogatory remarks about him or showing evidence of disliking him. It is not a false perception in that he does not actually hear people speaking against him, nor is it a delusion in that he is not absolutely convinced of any particular thing that has happened, but just aware of a general atmosphere of opposition. Such ideas are frequently associated with abnormality of personality, of sensitive or anankastic type (Chapter 13).

The distinction between *primary* and *secondary delusions* is complicated by the terms 'primary' and 'secondary' being used in different ways by different authors. It is best to reserve the term '*primary*' for the implication that delusion is not occurring in response to another psychopathological form such as mood disorder. It is ultimately, therefore, not understandable in the sense that we can put ourselves into the position of a single woman with concerns about sex and violence, but we cannot understand how the *form* of her experience is delusion: 'that people are coming through the locked door at night, when I am asleep, and raping me'.

Secondary delusion implies that the false idea is understandable in terms of the mood state or the background cultural context; so when a detailed psychiatric history and examination is made, one can understand the delusion. A depressed clergyman believes himself to be eternally damned. The belief becomes understandable in terms of the mood state and the background cultural context. Secondary delusions can be seen to have their origins in the life circumstances of the individual, their current mood state, the beliefs of their peer group and the characteristics of their personality. There is no difference in subjective experience, as far as the individual sufferer is concerned, between primary and secondary delusions. It is a psychopathological distinction.

Delusion is an idea or an intuition that arises in the same way as any other idea; that is, it may appear to occur spontaneously, it may arise as the result of perception, or as a result of mood, or from memory. *Autochthonous delusion*, delusional intuition (sudden delusional idea), is a delusion which seems to arise suddenly, out of the blue. For instance, without any obvious cause a patient quite suddenly came to believe that he had stumbled upon a plot to overthrow the world. A *delusional percept* occurs when the patient has a normal perception but this is interpreted with delusional meaning which has immense personal significance; that is, abnormal, personal meaning attached to a real, external percept. It is self-referent, momentous, urgent and carries overwhelming personal significance. A single man was offered a sausage for breakfast in a boarding house. He

immediately knew when he saw the sausage that everybody else regarded him as homosexual. In *delusional atmosphere* the patient believes that everything in his environment is sinister, peculiar and altered in a subtle way. He has a feeling of anticipation and misinterprets his surroundings. Sometimes this is called 'delusional mood' as it is the mood of anticipation, excitement or foreboding which is the prominent feature. *Delusional memory* describes the situation where the patient 'remembers' an event or idea that is clearly delusional in nature; these are sometimes called 'retrospective delusions'.

Delusions vary enormously in their content, but some types occur regularly. The content is determined by the emotional, social and cultural background of a patient. Soon after the first, actual moon landing psychiatrists began to see patients who believed that they had been sent to the moon and back! Some of the commonly occurring contents are listed in Table 2.1. Delusions of *persecution* are probably the most frequently described of all delusional contents. *Morbid jealousy* is the pathological development, most often in the form of an over-valued idea, of a normal human emotion; the psychotic form of morbid jealousy is a delusion of *infidelity*. Amongst delusions of love, *erotomania* describes the patient loving a person in a delusional and destructive way, *De Clérambault's Syndrome*

Table 2.1   *Content of delusions*

Delusion of perception
   delusion of prejudice
Morbid jealousy
   delusion of infidelity
Delusion of love (erotomania)
   De Clérambault's Syndrome
Delusional misidentification
   Capgras Syndrome
Grandiose delusion
Religious delusion
Delusion of guilt and unworthiness
Delusion of poverty
Nihilistic delusion
Hypochondriacal delusion
Delusion of infestation
Shared delusion
   folie à deux
Delusion of control

describes the situation when the patient has a delusional belief that a person, usually older and of higher social status than herself, is in love with her. In delusional *misidentification*, or the Capgras Syndrome, the patient believes that someone close to him has been replaced by an impostor, perceptually identical with the real person, and pretending to be that person.

In *grandiose delusions* the patient believes himself to be a famous person or to have enormous powers; a variant of this is delusion of *special purpose* in which the individual believes himself to be called to some quite extraordinary feat of intellect or valour. In *religious delusions* the content of the belief clearly arises from the patient's background, social context and religious experiences; they are, therefore, more frequent in a devout than in a secular society.

Delusions of *guilt* and *unworthiness* are particularly associated with depressive illness. They often totally dominate thought and may result in suicide. Delusions of *poverty* are also characteristic of depressive illness, as are *nihilistic* delusions, in which the depressive tendency to see everything as negative is taken to its ultimate limit and the patient believes that he himself, a part of himself, or other parts of his surroundings, do not exist (see Chapter 5). *Hypochondriasis* is a description of content, preoccupation with health or symptoms of illness. When this takes the form of delusion it is a *hypochondriacal* delusion.

In delusional *infestation*, the patient believes that he is infested with small but macroscopic organisms; this may be associated with tactile hallucinations in some cases. *Shared delusion* (*folie à deux*) occurs when a delusion is transferred from one person who is undoubtedly psychotic (the principal), to another (the associate) who lives in close association with the principal. Whether this delusion persists depends on the mental state of the associate; if that person is not psychotic, the symptom is likely to remit on separation from the principal. Delusion of *control* (passivity or made experiences) is an important indication of the presence of schizophrenia. The patient believes that his thinking or his activity is influenced from outside himself.

Thought disorder

Three types of disorder of the thinking process are different phenomenologically: formal thought disorder, disorder of language and speech, and intellectual retardation. *Formal thought disorder* is the subjective experience of the patient himself that his thinking processes are in some way disturbed. Disturbance in thinking may be described in the speed or flow of thought or, alternatively, in insertions into the thinking process. The speed of thinking may be speeded up as in mania, or slowed down as in depression. The flow of thoughts may appear interrupted as in derailment, or stopped altogether as in thought blocking. The thinking process may be described as being interfered with from outside the patient in schizophrenia; for example, *thought withdrawal* where the patient believes thoughts are being taken out of his mind, or *thought insertion* where the patient believes they are being put in.

The two ways that we can know about the thinking processes of our patients are to ask the patient to introspect on his mechanisms of thinking and to analyse the products of thought that are manifested in speech. In considering this latter, there is a need to make a clear distinction between speech and language. Speech is the production of communicated sound, whilst language is the message which is actually conveyed; these two obviously overlap to a considerable extent. The *speech disorders* which are commonly encountered in psychiatry include *aphonia*, where there is a loss of the ability to vocalize and the patient therefore whispers; *dysarthria*, where there is difficulty in articulation; and *stuttering*, where the syllables are not produced in an even flow. *Echolalia* is the repetition by the patient of words or parts of sentences in a meaningless rather than an emphatic fashion. *Logoclonia* is the spastic repetition of syllables which sometimes occurs in Parkinsonism. *Aphasia* implies the loss of language, impairment of, or difficulty with, language. It is usually divided into receptive or sensory types, and motor or expressive types. Very often these are mixed. Aphasias normally occur associated with organic lesions of the brain, and determining the type of language disorder may enable localization of the lesion to be made.

Schizophrenic language disorder is a highly complex subject and research has been conducted in a number of different ways. Suffice it to say that schizophrenic patients tend to use unusual words in unusual sequences or sentences and there are certain patterns of deviation from the norm which occur frequently; for example *neologism* or creating new words, and *stock words* and *phrases*, using known words with a greater range of meaning than they normally carry. There are various other types of destruction of language which occur. Impoverishment of language may, of course, indicate that the patient has intellectual impairment or difficulty with learning. Although inheritance and organic factors in early life are important causes of intellectual impairment, sensory and social deprivation may also impair subsequent intellectual performance.

Disorder of the boundaries of self is the inability to know where *I* ends and *not I* begins. This is highly characteristic of the first-rank symptoms of schizophrenia (Chapter 6), in which loss of boundaries of self may be seen as fundamental. There appears to be invasion of self from influences outside and the ability to influence what is outside from inside the self.

Depersonalization is a change in the awareness of self in which the individual feels as if he is unreal or altered. It is often accompanied by *derealization*, which denotes a similar change in the awareness of the external world, things outside the self or a specific object in the external environment. The *'as if'* feeling is a very important part of depersonalization and derealization. The patient has extraordinary difficulty in describing the symptom and is very embarrassed to do so because he often feels that the symptom is unique and indicates madness. It is subjectively extremely unpleasant. One patient described this as 'a horrible feeling that I am outside myself and seeing myself on a video film'. Depersonalization is often associated with the mood states of anxiety or depression.

Disordered body image

As well as disturbances which affect the whole of the way the sufferer sees himself there are also specific disturbances of body image, and of parts of the body. These are represented in Figure 2.3. *Hypochondriasis* is morbid preoccupation with the body or state of health. *Narcissism* is undue concern with appearance, often associated with a pathological fear of growing old. *Dysmorphophobia* is an over-valued idea that the body, or more often a part of the body such as the nose or the breasts, is unattractive, and this is coupled with an intense dislike of the body. *Distortion of the body image*, in which it is perceived as fatter or wider than it actually is, occurs in both anorexia nervosa and in obesity. An over-valued idea in which the individual has come to believe that his 'true' identity is opposite to that suggested by his biological gender occurs in *transsexualism*. There are also abnormalities of the body image resultant from organic lesions in the brain.

Pain is ultimately a subjective experience. All pain, therefore, occurs in the brain, or in 'the mind', and there is no simple distinction possible between organic or psychogenic causes of pain. In psychogenic pain there is disturbance of mood and no clear organic cause for the pain.

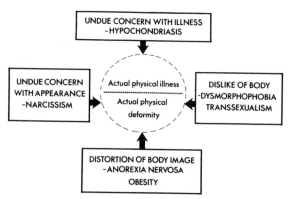

Figure 2.3 Disorders of bodily complaint

Disturbance of mood and volition

The abnormal moods that occur in psychiatric illnesses are mostly described in later chapters with the affective disorders (Chapter 5) and with the anxiety disorders (Chapter 10). However, at this stage it is important to realize two important facts about morbid mood: (1) The range of different sorts of mood experience is infinitely great, very much more than simple severity of depression or anxiety; we simply do not have language for all the finer nuances of disturbed mood that patients attempt to describe. (2) There is a qualitative difference between the unpleasant mood of which patients complain and the occasional miserable or worried mood of which we are aware in normal everyday life. It is important to appreciate the mood state of our patients: I am only able to understand how my patient is feeling by going through the process, 'If I felt as he looks to be feeling, I would be feeling ———'.

Similarly, *anxiety* is much more than a straightforward, more or less quantitative phenomenon. *Irritability* is a related but subtly different affect. There is situational mood – that is, *phobia* – in which anxiety occurs in specific situations or with specific provocation. There is also episodic anxiety as exemplified by *panic attacks*, in which anxiety occurs with great intensity for a short time and then clears completely. There may also be *free floating anxiety*, in which there appears to be no obvious external precipitant.

The phenomenology of *volition* is not easy to categorize. There is, for instance, *compulsive behaviour* as part of an obsessive-compulsive disorder in which the patient knows that the repetitive act is at his own volition, he tries not to carry it out but is still unable to prevent its repetition because of this feeling of subjective compulsion (Chapter 12). This is phenomenologically different from the *impulsive* act of repeated drinking in an abuser of alcohol, who knows that he should resist his behaviour, but does not in fact do so. Observation of *motor activity* and distinctive patterns of behaviour also forms part of the examination of the mental state.

Uses of descriptive psychopathology

Descriptive psychopathology and the method of

Table 2.2 *Uses of descriptive psychopathology*

1 Diagnosis
2 Research
3 Therapy
4 Legal

empathy needs to be learnt as a clinical tool. It can be used diagnostically in the common but difficult clinical syndromes, hair splitting and hare chasing for the minutiae in the common but difficult clinical distinctions that need to be made in everyday practice (Table 2.2).

Descriptive psychopathology is essential for research in psychiatry as it is based upon observation and deduction. Detailed psychopathological enquiry allows a therapeutic relationship to be established. It is a most useful first step in understanding the patient, helping him to realize that the doctor is beginning to understand the symptoms and problems.

It is very difficult for psychotic patients with apparently unique experiences to explain their internal state. There is often great relief when the doctor appears to be able to understand what is going on. It is also useful for neurotic patients for their internal experiences to be explored without attaching theoretical explanations for their behaviour. Phenomenology has also always formed the basis for legal definitions of mental illnesses.

Further reading

Jaspers, K. (1963) *General Psychopathology*, 7th edn, J. Hoenig and M. W. Hamilton (trans.), Manchester: Manchester University Press.
Sims, A.C.P. (1988) *Symptoms in the Mind*, London: Baillière Tindall.

3

Psychiatric interviewing

In psychiatry the initial interview with the patient is considered important and requires time and effort. For example, senior psychiatrists will usually allow one hour in the outpatient clinic for each new-patient appointment, and doctors in psychiatric training usually spend an hour or more in the first interview with a newly admitted patient. It is intended that an initial interview, if it does not arrive at the whole truth, should narrow possibilities, suggest differential diagnoses and begin to answer basic questions:

- what is the nature of the patient's illness?
- why has it taken this form?
- why has it arisen at this time?

For most patients there will be further consultations; a single interview is rarely complete. In order to address these questions, an initial interview has a number of specific objectives:

- setting the scene;
- collecting information;
- examining the mental state;
- making a provisional assessment;
- alleviating distress.

Setting the scene

The early stages of a psychiatric interview should be directed at putting the patient at ease and should never be neglected or hurried.

Indeed, the beginning of an interview may govern the whole of its subsequent success. It needs some experience to strike a satisfactory blend between formality and informality. An unduly formal attitude may lead the patient to feel that the psychiatrist is unlikely to be sympathetic; as a result, the patient may not be forthcoming. Conversely, if the interviewer assumes an air of undue informality, there is a risk of appearing casual or uninterested.

Apart from the obvious need for sympathetic interest, getting an interview off to a good start may be enhanced by several kinds of manoeuvre. Where the psychiatrist has some foreknowledge of the patient's problem, such as may have been gleaned from the referral letter, discussion of this information may be a useful opening gambit. If, as sometimes happens, prior information is completely lacking and the patient fails to respond to an open invitation to proceed, the interviewer may have to fall back upon other tactics, such as collection of factual information.

Patients are sometimes embarrassed by the prospect of having to give accounts of themselves, but there are other important reasons why they may be unwilling to be interviewed. In the case of some psychotic patients, complete lack of insight may lead them to believe that there is nothing wrong at all. Alternatively, those who are suspicious or deluded may suspect a trap. Some patients who see a psychiatrist only at the instigation of their relatives, or as a result of pressure by some other person, may transfer their resentment of this circumstance to the psychiatrist. This is quite common among disturbed adolescents who may be among the most difficult of all patients with whom to make an initial rapport. The patient who believes symptoms are due to some physical cause may, also, resent having been referred to a psychiatrist either because it seems a futile waste of time or because such referral implies that others think the symptoms are 'merely imaginary'. This situation can be made worse if the referring doctor omits to tell the patient that the referral is to a psychiatrist, using perhaps the euphemism 'nerve specialist' or something seemingly even more innocuous. By the time the patient meets the psychiatrist he is likely to feel he has been deceived and is likely to project his indignation upon the luckless psychiatrist.

There are many other possibilities and probably no specific ways of dealing with any or all of them. However, as a general rule, as soon as an interviewer becomes aware of some trouble of this kind – the sooner the better – the matter should be brought into open discussion. To a hostile patient, it may be helpful to say, 'I can see that you are not happy to have been asked to come today'. It is also sometimes important to give the patient some idea of what a psychiatrist is and does. Many people have misconceptions about psychiatrists, ranging from regarding them at one end of the scale as quacks, to suspecting, at the other, that they have quite remarkable powers. It is wise for the psychiatrist to be identified in the patient's eyes as a doctor concerned with both physical and psychological ailments but perhaps having some special experience in the evaluation of the latter. If the patient is convinced that symptoms are purely physical and that mind plays no part in them whatsoever, then the psychiatrist should indicate respect for this view while perhaps providing an illustration of just how psychological experiences can produce physical symptoms, stressing at the same time that such symptoms are by no means imaginary. It is not uncommon for patients to resent psychiatrists. This may be because they feel ashamed at being unable to control emotions or think that being

seen by a psychiatrist is equated with being 'insane' or something of that kind. This too may need an airing, for until it has been aired, reassurance may be impossible.

Collecting information

In most cases the first information a patient wishes to convey to the interviewer concerns the current problem. Many psychiatrists, therefore, regard this as the most favourable time to discuss in detail the 'presenting complaint'. However, the current problem needs to be considered in the context of past events and background. Accordingly, some psychiatrists prefer to discuss the presenting complaint only briefly at the start of the consultation, moving quickly on to collect background information before returning to the present problem in more detail. This latter approach is the one favoured in this book, although both strategies have advantages and drawbacks.

The order in which the interview is conducted is not in itself fundamental; effective doctors in all disciplines usually develop a systematic approach which they use flexibly. However, thoroughness is important.

After the patient has been invited to speak about recent difficulties, but before a full account of them, the interviewer may perhaps say, 'I wonder if I could stop you there for a short time and just find out a little more about your circumstances and past life. We will come back to the main problem a little later'. Most patients are willing to halt their narratives, understanding why the interviewer wishes to know more about personal and family history.

Personal history

After a short introduction to the nature of the current problem, brief enquiry into the patient's life and social background is an acceptable and useful way to proceed. Table 3.1 sets out the potential areas of interest in some detail. Not all aspects are necessarily enquired into – indeed, at a first interview, some may be deliberately avoided. Nevertheless, to gain even

Table 3.1 *Personal history*

Early development	• Date and place of birth, any abnormalities concerning birth • Achievement of milestones, physical health • Temperament as a child – confidence, fears, relationships, behaviour
Immediate family	• Father, mother and siblings: present whereabouts, health, age, occupation, degree of contact with patient
Home	• Atmosphere, and the relationships within the family
School	• Types of school attended, with dates of starting and leaving • Academic ability and achievement • Relationships with other pupils and staff • Attitude and attendance
Adolescence	• Difficulties in growing up, rebelliousness, drug taking, unlawful behaviour
Work	• Jobs held, in chronological order with approximate dates and duration, together with reasons for changing jobs • Present job – nature, responsibility, satisfaction, stresses, competence, relations with colleagues; any association of these factors with onset of symptoms
Sex and marriage	• Sexual development: *puberty* – timing and any difficulties 　　　　　　　　　*sexual knowledge and experience* 　　　　　　　　　*sexual orientation* • Pregnancies, abortions and childbirth • Important relationships, cohabitation, marriage • Partner's age, health, occupation • Details of current partnership: satisfaction and problems in general and sexual relations – including those related to intercourse (consider sexual practices, contraception, extra-marital affairs)
Housing	• Nature and adequacy of current housing and neighbourhood
Finances	• Income and debt
The law, courts and tribunals	• Problems with the police or courts or other legal action (civil cases, industrial tribunals, compensation)
Medical history	• *Physical*: serious or chronic illness, current treatment • *Psychiatric*: occurrence, nature and treatment of any disorders – including untreated episodes and those handled by GP

a rudimentary understanding of a current problem, some such background material is essential. It is a matter of judgement whether matters which are difficult to discuss, or even embarrassing, are best left to another occasion or dealt with early so that they may be pursued further or laid to rest. Enquiry of this kind may be carried out efficiently and sensitively, so that the occurrence and sequence of important past events and difficulties is established, together with an understanding of the current social setting.

An attempt should be made to answer the question, 'What kind of person are we dealing with?'. Some patients are able to give a good account of their own disposition and characteristics, whether they are habitual worriers, sensitive to criticism, or usually emotionally robust. Some patients are well able to draw contrasts between their usual state and their current one since the start of the present problem; not so other patients. This judgement is always a difficult task and is necessarily subjective. Separate interviewers may form quite different impressions of the same patient; each may be coloured by the interviewer's own experience and outlook.

Often, little information about the first few years can be gleaned at first hand though it may be available from parents or siblings. However, simple information relating to the circumstances of the patient's birth, early development and so-called milestones is of value – for example, in relation to possible impairments of higher functions. A history of separation in infancy from one or both parents may also be relevant. For most people, recall is more reliable after the age of 5, although some still seem to remember little until adolescence. In such cases it may often be correctly inferred that childhood was so unhappy a time as to have been forgotten. However, even when earlier years are remembered, feelings may be more important than facts. It may matter little where a patient went to school or even, within limits, with what success. What matters more is whether he enjoyed it, how he got on with his school-mates, whether he was away much of the time and if so, why; whether he was popular or not, a leader or a follower; whether his life was made a misery by teasing or bullying. So it is through childhood; while achievement or failure is not unimportant, it is the feelings which surround them which may be more significant; not only the subject's own feelings but also the feelings of those close to him.

In adult life some account should be taken of later educational attainments and occupational history. Once again, what is important is how the patient feels about progress. If the record of attainment is only modest, is he relatively content or bitter and frustrated? If the latter, does he blame himself, claim lack of opportunity, or does he blame others?

A chronological account of the patient's previous physical and mental health, accidents, operations, births, miscarriages, hospital admissions and previous treatments should be discovered; who carried them out and where? Important information should, in due course, be corroborated by means of letters, specialists' reports and case notes obtained from other hospitals where the patient may have been treated.

If the interview is proceeding smoothly and the rapport between the interviewer and the patient seems to be sound, attention may be turned to the patient's sexual history. If, for some reason, there are signs of unwillingness, the matter may often be deferred. In such enquiry it is often valuable to indicate recognition that the discussion of such highly personal matters may be a source of embarrassment. If the psychiatrist can talk calmly on the importance of a discussion about sex, without showing any embarrassment, the patient's cooperation will often be obtained. The list of items in Table 3.1 indicates just some of the many possible topics related to sex. Once again, relevance and importance of such discussion, and its timing, is a matter for the judgement of the interviewer.

Family history

Psychiatrists are interested in family histories because of the longstanding observation that patients with psychiatric disorders frequently report other family members with current or past psychiatric problems, often of broadly similar type. In short, whether due to genetic or environmental factors, many psychiatric conditions are familial. Because we believe there to be an important genetic component to some conditions, particularly more severe ones, family information is important. It is also valuable to obtain an account of upbringing which has been affected by close proximity to relatives who themselves suffered from mental illness.

In practice, the family history obtained is often unsatisfactory. Facts elicited may be unreliable, and information about feelings and relationships are prone to distortions due to conflict or loyalty. Nevertheless, even a small amount of accurate information about close relatives helps paint the picture of the patient's background.

Present complaint

Much of the first interview with a patient will be concerned with the current problem. The interviewer attempts to obtain a clear account of the onset of the problem, the development of its main features or symptoms, and the subsequent course of events. Difficulties and events prior to onset of symptoms are important, also similarities or contrast with past episodes, and any interventions or treatments undertaken.

This part of the interview usually includes detailed enquiry into the symptoms described and into aspects not described. Just as in physical medicine where there is, for example, a complaint of abdominal pain, the doctor enquires about quality, site, intensity, timing of pain, but also about bowel habit, urinary symptoms, menstruation and so on; so with psychiatry. With a complaint of anxiety, for example, its character and its circumstances are elicited in detail, but questions about depression, obsessions and physical symptoms are also important. This kind of enquiry into the patient's experience is part of what psychiatrists term the 'examination of the mental state'. A later section of this chapter deals with that part of the interview in more detail.

Case records

The complexity of the material elicited during a psychiatric interview and in the later, more formal, assessment of the patient's mental state necessitates the keeping of detailed records, at least of the initial interview and mental state examination. There are no adequate short-cuts. Tape-recording, while useful for research purposes, is of no value in routine practice, as it takes as long to replay and listen to the tape as to make the recording.

Some patients may become concerned or suspicious when the interviewer starts writing down what they say. If so, the interviewer should bring the matter into the open at once, and refer to the need to obtain as exact and complete a record as possible for the patient's sake. The extremely private nature of psychiatric case records should be emphasized, together with measures taken to preserve their confidentiality. Sometimes, when a very delicate matter emerges and the patient appears particularly uneasy at the possibility of its being written down, it may be wise for the interviewer

deliberately to lay down the pen for a time and make no record. In subsequent interviews, it is often unnecessary to make any notes during the interview, instead recording a brief précis of what seems important once the patient has left. Remember also that, except under unusual circumstances, patients and their representatives have a legal right of access to their case notes (all material after 1 November 1991).

One or two other points deserve mention. Often it is valuable to write down verbatim the patient's statements, particularly those concerning his relationship with others and his attitudes towards them. Such statements, especially if vivid, may in a few words convey more than half a page of description. Furthermore, they are examples of what the patient actually said and not merely a subjective and sometimes mistaken interpretation by the interviewer. The same may be said of the benefits of exact statements made by the patient concerning delusional beliefs, hallucinations and the like.

Mental state examination

Having taken the history, the way in which the doctor determines how the patient is currently is usually termed 'the mental state examination'. In a number of senses this task is analogous to a physical examination. Each is a systematic description, mentioning the presence or absence of abnormalities; each is recorded using technical terms. Physical examination and mental state examination are, however, carried out differently. Whilst the patient's cyanosis and breathlessness are noted during the history-taking interview, nevertheless it is usual for most of the physical examination to take place during a particular stage of the consultation. In psychiatry this balance is reversed; although most of the assessment of the present mental state is usually noted during the interview, there is a stage in which the patient is asked specific questions and sometimes set tasks in order to elicit abnormalities.

What are the components and terminology of this systematic description? How are abnormalities elicited?

Appearance and behaviour

A sensible first step in the description of a patient's mental state is to record prominent features of appearance and behaviour. For example, a patient may be calm and composed or hand-wringing and agitated, or expressionless and retarded. Attire and make-up may be sober or quite bizarre. A patient's attitude to the interview may be worthy of comment if, for example, it is hostile or suspicious. It may be useful to describe the degree of rapport established. In short, all relevant aspects of appearance and behaviour are described briefly, usually including reference to attitude and activity.

Talk

Speech may be spontaneous, copious or sparse and limited to brief replies; it may even be non-existent. It may be concise and relevant or circumstantial and rambling. It may be over-loud or excessively quiet, even whispered. In certain conditions the structure of speech may be abnormal: the flow is interrupted in thought blocking and in disorders of the form of thinking. Neologisms, aphasia or dysarthria may be present. It is worth commenting on the spontaneity, quantity and structure of speech, together with any abnormalities noted.

Mood

Direct enquiry should be made about mood, asking whether the patient is able to remain cheerful or rather becomes depressed or low-spirited. The result of such an enquiry is noted, together with the interviewer's impression of the patient's current appearance of mood. In addition, it is important to ask about hope and plans for the future. It is often relevant to enquire about feelings when life no longer seems worth going on with. If indicated, patients should be asked frankly about suicidal thoughts, intentions, plans and attempts. Once again, although this area of discussion is a difficult one, if approached sensitively in a logical order and without concealment, most patients respect the need for enquiry. On many occasions patients are thankful for an opportunity to discuss such feelings.

Other mood-related features include feelings of guilt, blame or unworthiness, ranging from comments which are understandable in the light of the current circumstances across to severe self-denigratory ideas which may be preoccupying or even delusional. Comment should also be made about morbid preoccupations concerning ill health, shame, poverty or ruin, all of which may occur in severe depressive illness. Conversely, enquiry should also be made into episodes of excessively cheerful mood or elation. Many patients are aware if they have been over-cheerful and they may report such feelings with vivid descriptions. A description should also be given of the interviewer's assessment of mood.

Thought

The stream or flow of thought has already been mentioned when considering the patient's talk. Abnormalities of this kind may occur when there is disorder of the form of thinking, as in schizophrenia, mania and certain neurological disorders. In addition, abnormalities of the possession of thought should be identified – whether thoughts are influenced, inserted, withdrawn, broadcast, echoed or otherwise shared. These experiences are termed 'passivity experiences' (see Table 3.2). Abnormal ideas in the form of delusions should be elicited and recorded. It may be important to ask specific questions in some of the areas referred to in Table 3.2, in order to establish precisely what beliefs and experiences have occurred. Further explanation about these delusions is given in Chapters 5 and 6.

Obsessions and compulsions should be considered and the patient asked about repetitive behaviours such as checking, washing or having to carry out procedures in a certain order.

Perception

Enquiry should be made into whether there is

Table 3.2   *Abnormalities of thought: delusions and passivity experiences*

Delusions

Delusions of persecution
Delusions of assistance from an outside person or force
Delusions of control by an outside person or force
Delusions of grandiose ability or identity
Religious delusions
Delusions of jealousy
Sexual delusions
Delusions of guilt
Delusions of self-denigration
Delusions of poverty, ruin or catastrophe
Nihilistic delusions
Hypochondriacal delusions
Delusional explanations: delusional experiences explained by *paranormal/occult* (e.g., telepathy, extra-sensory perception, black magic) or *physical* forces (e.g., electricity, X-rays, machines)

Passivity experiences

Thought insertion
Thought broadcast
Thought echo
Thought withdrawal

anything unusual about the way things sound, look, taste or smell. The various abnormalities of perception are described in Chapter 2.

Hallucinations are the most important abnormality of perception in psychiatric illness. It is important to establish when abnormal perceptions occur, whether, for example, in specific situations and if they are in clear, wakeful consciousness.

Auditory hallucinations may include sounds other than voices – such as machinery noise, tapping, music, crying or indecipherable muttering or whispering. Where there are voices it is worth making certain distinctions: whether the voice says single words (such as calling the patient's name) or if the content is more complex; whether a voice comments on the patient's thoughts or actions in the third person (for example, 'She's sitting at the table writing a cheque, now she's going towards the bathroom, going to have a wash'); whether two or more voices are involved – do they discuss the patient between themselves; whether the content is derogatory or otherwise unpleasant; whether voices are recognized.

Visual hallucinations, similarly, may be relatively formless – sometimes just flashes of light or shadows – or they may be complex and seen with clarity. Hallucinations of smell may be described as unique, not like any normal smell, or alternatively, may be ordinary but inexplicable. For example, one patient described a smell of food when there was none around, citing the smell as evidence of his persecution by people in 'another dimension'. Sensations of touch may be generalized itch or 'crawling' feelings, or more specific experiences; one patient described the repeated sensation of a woman's finger running up and down the skin of his back.

With all abnormal perceptions it is important to seek the patient's explanation of the experience, as well as to obtain details of the perception.

Cognitive function

For some patients enquiry should be made into higher cognitive functioning in an attempt to detect and document any impairment in performance. The way in which this may be carried out is described in Chapter 7. Systematic testing may be unnecessary in those whose predicament is unlikely to be related to impaired cognitive functioning and who show no kind of deficit during the preceding interview.

Finally, it may be possible to comment on the patient's own view of his problems and present state. Whether, for example, he recognizes a pervasive change in mood and sees this as an appropriate target for psychiatric treatment, or conversely whether he believes himself to be the focus of persecution with the consultation merely another component of a complex plot. It may be relevant to record patients' views about their outlook following psychiatric care; some, even while appreciating that they may be ill, consider that nothing can or should be done for them. Conversely, some patients have unrealistically high expectations from treatment.

Making a provisional assessment

At the end of an initial interview a brief account

of the case should be prepared. This account may fulfil a number of functions. In the setting of the clinic it will contain adequate information to inform the general practitioner about the consultation and a record of the assessment. For inpatients, it provides the necessary material for the case discussion which takes place in multidisciplinary ward rounds. For the student in training, preparation of this brief account of the case helps them to practise the clinical skills of summarizing material elicited, making judgements about the patient's predicament and planning for management.

The content of a brief account of the case is summarized in Table 3.3 The first three items are a shortened version of the more complete history and examination. They are, however, not merely a summary in a conventional order. The most pertinent facts are selected and arranged clearly, to provide the basis for conclusions about diagnosis and management. The whole process is analogous to the description of a case of acute appendicitis or diabetic peripheral neuropathy, where the accomplished clinician will briefly describe any relevant background factors, the evolution and progress of the symptoms, any relevant past history, the absence of certain key symptoms indicative of

Table 3.3 *Brief account of a case*

A brief account of the case should be given in the following terms (although not necessarily in this order):

1 Important aspects of the patient's personal background (age, sex, occupation, social background, etc.)

2 Major features and the development and course of the disorder; previous episodes of similar or other psychiatric disorder

3 Present mental state: positive findings

4 Differential diagnosis

5 Probable aetiological factors of the present illness

6 Further information required which may help in planning management

7 A broad outline of management

8 Prognosis

---

other conditions, the physical examination, initial diagnosis with other possibilities and further tests and interventions to be carried out. So it is in psychiatry. Straightforward cases may be described fairly easily in this manner, but even the most complex cases are best understood through this kind of process.

Those trained in medicine will be familiar with the construction of a differential diagnosis – a listing of the possible diagnoses, usually in descending order of likelihood. In psychiatry, it is useful to separate description from aetiology. As a first step it makes sense to decide whether the clinical state characterized by delusions and hallucinations and a degree of agitation and over-activity is most typical of schizophrenia, mania or depression. If the patient has also suffered from epileptic seizures and been involved in the misuse of drugs, these matters also need to be discussed in the differential diagnosis, although they are put forward as underlying factors rather than alternatives to the *descriptive diagnosis*.

The complex matter of aetiology is discussed more fully in Chapter 4. In an account of a clinical case it is usually worthwhile to make brief comment upon the reasons why the patient may have become unwell in this way at this time. As well as physical factors such as drug ingestion or endocrine disorder, there are often things that should be included about social and psychological matters. If enough is known about the patient's background and personal history, then it may be possible to comment upon how events and difficulties in the patient's life are associated with the current problem. First, the relationship of the timing of such events and difficulties to the onset of symptoms is important. Second, events and difficulties sometimes seem to bear a striking relation to the nature of the current symptoms. For example, an elderly man with severe depression complained that he was unable to swallow and he had stopped eating and drinking; his wife had died following an obstructive carcinoma of her oesophagus just one year before.

In medicine as a whole there are often a number of specific tests which may be carried out following an initial clinical assessment. In psychiatry there are relatively few tests of this kind which are valuable in practice. Of course, adequate physical examination is important, together with any biochemical or haematological, blood or urine tests indicated from the history or examination. From time to time it may be valuable to arrange detailed and specialized psychological testing, particularly where there is doubt about higher cognitive function. Most often, however, there are few special tests which are likely to have a major impact on the assessment of the case.

On the other hand, it is almost essential in psychiatry to obtain an account from someone who knows the patient well. Full understanding of the case arises when the current problem is understood in the setting of the patient's background and difficulties. Many patients are unable, particularly when unwell, to provide such a picture. Information from key informants such as parents, spouses, children or close friends is invaluable, and most patients will be quite willing for the psychiatrist to talk with such people. Different information is obtained if key informants are seen with the patient or on their own. Both may be valuable, but it is important to respect the patient's own wish on this matter.

The preparation of a brief account of the case is usually carried out in the early stages of care. For that reason management will usually be outlined briefly, suggesting the initial options. An important issue is the setting in which any work will be carried out: outpatient, day patient or inpatient. Management options do not include only physical treatment such as the use of drugs; there are often important social interventions. For example, psychiatrists need to be aware of agencies such as social work, Citizens' Advice Bureaux, crisis teams, facilities at the Department of Employment and in Housing departments. Where psychiatric illness has been long-term, social interventions may be much the most important elements in management. These matters are discussed further in Chapter 22. Similarly, many psychiatric conditions are amenable to psychological treatments, often involving various forms of psychotherapy or counselling. In almost all cases there is a place for some such psychological process. The various approaches are described in Chapter 21.

Alleviating distress

The first psychiatric interview with the patient is not only concerned with the collection of information, drawing of conclusions and setting up a plan for management. Patients are often distressed by their current predicament and such an interview will often provide a much-needed opportunity to give vent to feelings. Effective psychiatric interviewers use an *empathic* approach, trying to understand how the patient feels by imagining how one would feel in the same situation. Other important components of interviewing style include genuineness evident to the patient, and a degree of warmth – as opposed to a cold, aloof style.

There is often benefit from the sharing of distressing matters with other people. Their response is all-important. Most patients hope that the doctor, by virtue of experience and skill, will help with the current problem. Listening and questioning in a direct yet sensitive manner will often help to fulfil expectations of help.

Further reading

Wing, J.K., Cooper, J.E. and Sartorius, N. (1974) *The Measurement and Classification of Psychiatric Symptoms*, Cambridge: Cambridge University Press.

4

Aetiology and classification

When any human situation is identified as being unusual, different from normal or a problem, the automatic next step is to ask the questions, how did this happen? what makes it so? The study of causes and classification are inextricably linked conceptually. For any human problem to be solved it must first be categorized in a meaningful way and then its causes elucidated. This is as true for medicine as it is for other problem-solving professions. Aetiology and classification are interrelated; ideally, classification is based upon aetiology, but the classifications we use in medicine are necessarily also based upon course of the illness, symptoms, even the method of treatment, and sometimes theoretical concepts.

General comment on aetiological factors

In psychiatry we still know relatively little about the causation of the quite different conditions we are able to classify and diagnose. Although a condition such as neurosyphilis with general paralysis (GPI) may be categorized on aetiological grounds, for the majority of conditions causal explanations are much more tentative. The ideal for the organic model of causation is to give a name to a consistent pattern of symptoms with a known clinical cause and clearly recognized histopathological findings. In psychiatric practice, apart from some organic

states, this is a rare situation. Contributions to our understanding of psychiatric aetiology come from a number of different scientific backgrounds, and these are discussed later in the chapter under the general headings of social, individual psychological and biological causes. The condition of an individual patient requires separate consideration for each of these three broad areas of causation.

It is fundamental in psychiatry to realize that *multifactorial* causes are the norm, and single causation from one overwhelmingly predominant factor is extremely unusual. Thus, for a middle-aged man who has recently developed a severe depressive illness there may be genetic causes in that his mother also suffered from a manic-depressive illness, other constitutional causes such as his recently having suffered a viral illness, psychodynamic causes such as the death of his mother through suicide when he was aged 9, and social causes with the threat of redundancy due to his firm's relocation to another European country. These, and many other factors, may all be operative and influential in determining the manifestation of symptoms, their onset and duration, and their severity.

Causes of psychiatric illness may be remote in time. So, though this man did not develop depression until more than thirty years after the death of his mother, it may have been an aetiological factor. A single factor may have many different psychiatric effects; for example, the experience of parental deprivation in childhood has been evoked as causal in adult antisocial behaviour, for suicide and also depressive illness. Many different causes may have one single common effect; thus Down's Syndrome, phenylketonuria, tuberose sclerosis and many other pre-natal or early childhood conditions may all result in learning disability and, as far as the mental state is concerned, there is no difference between these various causes.

Causes of mental illness may be categorized as *predisposing*, *precipitating* or *perpetuating* factors (Table 4.1). With predisposing factors, cause is seen to lie in the background constitution of a patient. Thus, when an individual develops a schizophrenic illness, the predisposing factors looked for might be *genetic* in terms of a family history, *intra-uterine*, with evidence of being born following a difficult delivery perhaps with birth injury, and *early childhood* influences with perhaps problems in the bonding relationship with the patient's mother. Abnormality of personality is often considered a predisposing factor which may, for instance, be influential in the development of subsequent neurotic disorders or alcohol abuse.

Precipitating factors are those causes which can be seen to be immediately related in time to the development of illness; for example, breakdown of marriage may be followed within a few months by depression, or involvement in a major disaster may give rise to the symptoms of post-traumatic stress disorder. With perpetuating factors, the psychiatric disorder is caused to continue; for instance, in depressive illness there is frequently loss of self-esteem, a state of demoralization and consequent social

Table 4.1   *Aetiological factors in mental illness*

Predisposing factors	genetic influences
	intra-uterine influences
	early childhood influences
	abnormality of personality
Precipitating factors	bereavement
	disaster
	divorce, etc.
Perpetuating factors	permanent organic damage
	loss of self-esteem
	social disadvantage

withdrawal from previous interests and activities. This social withdrawal is likely to result in the prolongation of depression to a chronic, depressive illness.

Understanding and *explanation* have been discussed in Chapter 2. Explanation is the accounting for causation within the terminology of the natural sciences. For example, from knowledge of immunology, neuropathology and so on, the causes of AIDS dementia may be explained and the aetiology of the individual patient's condition becomes clear. Understanding in this other sense involves putting oneself in the position of the patient and thereby understanding how this behaviour or this mood state could arise from his previous state and from environmental causes. For example, when a man is promoted at work with an increased salary we would expect him to be pleased. When our individual patient becomes miserable and develops a depressive illness on promotion, it becomes understandable when we empathize with his subjective condition, and when, on ascertaining the history, we discover that his promotion involves moving to another city with much more expensive housing than where he lives now, his wife is threatening to leave him and will not consider moving, he has two children of whom he is very fond and he knows that his wife will gain custody if they divorce, and so on.

Clinical studies in aetiology

There are two main types of clinical study that give useful aetiological information: (1) *descriptive psychopathological* and (2) *longitudinal* studies. In practice these two types of study are often combined. In descriptive psychopathological studies a detailed investigation of the symptoms is made and individual symptoms and constellations of symptoms are related to cause of illness and also to factors present in the patient before development of the illness.

Longitudinal studies involve the follow-up of homogeneous groups of patients, preferably over a relatively long time, and a detailed assessment, both of the initial state and of the mental state after many years of follow-up. Such studies give both useful information of what does happen, such as the increased risk for suicide in anxiety disorders, and also negative information – for instance, that a previous diagnosis of severe anxiety disorder does not predispose to the subsequent development of a schizophrenic illness. Scrupulous clinical description is, of course, essential for making progress in any type of aetiological investigation; one cannot investigate the molecular genetics of schizophrenia without having a satisfactory descriptive psychopathological method of making a diagnosis of schizophrenia. In psychiatric research increasing sophistication of basic scientific methodology demands an accurate and reliable method of description of symptoms.

Epidemiology (literally, 'on the people') is the quantitative study of the distribution and determinants of disease in a defined population (that is, one limited by space and time). Epidemiology is concerned with varying rates of disease; for example, *prevalence*, which is the rate of established cases at a defined time in that population. Prevalence studies include rates for schizophrenia in different parts of the inner city, and such findings have aetiological implications. The clinical and social features of illness and behaviour may be studied epidemiologically; for instance, it has been shown that the highest risks for suicide are in elderly men, especially if they live alone, abuse alcohol and have a family history of depression.

Epidemiological studies may be designed to demonstrate particular aetiological factors; for instance, the numerous twin studies which have been carried out to demonstrate the relative importance of genetic and environmental factors in the development of schizophrenia. The findings are controversial or even meaningless unless the study has been designed with scrupulous attention to method. Age, sex and marriage have been investigated as aetiological factors; for example, increased maternal age is known to be associated with an increased incidence of Down's Syndrome (*incidence* is the rate of *developing* a disease in a defined time for a population); some conditions, such as anorexia nervosa, are known to be associated with female *sex*, and some, such as schizophrenia, are likely to develop at a younger age in males; the risk for suicide is greater amongst *divorcees* than for those who remain married.

Social causes of psychiatric illness

An important part of the recognition of multifactorial causation in psychiatric disorder is the importance given to social determinants. In general, organic theories of aetiology have tended towards over-simplifications, such as the statement: 'schizophrenia is caused by dopamine over-activity in the brain'. Social theories, on the other hand, have been at times so comprehensive as to be almost meaningless; for example, the statement: 'schizophrenia is caused in the family, a vulnerable member responding with symptoms to the destructive environment that has been established'. There is also a danger that terms derived from other disciplines will be used as metaphor; for example, 'a sick society'. Sometimes the testing of hypotheses in social investigations has not been as rigorous as in the natural sciences. This is hardly surprising because of the intrinsic difficulty of controlling variables and of quantification in human social groups. Despite these limitations, there have been many contributions to psychiatric aetiology from investigations of the environmental background and social situation. A few such factors are mentioned below, but others could also be cited.

There have been many studies in psychiatry and in other branches of medicine associating *poverty* and *social class* with varying rates for specific illnesses; for example, a child's malnutrition is readily associated with poverty and may result in higher rates for learning disability and epilepsy. Established schizophrenic illness tends to be associated with lower social class, but on further investigation it has been shown that development of the illness tends to antedate the individual being listed as of lower social class, rather than vice versa; the fathers of schizophrenic patients do not show the same marked lower social class skew. Depression has also been associated, especially in women, with lower socio-economic class. Social class and wealth also affect the availability of medical, and hence, psychiatric attention and the stage of development and severity at which the condition will be presented to a doctor, diagnosed and treatment initiated. Treatment and the availability of medical resources is also associated with social class and wealth. There are some conditions which have been associated in epidemiological studies with higher social class, an obvious example of this being anorexia nervosa which, in many studies, was found to be concentrated amongst girls with parents of higher social class and attending fee-paying schools.

Transcultural studies have often revealed interesting differences and similarities in the prevalence and in the presentation of psychiatric disorders. However, how to evaluate such studies aetiologically has often proved much more difficult. Patients of South Asian origin have tended to manifest more somatic symptoms in the presentation of depressive illness than British patients. It is not known whether they experience more of such symptoms or simply present these to the doctor as presenting complaints with greater frequency.

It is part of popular mythology that unpleasant mood results from the occurrence of untoward events. Thus, if somebody feels miserable, they will be asked what unfortunate happening has caused this. If a student fails an examination, he is expected to feel 'down' for a time afterwards. Over the last few years *adverse life events* have been studied in a methodical and quantitative manner. So the severity of life events has been quantified using the opinion of large groups of interviewees, not the interviewer, either rank-ordering or scoring particular life events such as 'death of spouse' or 'adolescent child leaving home'. Understandably, interviewees will score the former much higher as an adverse event than the latter. By aggregating life-event scores in the previous 6 months, a single score for adverse life events may be obtained which can then be related to the development of mental illness. It has been found that the onset of depressive illness is significantly associated with a high score for adverse life events in the previous 6 months and also for 'exit events',

which is where the individual has experienced a loss. The methodology of life-event research is highly complex, but it is likely that it will continue to be useful in psychiatric aetiology.

A particular type of adverse life event is involvement in *major disaster* such as a bush fire, or a bomb exploded in a civilian population. Over the past few years there has been increasing interest in the psychological outcome of the victims of disaster both in terms of the symptoms elicited and the treatment which might be beneficial. Involvement in such a catastrophe and its psychological sequelae may be seen as a collective form of exposure to stress (see below).

The study of *migration* and its association with mental health is also an area where social sciences have made a contribution to the understanding of the aetiology of mental illnesses. There was, for example, found to be an increased rate for schizophrenic illnesses amongst Hungarian refugees coming to western Europe following the uprising of 1956 as compared with rates in the native populations. The important aetiological question for this, as for other social transitions, is: did migration result in mental illness? or did the prior existence of mental illness result in the emigration of that individual with the mass exodus that was already taking place?

The social sciences have also made an important contribution to the study of *institutions*, their social networks, the power structure that exists within them, and their influence upon the development of symptoms and abnormal behaviour. Such investigations make comment upon corrective institutions such as prisons, coercive situations such as concentration camps and torture, and also upon more benign, but nevertheless institutional, environments such as schools and large mental hospitals. It has been claimed that the *total institution* will produce changes in behaviour and self-image in those who are exposed to it for any length of time.

Individual psychological causes

Ethology is the scientific study of behaviour, involving observation, description and comparison in different species. This science has made notable contributions in investigating infant-rearing practice and the formation of parental bonding. Comment on the aetiology of childhood emotional disturbance following maternal deprivation – for instance, when the child is admitted to hospital without its mother – has been based on ethnological experimental work, especially the separation of primate infants from their mothers.

The term '*stress*' is used regularly in everyday life, but often very imprecisely; it is an important factor in the generation of many types of psychological disturbance. It is discussed further in Chapter 9, and Figure 4.1 may clarify some of the confusion in the current use of the term. A stressor is an outside object or situation which causes the person to experience stress; such stress might be exemplified by examinations, or the anticipation of examinations, provoking acute anxiety. We also talk of a person under stress or being stressed. This *stress reaction*, which is common experience with a number of different provocations, may manifest itself with tachycardia, hypertension, raised circulating levels of adrenalin and noradrenalin, the feeling of being tense and on edge, and a number of other somatic and psychological symptoms. Probably the best way of using the term 'stress' is in the sense that there is a lack of fit between the individual and the environment. Thus, a concert pianist might well complain of feeling stress if compelled to work an eight-hour day in a confectionery factory, whilst the factory worker would undoubtedly feel stressed having to go on stage to play in a concert. This model of stress includes both individual and environmental characteristics.

A behavioural model for disturbance rather than a disease model is characteristically used in *experimental* and *clinical psychology*, so the factors that determine normal human behaviour, such as drives, reinforcements, cultural influences and so on, are explored and these determinants of normal behaviour are extrapolated to explain the abnormal behaviour of the group under consideration. For example, there is a small group of people, usually young, who regularly cut their wrists. The *disease model* would try and explain this in terms of the underlying psychiatric illness or personality type. A *behavioural model* might explain it in terms of drives, relief of tension, reinforcements, or cultural influences such as a piece of non-verbal communication understandable within the individual's sub-group. In the aetiology of depressive states, whereas organic aetiology might ascribe depressed mood to an underlying biochemical disturbance in brain monoamines, psychological aetiology might implicate cognitive theory in which primacy is given to depressive thoughts which are based upon previous experience of low self-esteem and cause depression of mood, rather than resulting from it. Another area in which psychology has contributed to our understanding of aetiology is in the study of *coping mechanisms* and how a bereavement reaction, for example, may be the method used by the patient to cope with his current situation.

Psychoanalytic *theories*, such as those propounded by Sigmund Freud, are developed in more detail in Chapters 9 and 21. Such theory is particularly rich in explanations for current mental symptoms and abnormal behaviour; the major problem is that it is extremely difficult to formulate such hypotheses in such a way that they may be proved or falsified. Because they are not available in this way for scientific proof they command less respect than they did previously.

From the highly complex psychoanalytic theories, three important aetiological principles may be highlighted: *unconscious* mind, *Oedipal*

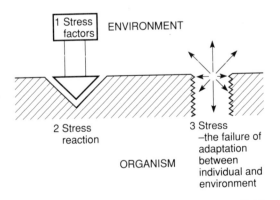

Figure 4.1 Stress, stress reaction and the individual

causes of adult symptoms and *sexual* conflict. It is considered that a large part of mental activity is unconscious and cannot be returned to consciousness unless it be subtly altered in acceptable and symbolic form. Thus, the mental mechanisms listed in Chapter 9 are ways in which the conscious self may defend itself against the discomfort of conflicts taking place in the unconscious part of the person. Much of adult neurosis and psychological disturbance is ascribed to conflicts associated with early relationships with the patient's mother and unacceptable desires which the individual has experienced at the Oedipal stage, round about the age of 3. This stage of development is followed by a later phase which is thought not to be so significant in the development of later disturbance. Sexual conflict is the concept which links these two ideas with the development of mental illness. All conflict is considered in psychoanalysis to be ultimately sexual in nature. The young male child seeks sexual gratification from his mother. This is unacceptable both socially and to the individual and is therefore repressed into the unconscious to become manifest in altered form as psychological symptoms and disturbed mood in later life. Thus, psychoanalysis makes eloquent but unproven comment upon the aetiology of adult psychological, and especially neurotic, disturbance.

Biological causes

There has been a considerable increase in biological research in psychiatric aetiology over the last few years. Only a brief summary is possible here, and this area of interest is changing rapidly.

Genetics

The genetic study of any individual psychiatric illness is concerned with whether a link can be found between symptoms and inheritance, and what is the precise nature of inheritance. The first family study of schizophrenia was carried out by Rudin in 1916, and the contribution of genetics has been explored using such methods as *family risk studies, twin studies* and *adoption studies*. For example, the lifetime risk of developing schizophrenia for first-degree relatives (those who share 50 per cent of their genetic material, such as parent, sibling, child) of schizophrenic patients is about ten times that of first-degree relatives of healthy controls. For the siblings of schizophrenic patients the lifetime expectancy of developing the condition is 10 per cent, for the children of a schizophrenic parent 14 per cent, and where both parents are schizophrenic, 46 per cent. This compares with a lifetime risk of about 0.85 per cent for the whole population. Many twin studies have been carried out for schizophrenia, and in general there has been found to be about 50 per cent concordance for monozygotic twins and 17 per cent for dizygotic. The concordance rates for monozygotic twins reared together and apart is generally similar, indicating a major genetic component. Adoption studies have tended to confirm this genetic contribution to the aetiology of schizophrenia in that biological relatives have been concordant for schizophrenia, whilst those in the adopting families have not.

The *mode of inheritance* has been investigated in major psychiatric illnesses, but in both schizophrenia and manic-depressive psychosis results are at present equivocal. There are four possible modes: on a single major locus inheritance may be dominant, recessive or sex-linked, or alternatively the inheritance may be polygenic. An example of a psychiatric condition with dominant inheritance is Huntington's chorea, in which the condition is inherited as autosomal dominant with high penetrance. The condition usually develops at about the age of 40, when procreation has often been completed, and of course males and females are equally affected.

Linkage studies to identify the gene locus have been carried out; for example, in Huntington's chorea using genetic markers. Cytogenetic studies have also been used aetiologically in psychiatry; for instance, in Down's Syndrome, in which the two most frequent abnormalities of chromosomes are trisomy, most frequently of chromosome 21, or translocation, also involving chromosome 21. *Molecular genetics* is still at an early stage in its development in the unravelling of causes of psychiatric disorders, and it is probable that this topic will receive more space in future editions of this book.

Biochemistry

Neurochemical studies have been carried out using the post-mortem brain. For example, an increase in density of dopamine receptors has been demonstrated in the nucleus accumbens and the caudate nucleus in the brain of deceased schizophrenic patients. The interpretation of such findings is difficult, as it may either be due to the condition itself or to the treatment, in this case psychotropic drugs, used for the illness.

Extensive chemical investigation has been carried out on a variety of body materials, such as blood, plasma, urine and cerebrospinal fluid. There have been a number of studies of tryptophan and 5-hydroxytryptamine in plasma and cerebrospinal fluid. In depressive patients it is thought that low concentrations of 5-HT in the brain are important in the development of depression. However, the studies are ambiguous at the moment. Phenylketonuria is an example of a condition which may be diagnosed from biochemical analysis of the patient's urine.

It is to be hoped that current developments in *brain imaging techniques* will make contributions to the biochemical understanding of the causation of mental illness in the future. Nuclear magnetic resonance imaging (MRI) allows the pictorial demonstration of areas of high metabolism in the brain. Single photon emission computerized tomography (SPECT) shows the distribution of radioactively labelled substances in the brain and therefore the site of chemical reactions involving these materials. Positron emission tomography (PET) demonstrates cerebral blood flow and metabolism in the brain and is able to localize areas of high activity. Much preliminary work has been carried out involving these various techniques, not only in organic states and major psychoses,

but also in anxiety states and other neurotic conditions.

Other neurosciences

Endocrinological studies often involve chemical assay in the study of psychiatric disorders. Such investigations have included finding high levels for free and total cortisol in plasma in depression, and marked abnormalities in the dexamethasone suppression test have been found in many studies of depressive illness. It has also been found that in depression there is diminished growth hormone response to the drug clonidine, which is a noradrenergic agonist. The interpretation of these various findings is still not clear.

Numerous *physiological* measures have been carried out in psychiatry, including measurement of pulse rate, blood pressure, blood flow and skin conductance, and the more elaborate techniques of measuring muscle activity, cerebral blood flow and electro-encephalography. Measurement of skin conductance has proved useful in investigating the antecedents of anxiety, whilst the electro-encephalogram has been used in investigating symptoms of schizophrenia using evoked potentials.

The use of *pharmacological* techniques holds promise in psychiatric disorders in that active pharmaceutical agents may be studied for their neurochemical actions in animal experiments. For instance, it has been demonstrated that some of the more commonly used antidepressant drugs such as the tricyclics are capable of altering the post-synaptic noradrenergic receptors. A drawback of pharmacological work in psychiatry is that there are no true animal analogues for the human psychiatric syndromes.

Much of the early neuroscientific work in psychiatry involved macroscopic and microscopic *neuropathology*; for example, demonstrating neurosyphilitic changes in the brains of those who have died with dementia in general paralysis. Another important finding has been the pathological damage to the mamillary bodies in the brains of those suffering dysamnestic syndromes such as those associated with Wernicke's encephalopathy.

Classification of psychiatric disorder

The most satisfactory method of classification for medicine involves both aetiology and demonstrable pathology; for example, tuberculous peritonitis in which the causative organism forms part of the classification, and the pathological changes, which may be seen both macroscopically and microscopically, forms the other part. It is unusual in psychiatry to have conditions where the aetiology and pathology is so clearly known.

Classification, and hence diagnosis, is required in medicine in order that communication may take place between doctors. It is a necessary basis for rational research; for example, any meaningful investigation of the biochemical changes in what we refer to as depressive illness requires a reasonably consistent classification of depressive illnesses. Rational treatment also can only be based upon a satisfactory system of classification of diagnoses.

Three types of classification are currently in regular use in medicine. (1) *Categorical* classification uses the patterns of symptoms, their course and outcome to place patients into different diagnostic categories; for example, this is the basis of the diagnosis of anorexia nervosa; (2) *Dimensional* types of classification imply that the individual can be measured for various characteristics, and diagnosis is determined by the position represented graphically in space; for example, the Eysenck Personality Inventory measures personality characteristics in any population with axes of extraversion/introversion and neuroticism/stability. With these two dimensions a patient may be placed in any of the four: neurotic extravert, stable extravert, neurotic introvert, stable introvert. (3) With *multiaxial* classification the patient is classified for a number of different qualities which are considered to be in different axes. These might, for instance, be (a) syndrome, (b) personality, (c) physical condition, and so on.

Systems of classification in psychiatry

One of the simplest and oldest distinctions in psychiatry has been that between *psychosis* and *neurosis*. This still has some usefulness in clinical practice, although it takes time and experience to be clear about the differences between them. Psychosis implies loss of reality judgement, loss of insight and especially such positive symptoms as delusions, hallucinations and thought disorder. In neuroses, the symptoms are out of proportion to the stimulus, they may persist after the stimulus has been removed, and they are disabling; however, the experience of a neurotic patient is on a continuum and therefore within the powers of empathy and identification of a normal person. A highly simplified form of categorization for psychiatric conditions is shown in Table 4.2. It is perhaps useful to consider these very limited categories on starting psychiatry, although with increasing sophistication a more elaborate system will be required.

As the range of treatment in psychiatry has increased, so the specificity of treatments for diagnostic groupings has become more

Table 4.2 *Simplified system for psychiatric disorders*

Mnemonic key	
M	Mental handicap (learning disability)
N	Neurosis and personality disorder – neuroses
O	Organic state
P	Psychosis { Manic-depressive psychosis / Schizophrenia
C	Psychiatric disorder of childhood

important and there has been a more pressing need for a satisfactory system of classification. Over recent decades the International Classification of Diseases has been the official document used for recording psychiatric diagnosis in the United Kingdom and Ireland, and the 9th Revision (ICD-9) which was published in 1977, had significant improvements on previous versions. This included a glossary of mental disorders with descriptive paragraphs for the different conditions. ICD-9 is still, in 1993, the official classification for psychiatric disorders in Britain, but will soon be replaced by ICD-10 (see below).

The American Psychiatric Association has published successive editions of their *Diagnostic and Statistical Manual* for mental illnesses. The 3rd edition (DSM III) was published in 1980 and was intended to provide a comprehensive classification for use in research, as well as the recording of health data. DSM III contains operational criteria for diagnosis with rules for inclusion and exclusion for diagnosis. It also uses a multiaxial classification with the following axes: (1) Clinical syndromes; (2) Personality disorders; (3) Physical disorders and conditions; (4) Severity of psychosocial stressors, and (5) Highest level of adaptive functioning in the last year. DSM III contained a number of alterations to the terminology used in previous editions of the American Classification, and also from ICD-9. More recently, a revised version, DSM IIIR, has been published.

The World Health Organization has introduced the 10th Edition of chapter V of the International Classification of Diseases (ICD-10), and this edition is entitled *The ICD-10 Classification of Mental and Behavioural Disorders*. The major categories are listed in Table 4.3. ICD-10 takes advantage of the improvements introduced both in ICD-9 and DSM IIIR. It includes a multiaxial system of diagnosis and a detailed glossary of the conditions listed. There are also diagnostic criteria for research. It is to be hoped that ICD-10 will be easier to use internationally than DSM IIIR, which creates some difficulties when used outside the United States. In particular, the conceptualization of schizophrenia and of neurotic disorder in ICD-10 is closer to previous internationally agreed definitions than to American usage.

ICD-9, DSM III and DSM IIIR have been mentioned above because medical undergraduates or postgraduates working in psychiatry in the 1990s are likely to hear these terms mentioned. However, the following chapters of this book are based upon ICD-10. We also aim to explain terminology commonly used in psychiatric practice, such as 'psychosis', as it is important to know to what such terms apply.

Table 4.3 *Major categories of ICD-10*

Key from ICD-10		Key from Table 4.2
F 0	Organic, including symptomatic, mental disorders	O
F 1	Mental and behavioural disorders due to psychoactive substance use	O
F 2	Schizophrenia, schizotypal, and delusional disorders	P
F 3	Mood (affective) disorders	P
F 4	Neurotic, stress-related, and somatoform disorders	N
F 5	Behavioural syndromes associated with physiological disturbances and physical factors	N
F 6	Abnormalities of adult personality and behaviour	N
F 7	Mental retardation	M
F 8	Disorders of psychological development	C
F 9	Behavioural and emotional disorders with onset usually occurring in childhood and adolescence	C

Effective treatment in psychiatry is dependent upon the application of appropriate remedies, and this in turn is dependent upon accuracy and consistency of diagnosis. Thus the classification of psychiatric disorders is important not only for understanding different mental illnesses, but ultimately for improving and refining the quality of treatment.

Further reading

American Psychiatric Association (1987) *Diagnostic and Statistical Manual of Mental Disorders*, 3rd edn, revised, Washington, DC: American Psychiatric Association.

Gelder, M., Gath, D. and Mayor, R. (1989) *Oxford Textbook of Psychiatry*, 2nd edn, chs 3 and 4.

World Health Organization (1992) *The ICD-10 Classification of Mental and Behavioural Disorders; Clinical Descriptions and Diagnostic Guidelines*. Geneva: World Health Organization.

5

Depression and mania

Psychopathology of depression

Depression is one of the commonest conditions encountered in psychiatry and one which may be very disabling. It may impair social and occupational functioning, sometimes severely and over long periods, affecting relationships and livelihood. At times, especially if untreated, it may lead to suicide. It is, however, highly amenable to treatment and, generally, it has a favourable prognosis. Depression also presents a challenge to medical diagnosis because it may present in a number of disguised forms, often resembling various physical conditions as well as other mental illnesses.

Almost all of us become 'depressed' at times. Usually, but not always, we recognize an association between life's events and difficulties and our depressed mood. Similarly, the commonest presentation of depression as an *illness* is one in which understandable reactions to circumstances are more prolonged and/or more severe than seems reasonable. On the other hand, again in common with everyday experience, depression in the illness sense sometimes occurs without any obvious provoking factors. This distinction has led some to classify depression according to whether it is 'reactive' (apparently emerging as a result of stresses) or 'endogenous' (arising from within, in the absence of clear precipitants). Unfortunately, this distinction is often difficult to make and is not very useful clinically.

The most obvious features of a depressive episode are *lowering of mood*, and *decrease in energy* and activity. These are usually accompanied by a reduction in the capacity for enjoyment – of simple, everyday pleasures or even of pleasure-evoking events; this altered experience is termed '*anhedonia*'. There is often *loss of interest*, not just in pleasurable matters but also in important aspects of life, such as self-care, family or work, together with *reduced concentration* when an effort is made. Depressed patients describe *inefficient thinking* – often feeling their thoughts to be muddled or slow – and frequently complain of becoming excessively *tired*, even if very little activity has been undertaken.

Sleep is usually disturbed and *appetite* affected, sometimes leading to marked *weight loss*. For many, depressed mood and these other symptoms vary little from one day to the next and are little affected by circumstances. One common exception to this unremitting quality is a characteristic rhythm through the day of mood and other symptoms; a so-called *diurnal rhythm of mood* wherein the patient describes (and relatives may report) being at his worst in the early morning, improving gradually as the day progresses, only to relapse into low mood again by the next morning. In depressive illness, although sleep may be delayed or broken during the night, it is very *early waking* which is the most striking and characteristic sleep disturbance; this early waking has a strong association with diurnal rhythm of mood.

It is not surprising, in the face of such feelings, that *self-confidence* may be low when faced with tasks normally accomplished with ease. One consequence is *low self-esteem*, frequently accompanied by guilt, perhaps about letting others down. The future may seem more uncertain than usual or, for some, very bleak. Feelings of *hopelessness* arise, and some patients say that they no longer feel like trying. Fleeting *suicidal thoughts* are common. More definite preoccupation with, or planning of, suicide is not infrequent, resulting in substantial mortality.

The following is the vivid retrospective account by one patient – a young doctor – of the progress of his depressive illness:

> In April the whole of life slowed down and time seemed to stand still. I had begun to worry and I was aware that I was grinding my teeth constantly so that my lower incisors became loose. I did not mind as eating had become a chore. I could not remember anything about my patients. … I had no power to help them. … I was waking early in the morning, listening to the hours pass through the chimes of my neighbour's grandfather clock. I would lie worrying, feeling physically ill, unable to get up and make use of the time, but dreading every moment of it. When it came to getting up I did not mind what I wore. If I looked like a tramp then that did not seem inappropriate. I remember trying to shave one morning. It took about 10 minutes – I could not keep my mind on it. The morning walk with the dog gradually became shorter and shorter although it seemed to take as long as ever. It gradually dawned on me that I might be dementing. Somehow this seemed to fit. My memory and thinking capacity had gone. I was a changed person. Of this I was aware, but I could not say how, it was altogether too vague. I knew that the only reason people had faith in me was that I had managed to fool them all these years. Any good things I had done had been a matter of luck and any bad things overlooked or unmentioned. The latter seemed more likely. I knew that while my boss was pleasant, he despised me for my incompetence. Every comment he made was a guarded remark related to my uselessness.

In addition to the clinical features of depression described above, there are a number of further symptoms which occur in some cases. These will be described under various headings, indicating how they cluster together in depressive illness.

Morbid preoccupations

One effect of low self-esteem and guilty feelings is the development of morbid preoccupations. For example, some patients become over-concerned about minor misdemeanours carried out in the past, which may become greatly exaggerated in importance. One patient, who was an active church attender, when depressed could not shake off a continual worry about a time over forty years previously, during World War II, when he mixed with fellow soldiers who used blasphemous language. He never joined in with them, he said, but he was now unable to forgive himself for being in their company – despite knowing that he had, at the time, no alternative but to mix with them. Over the forty intervening years, he had experienced this worry only during his several bouts of depression. Other examples of such preoccupations include fears about the safety of others and worries about having serious disease. The central features of such worries are that they are only strong during a depressive episode, and that they are recognized by the patient as excessive in some way, yet unavoidable.

Obsessional symptoms

Obsessional states are described in Chapter 12. In depressive illness, obsessional *symptoms* may occur, only to resolve when the depression has passed. Indeed, the morbid preoccupations described in the previous section have much in common with obsessions. In addition, depressed patients may develop fears and rituals like those seen in primary obsessional illness. One depressed patient began to fear that she would use swear words in conversation – something she had never done, and a notion which she found abhorrent. This fear was undetectable when she was no longer depressed. Another patient with depression began to fear that harm would befall his wife and children arising from some glass which had been broken at home. He began to check for glass fragments around the house and in his own clothing. He understood how unlikely such harm was, and he resisted the thought, yet it was not until the depressive illness was treated that the checking stopped.

Physical symptoms

There is a close association between depression and symptoms of physical illness. Pain, almost anywhere, is a frequent symptom in depression; it may occur in multiple sites. The attitude of patients towards such pain varies. For some the symptom itself, perhaps accompanied by a fear that it indicates serious disease, takes the person to the doctor. The doctor may then detect other depressive symptoms along with the physical ones. Some patients are so preoccupied by the possibility of some sinister physical disorder that fear becomes conviction and the initial symptoms are forgotten. The next paragraph describes how such beliefs progress in some patients to form the content of delusions.

Psychotic symptoms

A Delusions

In severe depressive states, excessive concerns may have such intensity that they are taken as true and justified, beyond the degree described as morbid preoccupation. False beliefs – delusions – are held, usually in keeping with the depressed mood. The most frequent topics of such depressive delusions are outlined in Table 5.1.

Some depressed patients have delusions about their health. One well-educated patient was quite certain that his metabolism had

Table 5.1 *Content of depressive delusions*

- Disease
- Nihilism
- Poverty and ruin
- Guilt and self-denigration

stopped; he cited as evidence that his fingernails had stopped growing. A day or two later he became convinced that his bowels had disappeared, and that his food was therefore passing down his oesophagus and pouring directly into his abdominal cavity. This belief, that parts of the body have 'gone', where they once existed, is sometimes termed a *nihilistic* delusion. In some depressive nihilistic delusions, the patient may believe that his whole body or person has ceased to be. One depressed patient, discharged not long before, was brought back to the hospital by his workmates; his attitude was one of terror and he claimed to be dead. He refused to walk, saying that 'dead people don't walk'. Some patients believe that other persons such as spouses or children no longer exist – perhaps even that they never existed. Some speak of themselves in the third person as if they did not exist; one woman, referring to herself, said: 'It's no good, take it away, wrap it up and throw it in the dustbin'.

A theme of many depressive delusions is that of *poverty* or ruin. The patient becomes sure that he faces penury, perhaps due to some false belief about squandering family money. An elderly patient with recurrent depression repeatedly developed the delusion that he would never again be eligible for his pension. He could not say why, yet he was not amenable to assurances that his daughter would continue to collect it for him, as she had done for many years.

Wickedness and *guilt* are among the commonest subjects of depressive delusions. One patient falsely stated that he had given his grandson's toys away; another that he had brought a deadly disease into the household, endangering others in his family. One patient, soon after admission to hospital, scribbled a 'last will and testament' in which he floridly confessed serious but false misdeeds against his family and signed the paper 'The Rotter'.

Of all the delusions of depression portrayed above, the common feature is how they seem to be determined by mood. Most but not all delusions in depressive illness are in keeping with the mood state. There are, however, other themes, such as persecution, which may or may not be so obviously associated with mood. For example, a patient who believes he is being persecuted may regard it as either a justifiable consequence of his wickedness or unjust, and so profess his innocence.

B   Hallucinations

Hallucinations are not a prominent symptom of depressive illness, but they do occur. As with delusions, hallucinations are generally in keeping with the mood. Thus, if a patient hears voices they will often accuse – perhaps alleging wrongdoings or making disparaging remarks. In other sensory modalities the relation of false perception with mood may be equally striking. One patient saw himself laid out in a shroud in an open coffin; another was continually aware of the 'smell of death' on her hands and persistently washed in antiseptic fluid to obliterate the smell. Some patients report that they are emitting a stench, which they smell and so believe that others must be able to smell it also.

C   Abnormalities of motor and psychic activity

In severe depression, movements, speech and thinking may be slowed, a state known as *psycho-motor retardation*. All degrees of severity occur, from the merest hint, confirmed when the patient is recovered, to complete loss of speech – *mutism*, or even loss of speech and movement – *stupor*. Mobility of facial expression may be greatly reduced, so that the patient may have an almost Parkinsonian appearance.

Patients who have become retarded may be difficult to interview because replies to questions, if forthcoming, may each take many minutes to emerge. A slow but painstaking examination of the mental state may reveal other psychotic and depressive features. Slow thinking may perhaps be inferred from slow speech, and some patients will describe a sluggish quality to their thoughts. On occasions, however, depressed patients who are retarded in movement and speech report that their thoughts are racing so fast that they cannot express them adequately.

One of the most striking clinical presentations of severe depression is one of extreme *agitation*. It is characterized by restless over-activity, sometimes leading to physical exhaustion. The patient may pace about and be unable to sit for long. He may be so unsettled that he fails to carry out even simple tasks such as dressing, eating or drinking. In such cases he may powerfully resist all attempts to help.

States of this kind arise particularly in elderly patients, in whom the combination of exhaustion and refusal to drink may lead rapidly to a life-threatening condition. Such patients also represent a high suicide risk. In addition to purposeless motor activity and resistance to the help of others, patients with agitated depression are usually wretched in their demeanour. One elderly man, who had recovered fully from several episodes of depression, rapidly developed a severely agitated state at each recurrence. He would begin to pace the room, wring his hands and mutter 'Oh dear', also developing a coughing mannerism and delusions of poverty. Within a day or so these two words were his only speech and it was impossible to persuade him to sit or lie down; exhaustion soon set in. It may be apparent that an agitated depressive state is one of the conditions to be considered in the differential diagnosis of excitement, over-activity and confusion.

Epidemiology of depression

While some of the symptoms of depressive illness, particularly the more severe ones, are specific to that condition, many are non-specific accompaniments of any state of distress: unhappiness, poor concentration, disturbed sleep and so on. One corollary of this observation is that depressive symptoms are continuously distributed in the population. At any time, some people have none of these symptoms, many have a few of them, and as the symptoms become more severe and more specific their frequency in the population decreases. For this reason, it is not possible to provide a simple and meaningful estimate of the incidence or prevalence of depressive illness – it depends where you draw the line between normality and disease. Little wonder, then, that research estimates of frequency have varied enormously between studies, not least because of differences in definition of the disorder.

As an illustration, let us consider one longitudinal investigation of the entire population of a small town in Sweden. During the fifteen years of study, among subjects who lived until age 70, 'clinically significant' depression occurred in 27 per cent of males and 45 per cent of females. If restricted to cases regarded as severe or medium-severe, rates were 16 per cent and 29 per cent respectively; however, rates for severe cases only were 2.9 per cent and 3.4 per cent respectively. These figures also illustrate another recurring observation: rates are much higher in females than males, but the disparity almost disappears when only the severe cases are considered.

Bipolar affective disorder

Although both mania and severe depression have been well known and well described for centuries, it was only a little over 100 years ago that it began to be fully recognized that the two were in some way connected. In 1896, Emil Kraepelin proposed the concept of manic-depressive insanity, in which some patients suffered recurrent attacks only of depression; others recurrent attacks only of mania; while some developed both kinds of episodes. This concept has survived the years and is still widely referred to as manic-depressive psychosis. In the latest terminology (ICD-10) both the term and the concept of manic-depressive psychosis have been abandoned; instead, a

distinction is drawn between *bipolar affective disorder* and *recurrent depressive disorder*.

Bipolar affective disorder, as the name suggests, is characterized by repeated episodes of severe mood disorder, sometimes mania (described below) and sometimes depression. Patients who develop recurrent mania but have no depressive episodes are comparatively rare and, because they are regarded as similar in many ways to patients who have depressive as well as manic episodes, they are included in the category of bipolar disorder.

Kraepelin noted that, during an episode of depression, no clinical distinction could be made between those patients who had recurrent depression and those who also became manic. For example, mild depressive episodes occur in bipolar patients, and severe, psychotic depressive episodes in patients who never become manic. Kraepelin therefore proposed a single disease. Although our latest classification has broken with this premise and put in its place two categories, there is still no way of distinguishing those with bipolar illness from those with recurrent depression except by the longitudinal course of their condition.

Recurrent depressive disorder is more common than bipolar disorder and, in contrast to bipolar states (where the sex ratio is almost equal), is noticeably more prevalent in women. Although a few patients develop chronic depression, a great majority make a good recovery, at least between episodes. Some patients, particularly while recovering from an episode of depression, and while receiving antidepressant treatment, become mildly manic yet never develop full-blown mania. These patients are included within the category of recurrent depression.

Classification

Of all the uncertainties in psychiatric classification, those related to mood disorders are perhaps the most troublesome. The latest internationally agreed classification, ICD-10, provides a helpful framework based mainly on description – avoiding as far as possible diagnostic statements based on aetiology or theoretical concepts. In Table 5.2, the main categories of mood disorder are set out. Diagnostic decisions are made according to whether there have been previous episodes; if so of what nature; and the nature and severity of the present episode. There are a number of additional categories and more specific sub-groups related to patterns of symptoms which, for simplicity, are not shown or discussed here.

Psychopathology of mania

The fundamental features of mania are *elevation of mood* and *increase in thinking, energy and activity*. The term 'hypomania' is not used in this chapter to denote a less severe form of the condition; such a distinction is largely arbitrary and there is great inconsistency in its definition.

Although mood in mania is elated, even exalted at times, it is often changeable and periods of depression are common; sometimes *lability* of mood is prominent. The elevated mood may be infectious, leading others to share in humorous banter. However, perhaps more often, manic patients may readily become *irritable*. This is particularly noticeable when other people – relatives, doctors, nurses – try to confine the patient's exuberance and plans.

Whereas depressed patients lose interest, those with mania develop new ones – sometimes

at great cost. Such interests may be linked with extravagant and unworkable projects and patients may part with more money than they can afford in trying to realize their schemes. *Grandiose thoughts* may range from an over-inflated self-opinion to clear delusions about ability or identity (see below). The increased energy which accompanies their expansive plans may develop into severe motor over-activity (see below). Often, *concentration span is reduced* and, despite the exuberance, many plans are not realized.

Another feature of mania is *disinhibition* of behaviour: caring little what others may think, and acting without thought for the consequences. In combination with other symptoms, disinhibition may have unfortunate effects. Some patients, believing themselves to be rich, or simply not caring about money, may give away property belonging to themselves or their family. Some may shout or sing or play music loudly or act in other conspicuous ways in a public setting. Less frequently, when accompanied by increased libido, disinhibition may lead to sexual indiscretions. Occasionally, disinhibited behaviour brings manic patients into conflict with the law. Unfortunately, all such actions may result in adverse public attention in the neighbourhood, at home or at work, and, despite full and often rapid recovery, there may be serious social repercussions.

Table 5.2 *Classification of mood (affective) disorders (from ICD-10)*

Manic episode

Bipolar affective disorder:
  currently manic
  currently depressed
  currently mixed
  currently in remission

Depressive episode:
  mild
  moderate
  severe

Recurrent depressive disorders:
  current episode mild
  current episode moderate
  current episode severe
  currently in remission

A   Delusions

The commonest delusions in mania are *grandiose delusions* about *ability*, *wealth* or *identity*. One psychiatric inpatient asked if one of the ward offices might be lent for his use so that he could interview the other patients – he said he had the skills of a consultant psychiatrist! Another patient stated that he was 'an avatar – a kind of super angel'. Yet another patient reversed normal experience, saying that when he felt cheerful the sun shone and when he felt sad it rained. Some patients experience *delusions of special mission* in which they believe themselves chosen to carry out some special task. Such beliefs often have religious content, but it is not usually difficult, with the help of family or members of the patient's religious group, to differentiate symptoms from well-grounded religious convictions.

B Hallucinations

Hallucinations are not common in mania. When they occur, they are frequently in keeping with the elevated mood. For example, voices may seem exalting and may instruct the person towards lofty goals. A few patients describe hearing music.

C Abnormalities of motor and psychic activity

Abnormalities of motor and psychic activity are a prominent feature of mania – more so than with depression. *Increased energy* is often accompanied by greater activity than usual. Once again this may have a wide range, from an almost enviable exuberance to uncontrollable *excitement*. When *over-activity* and excitement are severe and prolonged, there is real danger of exhaustion, dehydration and risk to life if left untreated. It is in such states of arousal that manic patients may become aggressive, occasionally even violent.

One of the most prevalent and striking clinical features of mania is an increase in the quantity of speech. Patients may talk incessantly and at greater speed than usual; it may be hard to interrupt. In one case, after the doctor had tried for more than an hour to obtain a narrative account of events, the patient patted the doctor on the hand and commiserated with him, saying that the trouble was that she was 'suffering from verbal diarrhoea'. The term '*pressure of speech*' is used to refer to these abnormalities. Sometimes speech is louder than usual for that person, and, depending on the prevailing emotion, laughter may also be conspicuous.

A common accompaniment of pressure of speech is an abnormality of thinking in which the patient's stream of thought flows very rapidly, sometimes referred to as '*pressure of thought*'. This may be apparent from the speech, and there are several degrees of severity. Some patients maintain their direction of thinking but bring in many details and become temporarily side-tracked on to irrelevant material; their talk is *prolix* but not without order and direction. Others lose the drift of their thought and become diverted onto entirely new thoughts and associations. It often seems that these diversions arise from one of two mechanisms. In the first the patient seems to be redirected by *associations of words or ideas*, such as chance rhymes, puns or 'clang' associations (in which two meanings of the same word are invoked – for example, one patient, talking of a relationship, said there was 'a great big barrier between us – not a reef'). In the second the patient is *distractible*; that is, he notices and is deflected from his course by insignificant events or objects in his surroundings – for example, by slight noises outside the interview room or by the name or appearance of the interviewer.

Few physical signs in medicine can be more striking and memorable than florid examples of this kind of thinking – usually termed '*flight of ideas*'. The combination of pressure of speech and flight of ideas often prevents the interviewer from writing down or even remembering examples of the abnormality. In the case of one patient, over a timed period of one minute he spoke about fourteen different topics, the headings for which could be written down; they varied from keeping budgerigars to his wife's physical attractions. Sometimes ideas flow so fast and the pressure to express them verbally is so strong that the result is incoherence. On the other hand, some patients whose speech is normal will nevertheless describe racing thoughts, perhaps accompanied by exciting ideas; this state is known as '*subjective ideomotor pressure*'.

Mixed affective disorder

Although bipolar illness is typically evident as separate episodes of depression and mania, sometimes patients show a mixture of depressive and manic symptoms. It is fairly common for patients currently manic to have phases where the mood is depressed; it is less common, but well recognized, for patients currently depressed to have manic phases. However, there are patients whose symptoms are so mixed throughout the episode that it is impossible to give one or other mood-state precedence in diagnosis. A few patients develop such *mixed affective states* repeatedly. One lady was, for several weeks, very distressed, weepy, hopeless and thinking of suicide; she also had pressure of speech, wore extremely striking make-up and was rather disinhibited in behaviour (at the end of the first interview, at her home, she gave the psychiatrist and social worker each a spray of orchids to wear). When well she was a composed and normally reserved person. The episode described here was the third in five years in which she had a similar mixture of symptoms.

Aetiology of depression and mania

In mood disorder, as with all psychiatric illness, many factors are likely to be relevant when answering the question: why is this person ill, in this way, now? In Figure 5.1, this idea is represented diagrammatically.

Constitutional factors are those which are biologically predetermined, by genetic make-up and any other pre-natal factors. There is good evidence that both depressive illness and mania tend to run in families. It is thought that bipolar

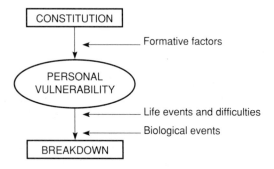

Figure 5.1 A model for the aetiology of psychiatric disorder

illness and recurrent depression may have separate inheritance and therefore tend to breed true in a family. It would be wrong, however, to place too much emphasis on genetics; certainly, single gene disorders seem unlikely to provide a full explanation. Inheritance has been shown to be more significant where severe psychotic symptoms are present. It is more important in bipolar disorder than in those states where depressive symptoms are close to the normal range of experience of mood.

It is a widely held belief that experiences, particularly in early life, are powerful *formative factors* in personal development. Psychiatrists and psychologists have been among those who have been most influential in putting forward such a view. It seems self-evident, and it is confirmed by investigation, that adverse experience may increase *personal vulnerability*. For example, we all know that deprivation or abuse of any kind, especially if severe or repeated and starting early in life, renders a person more likely to have emotional difficulties in adult life. We do not know what specific vulnerability factors are associated with later development of bipolar illness, but there have been many suggestions of childhood occurrences which make adult depression more likely. These include loss of parents through separation or death, childhood abuse and prolonged institutional care.

Having proposed why one person may be more vulnerable than another, the next step is to suggest why a state of long-term vulnerability might be triggered into a different state – one which the general public understands by the term '*breakdown*'. This expression is entirely non-specific. When patients use it to describe an earlier period of illness of their own or of a relative, it conveys no diagnostic information but does imply that an *episode* of difficulty in coping occurred. Often one correctly infers that the episode was one of mental illness; only by determining the character of the 'breakdown' can the interviewer speculate whether it was transient anxiety, prolonged schizophrenia, or indeed any other condition.

Why, then, does a 'breakdown' – in this case an episode of depression or mania – occur? It is widespread opinion that unpleasant events or persistent troubles may lead to 'breakdown'. In recent years it has been firmly established that *life events* and longer-term *difficulties* do indeed provoke the onset of specific psychiatric illnesses, including depression and mania. Perhaps because the condition is so common, this evidence is clearest for depression. Events recognized as precipitating episodes of depression are, not unexpectedly, usually ones which involve loss or threat: bereavement, other separations from a loved one, serious family conflicts, unemployment, failure to achieve some cherished ambition, debt and many more. Depression is also more likely in the face of chronic difficulties such as may be associated with poverty, poor housing, being the victim of racism, bearing the burden of caring for another person, social isolation, and a multitude of other hardships.

It is perhaps surprising that an attack of depression usually seems to be triggered by life events and difficulties even when depression is recurrent and the symptoms severe. It used to be supposed that it was mainly the milder (sometimes called 'neurotic') depressive episodes which occurred in response to events and difficulties, while the more severe attacks (sometimes called 'psychotic') arose without such provocation. The terms 'reactive and 'endogenous' were used to convey this notion; such a distinction is being abandoned and is absent from modern classifications. Nevertheless, a minority of patients are seen in whom there seems to be no clear precipitating factor; they tend to be those with severe and recurrent symptoms.

These social and psychological explanations of how depression is triggered by life events are not the only aetiological factors. There is a great deal of evidence that *biological changes* occur in affective illness. Patients with depression show *endocrinological abnormalities*. The hypothalamic-pituitary-adrenal axis is affected; for example, the normal diurnal rhythm of cortisol production is altered. In addition, in tests of function a substantial proportion of depressed patients show an abnormal pattern of cortisol suppression in response to dexamethasone. Changes in the hypothalamic-pituitary-thyroid axis have also been widely reported. It is also worth noting that both thyroid and adrenal disease have a strong association with affective illness (see Chapter 16).

For many years it has been apparent that drugs which affect *brain monoamine neurochemistry* have a link with depression. Reserpine was the first of several monoamine-depleting drugs observed to be associated with the development of depression. Both the tricyclic group of antidepressants and monoamine oxidase inhibitors have the effect of producing a relative increase in monoamine activity at central synapses. Theories linking depressive illness with a relative lack of monoamines therefore became established. Interest focused on noradrenaline and 5-hydroxytryptamine (5-HT), and the most recent evidence favours important roles for these transmitter systems. In the 1990s there have become widely available in the United Kingdom several antidepressant drugs with a specific 5-HT re-uptake inhibiting action. Their arrival has been accompanied by claims of high efficacy; their community effectiveness is, however, not yet established (see Chapter 23).

One adverse event in life which has social, psychological and biological impact is *physical illness*. It is therefore not surprising that physical ill health has a marked association with depressive illness. Although there are specific examples of this connection, some of which are described in Chapter 16, recent or current physical disease of any nature has a strong association with depressive illness. This is perhaps most evident among elderly patients.

Treatment

Depression

One of the reasons why Kraepelin, almost a century ago, put forward manic-depressive illness as a disease category was the observation that, for many patients at least, there was natural remission. This observation remains true. However, for most of those suffering depression or mania it is unacceptable simply to wait, and there are reasons why active measures must be taken. First, there are available treatments of proven efficacy which are likely to reduce the period of suffering. Second, there are at least three important risks to inaction: worsening of symptoms resulting in a severe and perhaps persistent state of depression, which may be accompanied by severe physical deterioration; disability arising from lengthy impairment of the normal social and occupational functioning; and, most important, the possibility of suicide. Practical management of depression has, therefore, various components.

A   Physical treatment

Physical treatments for depression are described in some detail in Chapter 23. They will therefore be dealt with only briefly here. Both electroconvulsive therapy (ECT) and antidepressant drugs are effective with depressive symptoms of all severity. However, where the condition is severe – and especially where there are delusions, hallucinations or motor abnormalities – ECT is widely regarded as the treatment of choice. Compared with drug treatment, it is more likely to be effective and to produce rapid results.

In most cases of depression the first line of physical treatment is a drug from the tricyclic and related antidepressant group (British National Formulary category). In addition to instructions about dose, patients are usually informed that there will be delay before benefit is noticeable, and about the common side effects (see Chapter 23); both these drawbacks to the drugs are so commonplace that it makes good sense to anticipate their occurrence. An adequate dose may need to be built up gradually. If after several weeks on a satisfactory daily dose there is insufficient response, there are several options in physical treatment. They include an alternative drug from the same general group, a monoamine oxidase inhibitor drug, and ECT. Each of these, separately and sometimes in combination, have their indications and adherents, as do various other compounds not discussed here.

B   Psychological treatment

Many of the available psychological treatments are suitable for use with depressed patients. Where symptoms include delusions, hallucinations or marked motor disorder, most psychiatrists would choose a physical treatment in the first instance – perhaps also where obsessional symptoms, morbid preoccupations, anhedonia or biological features are prominent. Specific psychological therapies are, therefore, more widely used in milder cases, in those which have been more prolonged, and in some cases where physical treatments have been unsuccessful. *Cognitive therapy* incorporates strategies directed at depressive illness and some patients will be offered *individual psychotherapy* (see Chapter 22). Neither behaviour therapy nor group psychotherapy are widely used in depressive illness.

C   General aspects of management

Depression may affect the patient's judgement. The physician needs to recognize when this has occurred; decisions must sometimes be taken on the patient's behalf. On occasions the over-conscientious depressed patient must be told, when he is clearly unfit for work, to take time off – despite any protests about letting workmates down. He may need to be told firmly that he is ill, not shirking, as he may insist himself to be. It is appropriate to tell the patient that, in the experience of the psychiatrist, cooperation with treatment is likely to result in recovery.

Risk of suicide is an ever-present danger in the care of severely depressed patients. The assessment of this risk, both in the initial and later stages of the illness, must not be neglected. It is important at times to encourage the patient to talk about any suicidal ideas. The doctor must be able to enquire about such feelings without embarrassment and without being fearful of the reply. Provided the patient feels cared for, discussion of the topic does not precipitate suicidal behaviour. There are many shades of ideas of hopelessness and self-harm. It is useful to be able to ask, when appropriate, one or more of a series of questions: whether the patient feels like giving up hope at times, like not carrying on, perhaps even feeling better off dead.

If indicated from what has been said, or from past behaviour, a direct enquiry should be made about whether the patient has felt like acting on such feelings – perhaps taking his own life. This may proceed to questions about whether plans have been made, if so what they have been, and if there have been any suicide attempts. Relatively few patients with depression will talk spontaneously about such matters, but, on the other hand, few will either resent being questioned or be evasive or untruthful as to their real feelings. Particular care must be taken when patients are deluded about guilt, worthlessness, ruin or bodily disease. These patients have high suicide risk and may be unable to give an accurate account of self-destructive thoughts; they are also changeable and therefore unpredictable in their actions. Usually, hospital inpatient care and close observation is indicated in such cases, occasionally on a compulsory basis (see Chapter 24).

Apparent improvement does not necessarily mean that the risk of suicide has passed. Indeed, where suicide is considered a possibility, periodic assessment of a patient's attitude to himself should be carried out. Some previously retarded patients may be at a greater risk when they have made some improvement – being then able to think clearly enough and find the energy to act on suicidal wishes. Many depressed patients can nevertheless be adequately cared for at home, especially where there are family members willing and able to help. Day hospital attendance can allow repeated and frequent reappraisal of both treatment and risk and permits much closer attention than can be provided at an outpatient clinic. In some cases there is a key role for the Community Psychiatric Nurse in close monitoring of treatment and mental state.

Two important aspects of treatment are attention to *nutrition* and to *sleep*. Many depressed patients lose a great deal of weight, and in most cases appetite does not return until recovery begins. Regaining weight may be an objective sign of progress; the converse is also true. All

depressed inpatients, and some who are outpatients, should be weighed regularly under the same conditions. Sleep is another barometer of recovery for some patients. Sedative properties of many common antidepressant drugs can be used to the patient's benefit. It is usual to prescribe these drugs in a single night-time dose which may help any sleep delay or early waking. Hypnotic drugs are used on occasions, but the only good advice is to avoid them where possible and to use them for as short a time as possible. In some agitated depressed patients, neuroleptic drugs are more effective sedatives than benzodiazepine drugs.

During recovery patients should be warned that they are likely to suffer *bad days* which arise out of sudden swings of mood. If not forewarned, patients who find themselves plunged once again into suffering may rapidly come to believe that all is lost. It is also important to help patients decide about *return to work*. Premature attempts to return to work by patients who have been depressed are common and should be resisted, if necessary enlisting cooperation from the patient's family. What depressed patients often fail to realize is that when away from work and from having to take responsibilities and make decisions, they may seem to themselves better than they really are. Exposed again too soon to stress with which they are not yet ready to cope, they may well relapse. In many cases, return to work should be accomplished by stages, if possible.

Preventing recurrence has as many aspects as does the initial management; only a few will be mentioned here. First, if there are events and difficulties considered to have played their part in precipitating the disorder, these should be addressed – some can be changed, perhaps with family help. Some others can be worked through, or at least a start can be made on such a process, to be continued over a longer time. Second, antidepressant drug treatment is known to protect from early relapse if continued after recovery; opinions vary on duration, but at least for several months. Third, lithium carbonate and carbamazepine are considered to have specific prophylactic effects and may be introduced for that reason in patients who have suffered repeated episodes (see Chapter 23).

Mania

There are two specific *physical treatments* used widely in mania: neuroleptic drugs and lithium carbonate – used separately or in combination. Even states of moderately severe disturbance are usually readily controlled by oral, or if necessary parenteral, sedative neuroleptic drugs such as chlorpromazine or haloperidol. In a few cases ECT may be used; many psychiatrists have been convinced by its effectiveness in severe cases but, because it is a second-line treatment when drugs are proving insufficient, hard evidence about efficacy in mania is lacking. Most manic patients will be well enough to leave hospital after a few weeks and a full recovery to pre-morbid mood and function is usual. Unfortunately, a small minority of patients swing, during the successful treatment of the manic state, across to marked and prolonged depression; transient depressive episodes are more common and self-limiting. In some patients who have had recurrent attacks, prophylaxis against return of mania is attempted, through the use of lithium carbonate or carbamazepine (Chapter 23).

As described above, manic patients suffer a lack of judgement, leading at times to eccentric, profligate, antisocial and occasionally violent acts. It is imperative that patients with manic illnesses are brought speedily under control. In severe cases, despite the utmost skill and tact, compulsory admission to hospital is usually necessary. An over-active, grandiose, exhilarated and energetic manic patient is a challenge for all staff involved. However, the usual complete and relatively rapid recovery more than repays the efforts made.

Further reading

Arieti, S. and Bemporad, J.R (1978) *Severe and Mild Depression: The Psychotherapeutic Approach*, New York: Basic Books.

Brown, G.W. and Harris, T. (1978) *Social Origins of Depression. A Study of Psychiatric Disorder in Women*, London: Tavistock Publications.

Gilbert, P. (1984) *Depression: From Psychology to Brain State*, London: Lawrence Erlbaum Associates.

Goodwin, F.K. and Jamison, K.R. (1990) *Manic-depressive Illness*, Oxford: Oxford University Press.

Paykel, E. (ed.) (1992) *A Handbook of the Affective Disorders*, Edinburgh: Churchill Livingstone.

6

Schizophrenia and delusional disorders

The concept of *dementia praecox*, now known as *schizophrenia*, dates back to the the work of Emil Kraepelin in the last quarter of the nineteenth century, prior to which the disorder does not seem to have been distinguished from the amorphous mass of mental disorder. However, the use of the term 'dementia' was misleading, since the type of deterioration which occurs is different from that due to organic brain disease. In schizophrenia, the formal intelligence of the patient remains relatively intact. What suffers is the capacity to use intellectual powers in a realistic and purposeful way.

The term 'schizophrenia' was first introduced in 1911 by Eugen Bleuler. Although this term means 'split mind', Bleuler did not intend this to be regarded as being split into two parts, as is commonly misunderstood. Instead, he was referring to 'fragmentation' leading to disconnection in the normal association of ideas, to the inappropriate expression of emotions in relation to thought and behaviour, and to detachment from reality.

It has remained unclear whether schizophrenia covers one disorder or several. Variability of course and outcome has led to suspicion that there may be several conditions having certain features in common. For example, a substantial proportion of cases emerge as acute short-lived episodes following some fairly clear precipitating event. In such cases complete recovery is not unusual. In contrast is that form of the disorder which begins so insidiously that a clear point of onset cannot be identified. In cases of this kind, the condition may run an unremitting downhill course towards an apparently irreversible state of disability. Although these two conditions are described as distinct, there are other schizophrenic disorders having a course and outcome lying somewhere in between; it may well turn out that these descriptions are no more than two end points of a continuum.

Clinical features

It may be evident from the above account that a great variety of clinical features arise in schizophrenia. It is convenient to describe the bulk of these signs and symptoms under the following headings, as disorders of

- possession of thought,
- thinking,
- perception,
- movement and speech,
- mood.

Possession of thought

A number of experiences related to the possession of thought are regarded as characteristic of schizophrenia. These *passivity* experiences are described in Table 6.1. Their common feature –

Table 6.1   *Passivity phenomena*

Thought insertion	The patient experiences thoughts which are not his own, intruded into his thoughts (very often the alien thoughts are believed to be inserted by a psychic process such as telepathy or a physical process such as a radio transmitter).
Thought withdrawal	The patient believes that thoughts are removed from his mind, usually by some external force or agency.
Thought heard aloud	The patient may hear his thoughts 'aloud', just before he thought them or at the same time; or they may be repeated or echoed immediately after he has thought them.
Thought broadcast	The patient may experience his thoughts as shared with other people – often with large numbers of others.
Other passivity experiences	The patient may experience his will, movements, speech or sensation as being replaced by that of some outside force or agency; for example, feeling controlled as if a robot or zombie, or that his writing is no longer his own.

whether related to thinking, personality or body – is the loss of a clear boundary between self and the external environment.

Thinking

Abnormalities of thinking in schizophrenia may involve disorders of *belief* or disorders of the *form* (or style) of thinking.

Disorders of belief

Disorders of belief in schizophrenia are usually delusions. Indeed, very often the diagnosis of schizophrenia will be arrived at because

delusions are prominent. The definition of a delusion has already been discussed in Chapter 2. Very often, although by no means exclusively, persecutory themes predominate in schizophrenia. Thus a patient may feel under some form of threat or attack, or the subject of surveillance or monitoring. A basic delusional belief of this kind may extend into ideas of explanation. Persecution may seem to be carried out by specific organizations such as police Special Branch or, in the case of one patient, a network of solicitors. A further explanatory process may result in the belief that physical forces such as X-rays, transmitters, even space satellites, are being used in the persecution. Some patients attribute the experiences to paranormal mechanisms such as hypnotism, telepathy or extra-sensory perception; others, to occult or similar forces.

A number of other delusional themes also arise in addition or as alternatives to those of persecution. Patients may be *grandiose*, believing that they have unusual powers or significance or a special mission to accomplish, or that they are related to prominent persons. Delusions of a *sexual* kind occur, as do those involving *abnormalities of bodily function*.

In addition to the subject matter of delusions, it is important how such beliefs arise. Two ways in which delusions emerge are characteristic of schizophrenia. First, there is the *delusional perception*, in which a seemingly innocent object or event is perceived normally but is immediately regarded as significant for the patient in a delusional way. For example, a patient, when she saw on the side of a bus an advertisement for soap powder, realized that it confirmed her fears about the existence of a plot against the life of her adult son. Second, on occasions a *sudden delusional idea* seems to arise quite without a clear trigger or explanation. For example, one patient realized one afternoon, whilst looking out of the window, that the university Department of Philosophy in his local city was organizing a conspiracy against him.

The delusional perception is an example of the *referring-to-the-self* quality so typical of delusions in schizophrenia. Delusions which arise in this way include those in which the patient may misinterpret apparently innocent words or actions of others as drawing attention to him or commenting about him. Sometimes this may occur on a grand scale; for example, when the gestures of a television newscaster are taken to indicate that news items are aimed specially at the patient. *Delusional misinterpretation* of this kind may extend so that unremarkable occurrences indicate that situations are specially set up as some sort of test: for example, when all patients and staff on the ward are reckoned to be actors or stooges, only there to test out the patient's reaction.

Thought disorder

A frequent, important and characteristic symptom of schizophrenia is a peculiar disturbance of the process of thinking. It is difficult to describe the character of this *thought disorder* briefly. In essence, it lies in an inability to focus on the main point of a statement or an argument. In general, the patient retains a given concept, but seems unable to suppress irrelevant associations, with the result that the concept becomes blurred and hazy. Consequently, productive conversation is impossible, the patient may lose himself in a cul-de-sac, or in elaborate irrelevancies, often by dwelling on the sound or visual appearance of a word. Patients are often aware of an inability to direct their thinking. One patient said: 'It is like a motor car stuck in the snow, the engine keeps running but the wheels turn round and round in the same spot'. Another patient found particular significance in numbers, for example, 'Five equals "The Holy Trinity" like a Roman V, like a snooker triangle'; the experience was particularly disturbing while attempting mental arithmetic.

Sometimes thought disorder is not immediately evident in conversation. The interviewer may attribute his failure to understand the patient to a deficit in his own concentration. In due course it may dawn upon the interviewer that the meaning is unclear because the structure of the patient's thinking is abnormal. Some psychiatrists ask patients to perform certain tests in order to elicit thought disorder. The patient may be asked to recite a story or a fable, and to give the moral; patients are invited to interpret proverbs or to state differences such as those between a child and a dwarf. While these may have a ready appeal to those eager for a sign, they are often hard to interpret. In the absence of standardized norms, it is difficult or impossible to assess the degree of abnormality of a given response; thus two interpretations may be equally valid, although one may be unexpected. For example, what is one to make of the following example, provided by a young patient with schizophrenia who had delusions of persecution, when he was asked to describe the difference between a fence and a wall: 'A fence you can see through; a wall has ears'?

The flow of thinking in schizophrenia is sometimes affected in another way. Some patients report a sudden stoppage of their thinking – because they feel that thoughts have been withdrawn from the mind, although they were flowing quite freely before.

Despite all these disorders in thinking, basic psychological functions such as memory, grasp of concepts and orientation usually remain apparently intact. Some patients in the acute phase of a schizophrenic illness may, however, show a degree of clouding of consciousness, whether in a first illness or an exacerbation or relapse.

Perception

The nature of hallucinations is discussed in Chapter 2, but they may be defined briefly as false perceptions without an adequate external stimulus.

Hallucinations

Regarding hallucinations in schizophrenia, those in the auditory modality are the most conspicuous and the most prevalent and have come to be regarded widely as the hallmark of schizophrenia. This view is misleading for three reasons. First, hallucinations in schizophrenia may occur in all modalities; second, schizophrenia may be present without hallucinations; and third, auditory hallucinations may occur in other disorders such as depression, mania and organic psychiatric states.

Patients with schizophrenia may report, when there is no one else around and nothing else to explain it, various noises and sounds. These sounds may be ill-defined background noise, specific sounds such as machinery or perhaps muttering or whispering. Often, the sounds will incorporate formed words. Voices of one or more persons may speak in whispers, normal tones or loud volume. Words spoken may be normal in quality or enunciated in strange tones. Some patients recognize these voices as those of specific people. Voices may address the subject directly and in a pleasant, neutral or derogatory fashion. On occasions patients are given instructions which they may or may not obey.

While hallucinations of the above description are commonplace features of schizophrenia, there are further hallucinations which, if they occur, are characteristic of schizophrenia. First is the experience of two or more voices discussing the patient between themselves, as if in a conversation – often in a derogatory way. Second, some patients hear one or more voices describing their actions and thoughts as if in a running commentary, as in the following example: 'She's sitting at the table, writing a cheque. ... Now she's getting up, she's going towards the bathroom, going to have a wash ...'. Third, there is an experience which patients often find difficult to describe in which the sensation is of hearing one's own thoughts spoken aloud, almost as if someone nearby were able to overhear them. These experiences may be particularly distressing, especially if, as is not uncommon, they continue over long periods.

Hallucinations of the other senses also occur in schizophrenia. Visual hallucinations may be unclear or fully formed images, fleeting or persistent. Smells and tastes also occur. For example, one 50-year-old patient regarded a 'sexual smell' around her room each morning as evidence that spiritual forces were tampering with her soul during the night. Tactile hallucinations are by no means rare: one patient described a very persistent tickling sensation in the perineum which he thought must be carried out by an invisible robot (there was no evidence of pruritus ani). Some patients describe halluci-

natory experiences which are usually labelled 'somatic'. This physical sensation is not tactile to the skin but internal, as in a patient who reported that the reason she believed herself to be 'riddled with cancer' was that she could 'feel it riddling' inside her. Another patient complained that she was disturbed by two young male lodgers knocking nails into the walls of a room in her house, not because of the noise or the damage, but because each time a nail was knocked in she felt it in her own body. One of Bleuler's patients complained of feeling the pain of an injection given to the patient in the next bed.

Movement and speech

From the earliest days of the concept of schizophrenia, it has been observed that some patients show abnormalities of movement and speech. There is an enormous range of such disorders. Patients may be slowed down, some even stuporose. A stuporose patient may stand, sit or lie in various attitudes which may be uncomfortable. Patients may adopt the fetal position or lie back with the head uncomfortably raised from the pillow. If untreated, patients may remain completely motionless for hours or days, mute and unresponsive to painful stimuli, showing both retention of urine and faeces, or occasionally incontinence. As part of such a state, or in pre-stuporose states, some patients will permit their limbs to be placed quite freely into awkward positions – rather as one might move an Angle-poise lamp; such movement is known as *catalepsy*. Muscle tone may be apparently altered in such circumstances so that the limbs exhibit a curious 'waxy flexibility' which the examiner can feel as the limbs are passively moved. In other patients, muscle tone may be increased, with resulting rigidity. Although at the time patients may appear unable to do so, they may well be able to comprehend clearly what is going on around and can sometimes give an accurate account of the experience on recovery.

In contrast, patients with schizophrenia may at times show severe excitement. It may arise as a presenting feature or may emerge suddenly from stupor. At times the condition may be mistaken for, and be difficult to distinguish from, acute mania. Typically, manic patients present a rush of mainly purposeful activity, speech characterized by flight of ideas and mood which is infectious and expansive, if somewhat irritable. In excitement due to schizophrenia, however, behaviour will often be absurd, stereotyped, purposeless, and accompanied by incoherent speech which may be so disordered that it resembles some forms of aphasia; mood is not typically infectious. Hallucinations are a common accompaniment of schizophrenic excitement. They are much less prevalent in mania.

States in between stupor and excitement may be observed, in which the subject may take up an almost statuesque position in a corner of a room, occupying himself with ceaseless repetitive (stereotyped) movements. Other patients may sit for hours covering countless sheets of paper with meaningless writing of words, symbols and other indecipherable characters.

Just as with movement, so are there disorders of speech. As alluded to above, these may range from mutism to incessant talking or shouting. The disordered language which is described in Chapter 2 can become so severe that speech seems entirely without meaning, just a jumble of words often called *word salad* (also known as 'verbigeration').

For many psychiatrists, the above features of schizophrenia are regarded as *catatonic* symptoms, or components of *catatonia*. Rather like the term 'schizophrenia' itself, this word has been over-used and abused. If employed at all, it is best reserved for describing movement and speech disorder in the presence of a diagnosis of schizophrenia.

Mood

Changes in mood of almost any variety have a recognized association with schizophrenia. Patients may become anxious, depressed or elated. However, there are a number of states of abnormal mood which warrant particular mention. *Blunting* of mood refers to a loss of range of mood, resulting in an inability to express deep emotion. *Incongruity* occurs when the expression of mood does not fit the content; for example, laughter where sadness seems the appropriate emotion. This process, when severe, may manifest in a persistent silly or facile mood and behaviour.

Delusional mood (synonym: *delusional atmosphere*) is identified from patients' reports of a feeling that 'something is going on' which cannot be explained, perhaps that familiar surroundings seem altered in some indefinable way. This state may end quite suddenly with the formation of a clear delusion (often arising as a delusional perception or sudden delusional idea). Some patients are in a state of *perplexity*, where their lack of touch with the world around is evident from their vague and puzzled attitude.

Forms of schizophrenia

Since the days of Kraepelin and Bleuler, schizophrenia has been categorized according to clinical features into four sub-types: *paranoid*, *hebephrenic*, *catatonic* and *simple*. They are not mutually exclusive, and mixed forms are so common that, in the United Kingdom at least, most psychiatrists pay little attention to sub-typing except where the clinical picture is strikingly similar to that of the classical case.

Paranoid schizophrenia, characterized by delusions, hallucinations and passivity phenomena, is much the commonest of the four sub-types. It is worth noting that the word 'paranoid' in this context refers to its more literal sense, used since before Kraepelin's time, of 'deluded'. Thus it is not restricted to the persecutory connotations of today's vernacular. Delusions in paranoid schizophrenia may well, for example, consist of themes of special identity or hypochondriasis rather than persecution – although persecutory delusions seem the most prevalent in practice. Passivity phenomena are also frequently evident.

Hebephrenic schizophrenia is described when the most prominent symptoms are thought disorder and mood change – particularly incongruity of mood. These features have always been regarded as particularly prevalent among patients with onset of illness in late adolescence or early adult life. Indeed, the term 'hebephrenia' is derived from the Greek: *hebe* – youth; *phrenos* – mind.

Catatonic schizophrenia seems to have been much more common in past generations. Certainly it is unusual nowadays to encounter patients in whom the prominent symptoms early in the disorder are of movement and speech.

Once again it is important to stress that even in the minority of patients who fit a sub-group stereotype, other symptoms usually co-exist. For example, delusions and hallucinations are often present in those who, because of the prominence of other features, might be described as hebephrenic or catatonic.

The fourth classical category – *simple schizophrenia* – is the least satisfactory. Its features are hard to define: gradual deterioration into eccentricity and poor social function in the absence of the clear-cut symptoms and signs which define the other sub-types. Quite properly, the category is used rarely if at all.

In more recent times, a category of *residual schizophrenia* has developed to encompass patients whose well-documented acute symptoms in the past have subsided, only to be partially or wholly replaced by features such as apathy, lack of self-care, poverty of thought and speech, blunted affect and conspicuous eccentricity.

A number of other categories of disorder, often linked with schizophrenia, are described later in this chapter.

Epidemiology

Schizophrenia seems to be about as common in males as in females. The onset may occur at any time from mid-childhood to old age, but the age of onset most often lies between 15 and 45 years. An interesting and repeated research finding has been that the peak age of onset for men (mid-20s) may be earlier than for women (mid-30s). There have been many attempts to measure incidence (annual rate of new cases); rates now widely accepted are in the order of 10 new cases per 100,000 per year. This is a crude

rate; age-specific rates for those aged 15–40 are higher. Large-scale international studies conducted by the World Health Organization have suggested, for strictly defined cases, similar incidences in many different countries including several developing nations. In the general population, the lifetime risk of developing the disorder is reckoned to be slightly below 1 per cent. Schizophrenia is a common disorder with high morbidity and a consequent high cost in care. It constitutes a significant public health issue on a global scale.

Aetiology

No characteristic pathophysiological abnormality has been identified amongst patients with schizophrenia. There are several reasons why the search for any such abnormality has been difficult. First, given the variability of clinical patterns described above, it is not surprising that research has been hampered by ill-defined samples of subjects. Second, acutely ill patients are usually very distressed and often disturbed in behaviour, so drug treatments which are established as being rapidly effective in reducing florid symptoms are often used early; few new patients remain treatment-free for long. Third, the relatively high prevalence of the condition is a result of chronic illness and relapses rather than high incidence, so many patients studied have had the illness for a long time. Those with chronic symptoms often remain on drug treatment for symptom control, and those whose illness remits often receive prophylactic drug treatment which has been shown to reduce relapse rate. Therefore, although there have been many reports of pathophysiological abnormalities, none has so far been found consistently. Some findings may also be a result of medication or non-specific consequences of the long-term effects of disabling illness, or of prolonged hospital care.

Genetics

Twin studies have usually shown high concordance rates of up to 60 per cent for monozygotic twins, even when they are raised apart; dizygotic twins seem to have rates similar to those found in siblings (8–15 per cent). The risk in offspring of affected parents is much higher than in the general population – estimates have ranged from 14 per cent to almost 50 per cent, depending on whether one or both parents was affected. *Adoption studies* suggest a high inception rate for schizophrenia among children with an affected parent but adopted and raised by non-affected adults.

Such evidence supports the notion of strong genetic influence, but the nature of any genetic disposition and mode of transmission remains unknown. The genetic picture is complicated by the strong possibility that our concept of schizophrenia encompasses more than one disorder and multiple pathological changes.

Biochemistry

For many years it has been evident that consumption of certain drugs closely related to endogenous neurotransmitters (especially amphetamines) can cause psychotic illness somewhat similar to schizophrenia; also that therapeutic drugs effective in schizophrenia block the action of certain neurotransmitters. This evidence has led to a widely held and sustained theory relating schizophrenia to dysfunction of *dopamine* and its *receptor system*:

- amphetamines cause schizophrenia-like illness;
- amphetamines increase dopaminergic activity;
- neuroleptic drugs are effective in reducing symptoms of schizophrenia;
- neuroleptic drugs block dopamine receptors in the nigro-striatal system, causing extra-pyramidal symptoms;
- neuroleptic drugs may therefore act by countering primary dopamine over-activity in the limbic system.

Neuropathology

The development and availability of computerized axial tomography (CT scanning) and more recently of magnetic resonance imaging (MRI scanning) have given a boost to attempts to find structural brain abnormalities in schizophrenia. Structural changes in limbic areas and increases in ventricular size have repeatedly been found in patients with residual schizophrenia. Abnormalities in cases of more recent onset are gradually being identified, but changes are not yet clearly established.

Psychology

Numerous psychological theories have attempted to explain schizophrenia; most have paid attention to families. The ways in which parents interact and communicate with each other and with their children have been the most frequent focuses of attention. None of these theories has become widely accepted and sustained; some have been based on thin evidence, and attempts to replicate the findings have failed. Unfortunately, some family-based theories have tended to apportion blame for the illness, usually pointing it towards the parents of the person affected.

Sociology

In both the United States and the United Kingdom, schizophrenia has been found to be more prevalent among lower socio-economic groups in the community. It is not, however, self-evident that poor living conditions are to blame for the disorder because there is also considerable evidence that the illness tends to bring about a slow and insidious downward drift in the social scale. The allied finding, that the condition is commoner in urban than rural areas, may also be a result rather than a cause of the illness.

It has been shown that, in the weeks immediately preceding onset of an episode of schizophrenia, stressful life events occur more commonly than would be expected in the general population. In line with a common clinical observation, it seems that environmental pressures may precipitate schizophrenic illnesses in some people.

Management

Investigation

First, it is important to consider whether an acute illness, although characterized by typical symptoms of schizophrenia, may be a symptomatic state due to another primary condition. A significant minority of patients for whom the *descriptive diagnosis* is schizophrenia have, for example, been taking amphetamine drugs or are being treated with corticosteroids, or are suffering from hypothyroidism, cerebral lupus or another condition (see Chapter 7). Attention should be paid to history and physical examination, together with judicious use of physical investigations – such as testing urine for amphetamines, or blood for thyroid function.

Physical treatment

Symptoms of acute schizophrenia often include delusions, hallucinations and passivity phenomena. In practice, however, disturbance of behaviour, perhaps secondary to these experiences, may be the most pressing target for treatment. Fortunately, *neuroleptic drugs* are effective in reducing symptoms, and the sedative ones (for example, chlorpromazine, haloperidol) are also effective in quelling disturbed behaviour. Adequate doses of these drugs are an important part of early management in many cases.

When psychotic symptoms are present but sedation is not required, neuroleptics which exert little sedative effect are indicated (for example, trifluoperazine, pimozide). Later, for continuation treatment – either to subdue persisting symptoms or in the prophylaxis against further episodes – neuroleptic drugs may be given in *depot* form. The depot neuroleptic is given by intramuscular injection at intervals of perhaps three or four weeks; the active drug is contained in another substance (often an oily base) and is absorbed into the bloodstream very slowly. Drug treatment is described further in Chapter 23.

Careful management of patients by way of depot clinics and community nurses has, over many years, proved beneficial to patients who would otherwise fail to comply with medication and thereby relapse. Decisions to recommend or accept depot medication are not taken lightly because it will often lead to a lengthy period of drug treatment; most patients receiving depot drugs will already have had more than one episode of acute illness.

ECT, generally speaking, is used in the treatment of affective illness. However, it is used to good effect occasionally in acute schizophrenia, especially where there are prominent symptoms of depression or elation, or in rare cases of acute catatonic schizophrenia.

Other aspects of treatment

In an acute episode, especially if behaviour is seriously altered, hospital inpatient care will often be appropriate. Where there is reluctance to accept such admission and there is risk to the health or safety of the patient or other persons, compulsory admission may be required (see Chapter 24).

For many acutely ill patients, good nursing care and neuroleptic drug treatment will result in early eradication of symptoms. During hospital care attention needs to be paid to the social environment after discharge. This is particularly true when illness is recurrent and when it does not fully remit, leaving residual symptoms.

For those returning home, families need preparation. There is considerable evidence to suggest that high levels of *expressed emotion* in families – especially 'over-involvement' of family members with the patient, and a critical attitude – are detrimental to the patient's health. Where there is a good deal of face-to-face contact, patients in such families have a high relapse rate. Community nurses, social workers and medical staff can all contribute to the preparatory and continued work with families and patients which is needed to reduce these problems. Some patients and their families are helped by contact with one of the many local and national voluntary organizations which set out to assist patients, family members and carers; the National Schizophrenia Fellowship is particularly active in this way.

Some patients have no family care available. In other cases the patient or family decide not to live together – sometimes after many past difficulties. A range of accommodation choices exists, varying from town to town. A few schemes offer warden-assisted, *sheltered*, single accommodation. More common arrangements include *group homes* in which, as in shared student houses, several people share the rent and live together but with a certain amount of privacy. A community psychiatric nurse or social worker may visit regularly to check how the whole household is faring.

Hostels offer more structure – usually providing meals and often other forms of care such as supervision or administration of money and medication; many such hostels are formally registered with the local Social Services Department.

Whatever the accommodation – single, family, group home, hostel – many patients benefit from *day care*. Some hospitals offer long-term day-hospital attendance, but psychiatric *day centres* provided by Social Services or voluntary organizations are the principle source of long-term day care. Companionship, assessment of need for welfare or skills, education and recreation are just some of the features of successful day-centre care.

Sheltered working, once offered in many hospitals, has diminished with the reduction in size of the large psychiatric hospitals and with generally high unemployment rates. On the other hand, there has been recent growth in educational provision for those with chronic mental illness – by way of special needs courses, and access to generally available courses at Further Education colleges.

Inpatient care, usually of short duration, is required when acute symptoms demand it. However, very few patients nowadays stay in hospital indefinitely and long-stay numbers continue to dwindle.

The outcome for patients with schizophrenia is better in those treated early than in those who are first treated after a long period of illness.

This may be partly because cases with insidious onset have an inherently more resistant and adverse course. Cases of sudden onset, especially where depression or elation are prominent, seem to have a better prognosis. Many patients with schizophrenia have a brief illness then remain symptom-free. In the long term, a majority have either few symptoms or infrequent recurrence. Only a small but important minority have continuous disabling symptoms and permanent handicap.

Other non-organic psychoses

Persistent delusional disorders

Some patients develop long-standing delusional beliefs without other symptoms and without prominent mood disturbance. It is unclear whether or not such disorders are a variant of schizophrenia.

The principle feature of such conditions is delusion. This may be single, as in certain *hypochondriacal* delusions or multiple or *systematized* into a complex web of persecutory ideas in those who regard themselves as being at the centre of a network of surveillance. *Jealousy* may be the main theme for some, while others become *querulant* or litigious (seeking legal protection or redress for minor or imagined wrongs). Occasionally the subject develops the belief that another person, usually of high standing or even well-known publicly, is in *love* with him or her; protestations to the contrary by the other party are ineffective and interpreted as a necessary subterfuge because the affair is a secret one. This delusion of love is sometimes known as 'De Clérambault's Syndrome' (see Chapter 2).

Among persistent delusional disorders, hypochondriacal themes lead to two well-recognized patterns. First, *delusions of infestation* tend to occur in middle-aged or elderly persons. The subject believes himself or his home to be infested by insects. Careful examination by dermatologists or pest control companies are to no avail; the belief persists. Some patients describe the creatures in detail and may draw pictures of them. Dermatologists have referred to the 'matchbox sign' referring to such patients who may bring various forms of household or skin debris in matchboxes, seeking microscopic analysis which they hope may finally identify the infestation. Sometimes it is believed that insects on the skin have become lodged in one or other body orifice; in some cases the infestation is internal, as in the case of a lady who believed she had a worm in her bladder. All such beliefs may be very persistent and resist treatment. Many patients will refuse to see a psychiatrist, regarding psychiatric attention as irrelevant and insulting in view of the physical nature of the complaint. One patient, when she discovered she was talking to a psychiatrist, walked out saying, 'If my finger hurts, I don't go and see an eye doctor'. In a substantial proportion of cases, judicious use of powerful non-sedative neuroleptic drugs in modest doses is very effective; pimozide has been the drug most widely recommended.

Second, some patients complain of *bodily deformity*, believing that some anatomical part is misshapen. The term 'dysmorphophobia' is often applied to this state. Breasts and genitals are sometimes the focus of the false belief, but the parts most often affected are noses and chins. The patient may be convinced that his nose is a constant subject of discussion by acquaintances, workmates or even total strangers. He thinks that they look meaningfully in his direction and at one another as he passes, making at the same time barely overheard but clearly derogatory remarks. The disorder most often affects sensitive and socially unskilled young men, although women are not exempt. Some patients seek plastic surgery as a redress but surgical correction is notoriously ineffective in improving the state of mind of the patient. Once again, neuroleptic drugs are effective in some cases.

Induced delusional disorder (*folie à deux*)

A delusional disorder shared by two persons who have a close emotional bond is sometimes termed *folie à deux*. The most usual scenario is one in which the more dominant of the two persons develops a delusional disorder which is then induced in the other member of the partnership. The condition is uncommon, and often involves husband and wife, or parent and adult offspring, usually living in the same household. In some cases, both may recover when the more dominant partner with delusional disorder is treated.

Delusional jealousy

Jealousy is an emotion which, like so many, is distributed through the population. Some are rarely if ever jealous of their partner. Many may be mildly or transiently jealous when there is some provocation, but others may show marked and prolonged jealousy even with little or no cause. Although also seen in women, the most marked and dangerous jealousy is commoner in men.

Where a partnership is marred by severe jealousy, a great deal of misery arises. The jealous one of the two tends constantly to spy on the other, observing her every movement, subjecting her to perpetual cross-examination as to her daily activities. He may read her letters and go through her personal belongings for clues to infidelity. In the majority of such cases the jealousy is interrupted by periods of more rational thinking when the person acknowledges that the idea gets out of hand. Where there has been confrontation or even violence, there may follow apology and requests for forgiveness.

In some cases, however, no such change in belief occurs: jealous ideas are delusional. He believes unshakeably that his wife is unfaithful. Scrutiny of her underwear reveals what he is certain are seminal stains. Innocent encounters and remarks are interpreted as 'evidence'. Where there appears to be no such evidence, he believes only that she is covering her tracks well.

Certain characteristics are associated with states of morbid jealousy. The most important is alcohol excess and dependence, especially if complicated by erectile impotence; other forms of drug abuse, such as use of cocaine or amphetamines, and early dementia are also implicated in some cases. Sadly, as well as the unhappiness due to mistrust and confrontation, violence erupts on occasions; serious harm occasionally befalls the supposedly unfaithful partner, and homicide is a recognized outcome in a few cases.

Schizo-affective disorder

In this book the mood disorders and schizophrenia have been described so as to emphasize their differences. However, as with much classification in medicine, there are patients who show features of both conditions – whether at the same time in different phases of an episode or in separate episodes. Such cases are frequent enough to lead to a category of *schizo-affective disorder*. In keeping with attempts to define an intermediate form of illness, there has been much dispute about the disease status of schizo-affective disorder, and about which patients, if any, might be included in such a category.

In the latest International Classification (ICD-10), use of the diagnosis is restricted to patients showing mood and schizophrenic symptoms *at the same time*. Schizo-affective disorder is divided into manic and depressive types, according to which mood state predominates.

In each case, typical schizophrenic symptoms, such as passivity phenomena or commentary auditory hallucinations, also occur.

There has been a growing view that, in natural history and treatment response, patients who are regarded as suffering from schizo-affective disorder resemble those with affective psychosis more closely than they resemble patients with schizophrenia.

Schizo-affective disorder is treated as was described for the two disorders separately – according to circumstances; neuroleptic and antidepressant drugs are both used. Some consider mood-stabilizing drugs such as lithium to be of particular value.

Further reading

Cutting, J. (1985) *The Psychology of Schizophrenia*, Edinburgh: Churchill Livingstone.

Warner, R. (1985) *Recovering from Schizophrenia: Psychiatry and Political Economy*, London: Routledge & Kegan Paul.

Wing, J.K., Cooper, J.E. and Sartorius, N. (1974) *The Measurement and Classification of Psychiatric Symptoms*, Cambridge: Cambridge University Press.

Wing, J.K. (ed.) (1978) *Schizophrenia: Towards a New Synthesis*, London: Academic Press.

7

Organic disorders

There is no doubt that some mental disorders are organic in origin; for example, delirium due to septicaemia, alcoholic delirium tremens, dementia due to Huntington's disease, altered behaviour due to frontal lobe damage, and a great many more. It is important for all doctors, and other health staff, to know something about organic psychiatric disorders; because of the link with physical illness, such patients are frequently dealt with by non-psychiatrists.

Among the topics discussed in this chapter are some which are dealt with in other parts of the book. For example, both delirium and dementia are relatively common in old age and are described in Chapter 18; a number of organic conditions associated with substance use are described in Chapter 8. The chapter on general hospital 'liaison' psychiatry (Chapter 16) tackles some issues related to organic disorders. There will therefore be numerous cross-references to these and other chapters, and some repetition where it is deemed to be helpful.

Assessment of intellectual function

Although, as will be described later in this chapter, some organic psychiatric disorders may occur without cognitive impairment, most patients with organic mental disorders will have deficits in intellectual function. For example,

patients with delirium may be disorientated, and dementia is usually characterized by memory loss. It is therefore necessary for a clinician to be able to carry out a systematic examination of the intellectual functions. This task is analogous both to the physical examination of, say, the neurological system and to the examination of the general mental state (see Chapter 3).

Before setting out deliberately to test intellectual function, the interviewer should consider whether the preceding consultation has provided any hints or evidence about intellectual deficit. First, the patient's conscious level should be considered. Is the patient drowsy or fully alert? Is the patient aware of everyday events? Is the level of consciousness maintained or does it fluctuate? Second, has it been apparent during the interview that there are problems of grasp, memory, or any of the other components of intellectual function? Third, these functions are tested systematically, as set out in Table 7.1.

It is a matter of clinical judgement when to carry out systematic testing of intellectual function. The procedure set out in Table 7.1 takes at least 10 to 15 minutes and may be an unnecessary examination for many patients. If by the end of the interview and mental state examination the psychiatrist is reasonably satisfied that intellectual function is intact, it may be appropriate to omit formal testing or defer it to a subsequent interview – rather as, in other

Table 7.1 *Components of a brief assessment of intellectual function (brief cognitive testing)*

Function being tested	Test procedure
Orientation	Test orientation of: • *time*: time of day/day of week/month/year • *place*: present place/kind of place (e.g., house, hospital) • *person*: own name/names of relatives, staff, interviewer, etc.
Attention/concentration	Test ability to attend and to concentrate (choosing from several increasingly difficult tasks, as appropriate to patient's ability) • *counting* backwards from 10 to 1 • days of week in *reverse order* – Sunday, Saturday … • months of year in reverse order – December, November … • *serial subtractions*: first, 3 *from 20*: 20, 17, 14 … then, 7 *from 100*: 100, 93, 86 … • *digit span*: patient repeats digits delivered slowly by interviewer – for example, 3 5 9, 4 8 3 6, 7 6 3 9 1 … Increasingly difficult strings may be delivered, and repetition in reverse order may be tested in some cases
Memory	Test new learning, recall of recent memory and remote memory • *new learning*. Ask the patient to listen to a simple name and address and to repeat it at once; ask for further repetition 5 minutes later. To avoid rehearsal, the intervening time should be occupied with another task. More difficult and systematic is the use of standard sentences (see Lishman) • *recent memory*. Ask about events in news and current affairs, everyday occurrences such as visits, content of recent meals (as long as interviewer knows the answer) • *remote memory*. Ask about appropriate past events likely to be remembered by most people of the patient's age and background, such as past prime ministers, monarchs, wartime events, major sporting events, etc. With remote memory, and to some extent recent memory, it can be difficult to evaluate the patient's responses; new learning can be tested in a more systematic and reliable way
Language	Test several aspects of language • *motor aspects*: be alert to *dysarthria*; if suspected, try the patient's ability to pronounce tricky phrases such as 'West Register Street'. Look also for speech *perseveration* with repetition of words or parts of words • Test for *aphasia*: look for *expressive* problems such as word finding or naming difficulty; ask the patient to name common objects by, e.g. pointing to parts of a door – knob, hinge, lock, etc. Examine also for *receptive* difficulty: ask the patient to carry out simple and more complex commands (see apraxia, below) • Test *reading and writing*: ask the patient to read aloud; ascertain whether the material is understood. Ask the patient to write a sentence or two of his own choice; dictate a sentence

continued

Table 7.1 *(Continued)*

Function being tested	Test procedure
Visuo-spatial function	Test spatial orientation and ability to distinguish left and right • Ask the patient to hold up his left hand, to touch his left ear with his right hand, etc. • Ask the patient to judge which of two objects is nearer, to estimate the mid-point of a straight line, and similar spatial tasks. • Ask for a drawing of a square, triangle, circle. Ask the patient to copy more complex figures such as a box (see Lishman for further examples).
Apraxia	Test the patient's ability to carry out goal-directed actions • Ask the patient to carry out various complex motor tasks, such as: taking off and putting on a garment; making imaginary gestures such as waving goodbye, shaking hands; folding a piece of paper and sealing it in an envelope. *Note* that apraxia is only tested by the setting of such tasks if the patient understands the task and has no motor disability which impairs ability (for example, weakness or impaired coordination)

areas of medicine, further investigations are arranged electively. Sometimes a shorter version of the examination is carried out. The drawback of this short-cut is a failure to test important areas of function. If only orientation, and recent and remote memory, are tested – as is often the case – few patients will show deficits; they will usually be those whose impairments have already been evident during the interview. Put another way, very brief intellectual testing has very low sensitivity.

Organic psychiatric disorders

Despite the great many physical causes which may bring about organic psychiatric disorders, they lead to a relatively small number of important clinical syndromes – outlined in Table 7.2.

Dementia

Dementia (synonym: chronic brain syndrome) is a clinical syndrome resulting from disease of the brain, in which there is impairment of many of the identifiable components of higher cortical function. It is usually chronic and progressive. It may occur at any time in adult life, but it has a much higher incidence in old people, where prevalence is directly associated with age (see Chapter 18).

The clinical features of dementia are described in more detail in the chapter about old age psychiatry (Chapter 18). Neuro-psychiatric abnormalities are summarized in Table 7.3. In some patients there will be global impairment of all these elements but, especially in early cases, the deficits may be patchy. Unlike delirium (see below), it is not usual for consciousness to be diminished or fluctuating.

Table 7.2 *Clinical syndromes associated with organic mental disorders*

1	Dementia
2	Amnesic syndrome
3	Delirium
4	Organic hallucinosis
5	Organic delusional disorder
6	Organic mood disorder – depressive, manic or mixed
7	Organic personality change

Table 7.3 *Clinical features of dementia*

Orientation	Disorientation in time, place and person
Attention/concentration	Poor ability to attend to a task or manipulate information
Thinking	Impairment of comprehension, grasp of abstract concepts, and judgement
Memory	New learning and recall of recent memory are impaired. Remote memory is also affected, but may be relatively spared during the early phase of the illness
Language	*Aphasia*: characterized in the early stage by mild expressive problems such as word finding or naming difficulty; later, in more severe cases may include receptive difficulty. *Writing* and *reading* may also be affected. *Perseveration* may occur
Visuo-spatial function	Spatial disorientation; deficits in distinguishing left and right
Motor activity	Either restless over-activity or apathetic under-activity may occur (rapid fluctuation from one to the other is usually associated with coexisting delirium). *Apraxia* may occur, such that simple tasks like dressing or eating become impossible
Consciousness	Not usually affected unless there is coexisting delirium
Sleep pattern	Nocturnal wakefulness is common
Perception	*Recognition* of places and persons may be impaired. Distortions, illusions and hallucinations are not usually present unless there is coexisting delirium
Belief	False beliefs, if present, are usually directly attributable to failures of grasp and recognition
Emotion	Emotions may be relatively normal or increasingly labile; some patients become very distressed

Specific types of dementia

In old age, Alzheimer's disease, vascular dementia and a mixture of the two disorders account for most of those affected. Dementia in adults below the age of 60, although catastrophic in its effect, is mercifully rare. Alzheimer's disease is probably the most common condition; vascular cases occur but account for a much lower proportion of cases than in the elderly. The relative frequency of the other rare disorders described below is much greater in younger patients than in the elderly.

Alzheimer's disease is characterized by an insidious onset and a slowly progressive course. Localizing neurological signs are not usually evident until the disease is at an advanced stage. The pathological process is of unknown cause. There is substantial loss of neurones throughout the brain, especially in limbic, temporo-parietal and frontal areas. Neuroimaging has demonstrated in life what has been apparent for many years post-mortem – that there is clear shrinkage of brain substance with widening of sulci and enlarging of ventricles. Histopathological examination reveals neurofibrillary tangles and plaques of amyloid. There is also deficiency of cholinergic neurotransmitters. The condition is more prevalent at all ages in women than in men.

Vascular dementia typically occurs with an abrupt onset, is accompanied by neurological deficits even at an early stage, and tends to show step-wise rather than steady progression. The intellectual deficits are often more patchy than with Alzheimer's disease, and emotional lability may be a striking feature. Some patients show fluctuations in conscious level, particularly at night. In the typical case the patient will have established hypertension and will previously have suffered transient ischaemic attacks or completed strokes. The dementia usually results from multiple infarcts and is but one manifestation of more widespread vascular disease. The diagnosis may sometimes be confirmed when neuro-imaging reveals evidence of these infarcts.

Pick's disease is a rare condition of unknown cause which typically affects functions associated with the frontal lobes, although global dementia does gradually develop. The early clinical features are more often those of character change and loss of drive than defects of memory, concentration, grasp of concepts and so forth. Disinhibited behaviour – loss of normal manners, embarrassing actions, stealing, sexual indiscretion, fatuous mood and many other alterations in demeanour – may be the conspicuous abnormalities at first. Later, other cognitive changes occur and profound global dementia slowly emerges. Although there is usually generalized brain atrophy and ventricular enlargement, the characteristic pathology is differential shrinkage of certain lobes, particularly frontal and, sometimes, temporal lobes. Modern neuro-radiological imaging can sometimes identify the specific lobar changes. Neuronal loss, astrocyte proliferation and gliosis are usual; characteristic 'balloon cells' are sometimes seen at post-mortem. The typical plaques and tangles of Alzheimer's disease are largely absent. Pick's disease has often been described as a disorder with a clear autosomal dominant genetic transmission. Whilst transmission of this kind may occur in some families, this notion has probably been over-stated – most cases seem to arise in the absence of family history. It is, like a number of dementias, more prevalent in women.

Huntington's disease (Huntington's chorea) is a rare condition with clear autosomal dominant genetic transmission. The overall prevalence is around 5 cases per 100,000 population but there are localities where, for obvious genetic reasons, the prevalence is many times greater.

Typically, neurological signs, especially chorea, occur before dementia, although this pattern is sometimes reversed. Sadly, both are almost invariable, as the condition has nearly complete manifestation in those with the affected gene. The ever-changing, jerky, random movements of chorea in the limbs and face are, when severe, amongst the most striking physical signs in medicine – once seen never forgotten. Milder choreiform movements in the early stages of the disorder are easier to miss or mistake in importance. The pattern of dementia is one of slow intellectual decline. Dementia is not, however, the only psychiatric disorder in Huntington's disease. For many patients the first sign of the illness is a depressive or schizophrenia-like illness; only later does chorea or dementia ensue and the primary diagnosis become clear. Huntington's disease, despite its rarity, is an important condition; those interested are advised to read a fuller account in one of the general postgraduate texts recommended in Chapter 1, or in the book by Lishman (see below).

Creutzfeldt-Jakob disease (CJD) is extremely rare but worth mentioning because of several very important aspects to its pathology. First, whereas all the progressive dementias described so far tend to be slow in their evolution, the decline in intellect and function in CJD is typically very rapid. The intellectual deficits may worsen over weeks rather than months, and more than half of all patients have died within a year. Second, a mixture of severe neurological abnormalities is invariable. Ataxia, tremor, myoclonus, choreo-athetosis, rigidity, seizures – indeed almost any neurological sign – may occur at different stages of the disease before coma ensues. Third, CJD is regarded as a transmissible disorder. It has clinical and histopathological similarities with kuru (a transmissible disorder characterized by neurological symptoms and dementia, seen in a New Guinea tribe who until recent years practised cannibalism, eating the raw brains of their dead relatives), and with scrapie (a transmissible encephalopathy occurring in sheep and goats). Human transmission of CJD has occurred in the process of neurosurgical and ophthalmological procedures. One of the most noticeable histopathological abnormalities in CJD is spongy degeneration of grey matter. No wonder then that CJD became part of the concern, particularly in the United Kingdom, about bovine spongiform encephalopathy (BSE) and whether it might be transmitted to humans. At the time of writing, any such link remains unproven.

Normal pressure hydrocephalus is another rare condition but worthy of brief mention because, unlike any of the disorders so far described, it is potentially reversible. Usually for unknown reasons, cerebro-spinal fluid, although able to leave the ventricular system, is restricted in its flow over the cerebral hemispheres in the subarachnoid space. It is therefore unable to enter the superior saggital sinus in the normal process of absorption. Ventricular pressure is not high and headache is not typical as it is in obstructive forms of hydrocephalus. However, memory impairment and gradual global dementia may develop. The appearance at an early stage in the dementing process of two physical symptoms usually seen only in advanced states of dementia may help to alert the clinician to the possible existence of the disorder: *urinary incontinence*; and *abnormality of gait*, with shuffling, problems in turning, and frequent falls. The condition can be detected by modern forms of neuro-radiological imaging (CT and MRI scanning) and neurosurgical correction by means of a ventricular-vena caval shunt can arrest the progress of dementia and sometimes effect a striking recovery.

Human immunodeficiency virus (HIV) may bring about changes in intellectual function. The clinical epidemiology of the neuropsychiatric effects of HIV is not clear, but it does seem certain that a significant minority of patients show intellectual decline, sometimes accompanied by motor abnormalities such as clumsiness and other abnormalities such as agitation and hallucination. There is uncertainty whether deficits occur only after the appearance of systemic manifestations of Acquired Immune Deficiency Syndrome (AIDS), or whether they may develop in those who are asymptomatically sero-positive; the balance of evidence at present is against such early impairment. A minority of patients with AIDS develop frank dementia,

the course of which seems to be variable. Case reports suggest rapid deterioration in some patients but more prolonged worsening and even temporary improvement in others. There has been some suggestion from case reports and clinical trials that anti-viral drug treatment for AIDS may improve these neuro-psychiatric symptoms.

There are other underlying causes of dementia. For example, prolonged hypothyroidism and vitamin B12 deficiency may be implicated. More certainly, it seems that chronic neurological disorders such as multiple sclerosis or Parkinson's disease may ultimately lead to dementia. Chronic alcohol excess can also result in dementia (and of course, more typically, in the amnesic syndrome which is described in Chapter 8). It is incontrovertible that advanced neurosyphilis causes dementia – it was formerly the most frequent neuropsychiatric manifestation of the disease; however, the condition is now very rare in the United Kingdom and other western countries.

Diagnosis and investigation

Adequate history-taking and careful physical examination are essential when it is necessary to assess patients with possible or likely dementia. It is important first to ascertain that the intellectual impairment and other symptoms, behaviour and disability are part of the syndrome of dementia, and not due to delirium or other disorder – although both can coexist. Thereafter the focus is upon identification of reversible conditions and amelioration of disability and burden. These matters are considered further in Chapter 18; the principles are similar regardless of the patient's age.

Amnesic syndrome

The amnesic syndrome (synonyms: dysmnesic syndrome; Korsakov's psychosis) is a specific, chronic memory deficit associated with the vitamin B1 deficiency syndrome, Wernicke's encephalopathy. It is described in more detail in relation to alcohol problems (Chapter 8).

Delirium

Delirium (synonyms: acute confusional state, acute organic reaction, acute brain syndrome) is a syndrome, usually relatively acute in onset and potentially reversible, in which there is disorganisation of higher CNS function. It is a clinical manifestation of underlying brain dysfunction.

Clinical features

Delirious patients may show confusion, disorientation, poor attention and memory – indeed, any of the clinical features seen in established dementia. It can be seen, however, in Table 7.4 that abnormalities in consciousness and in mood, belief and perception help to differentiate delirium from dementia. Despite these additional clinical features, it is often the *history*, rather than the examination or special tests, which holds the key to diagnosis – as is so often the case throughout medical practice. Of all the features of the case, it is the short duration of confusion which most suggests a primary diagnosis of delirium.

A possible cause may sometimes be apparent, but even when it is not, the presence of some of the clinical features outlined in Table 7.4, together with a history of brief duration, may be enough to establish the presence of delirium. However, there will often be clear indications why delirium has developed. There are many causes, and Table 7.5 sets out some of the common or important ones.

Management

Identification and treatment of the underlying physical disorder is clearly the fundamental approach to care. This process will often require inpatient care, preferably on a ward where there is medical and psychiatric expertise and ready availability of laboratory, neurophysiological and radiological investigation.

Delirious patients should be nursed with particular care paid to the immediate ward environment. Motor over-activity holds dangers

Table 7.4 *Clinical features of delirium*

Consciousness and attention	From mild inability to focus or sustain attention through to severe drowsiness or coma: often fluctuating in severity
Perception	Distortions, illusions or hallucinations; in any sensory modality, but most noticeably visual
Thinking	Impairment of comprehension and grasp of abstract concepts
Belief	Transient delusions often occur
Memory	New learning and recall of recent memory are impaired. Remote memory may be relatively unaffected
Orientation	Disorientation, especially in time but also in place and person
Motor activity	Restless over-activity, apathetic under-activity and fluctuation from one to the other; perseveration of action; apraxia; visuo-spatial deficits
Language	Dysarthria, aphasia, perseveration of speech, comprehension deficits
Sleep pattern	Disruption of any kind, but especially nocturnal wakefulness followed by daytime drowsiness
Emotion	Distress – whether anxiety, fear, depression, irritability, hostility or perplexity; euphoria is less common

Table 7.5 *Some common or important physical causes of delirium*

Traumatic	head injury sub-dural haematoma
Neoplastic	primary cerebral tumour cerebral secondaries systemic non-metastatic effects
Vascular	stroke and transient ischaemic attacks sub-arachnoid haemorrhage myocardial infarction
Metabolic	uraemia hepatic encephalopathy hypoglycaemia anoxia porphyria dehydration and electrolyte disturbance thiamine (B1), vitamin B12 or folate deficiency
Infective	chest urinary intracranial (meningitis/encephalitis) viraemia and septicaemia
Epileptic	aura preceding seizure complex partial seizure post-ictal state
Endocrine	hypothyroidism and hyperthyroidism
Drug toxicity and withdrawal	anticholinergic drugs (including tricyclic antidepressants) all tranquillizers, especially benzodiazepines and barbiturates steroids L-dopa anticonvulsants antihypertensives digoxin diuretics *Substance use*: e.g., alcohol, cannabis, hallucinogens, solvents *Poisoning*: many substances, including carbon monoxide
Immune	HIV infection and AIDS systemic lupus erythematosis

for the patient and occasionally, when accompanied by delusions and hallucinations, for others too! Patients are sometimes best nursed in a single room with intensive nursing attention, preferably provided by a small number of familiar faces. Half-light is especially likely to promote visual illusions, so the room should generally be well lit, even at night when the patient's confusion is often at its worst. Sedation is sometimes necessary but carries considerable likelihood of increasing confusion even if it reduces risk of harm. In most cases, neuroleptic drugs are preferable – thioridazine, haloperidol or chlorpromazine are the most widely used (there are exceptions to this general rule; see next section). Elderly patients are especially likely to be rendered more confused by such drugs. When drug treatment is really necessary for elderly patients, doses should be much lower than in younger adult patients.

Withdrawal states with delirium

Substance withdrawal states which result in delirium have additional features and aspects of management. Much the commonest state of this kind is due to alcohol withdrawal – *alcoholic delirium tremens*. The condition may begin within a day or so of cessation of alcohol intake, or it may take as much as a week to develop; occasionally it may arise following a marked reduction of intake rather than abstinence. There may or may not be a prodromal phase of arousal and irritability, but the onset often seems sudden. The delirium is much as described above, and any or all of the clinical features described in Table 7.4 may occur. Three of these characteristics are, however, particularly prevalent: first, marked distress, fearfulness and motor restlessness; second, hallucinations, often visual and of a frightening nature – snakes, creepy-crawlies and the like; and third, delusions – often accompanying the hallucinations. In addition, there are important physiological changes. The popular name for the disorder, delirium tremens, indicates that tremor is characteristic. It may range from a mild, fine tremor which is easily overlooked, to severe, coarse tremor with ataxia. Dehydration is usual and fluid depletion may be profound. Autonomic over-activity is almost invariable, leading to pilo-erection, dilated pupils, tachycardia, sweating, and flushing or pallor.

The physiological changes require specific intervention. Autonomic over-activity, together with the presence of hallucinations and delusions, makes sedation essential. Risk of withdrawal seizures also calls for prophylactic treatment. Neuroleptic drugs however, are not indicated because they lower seizure threshold and make fits more likely. Benzodiazepines, often chlordiazepoxide in high and repeated doses (in severe cases as much as 30–40 mg four times a day), are the most widely used drugs; such a regimen achieves both sedation and anticonvulsant action. Fluid replenishment is essential, and is usually possible by the oral route. Thiamine (vitamin B1) should also be given, not to treat delirium tremens but to prevent the onset of Wernicke's encephalopathy (see Chapter 8). Prolonged malnutrition may have resulted in more general hypovitaminosis,

and large doses of multiple vitamins are usually indicated. Alcoholic delirium tremens and similar withdrawal syndromes with delirium are serious neuropsychiatric emergencies and have appreciable mortality. The patients at greatest risk are those with poor nutritional status, older patients and those with severe symptoms such as excitement, marked dehydration, intercurrent infections, seizures, delusions or hallucinations. Patients who are deluded and over-active are often best cared for on a psychiatric ward; those whose physical health is the more prominent concern are frequently treated on a medical ward.

Of the clinical syndromes associated with organic mental disorders, the three syndromes of *hallucinosis, delusion* and *mood disorder* (numbers 4–6 in Table 7.2) have one thing in common. Unlike delirium and dementia, they do not have clinical characteristics which identify them as 'organic'. Instead, they resemble, or are exactly like, psychiatric disorders which may have no obvious 'organic' cause. In any particular case, the condition is deemed to be 'organic' because a relation between the symptoms and signs and a physical condition seems probable.

Organic hallucinosis

Various physical conditions may cause a state characterized by hallucinations in clear consciousness, without any other features to suggest delirium. These hallucinatory syndromes are often transient, but may be recurrent or persistent. Hallucinations are often auditory but may be in any modality – including visual and tactile. The commonest cause of such a disorder is alcohol withdrawal, and 'alcoholic hallucinosis' is described separately in Chapter 8. Many other substances – for example, cocaine – may also produce hallucinosis of this kind. Sometimes the hallucinations are recognized as such by the patient, sometimes they are accompanied by delusions. It may be apparent from this description that an hallucinatory syndrome of this kind can closely resemble schizophrenia. Differentiating the two disorders will therefore usually depend more on evidence for a primary organic cause, and the timing and duration of symptoms, than upon psychopathology.

Organic delusional disorder

Some physical illnesses which affect cerebral function, some therapeutic drugs, and use of some psycho-active substances may produce delusional disorder in the absence of delirium or dementia. The delusions may focus on any matter, but as with other clear-consciousness delusional illnesses such as schizophrenia, depression and mania, the common themes are persecution, grandiosity, disease, guilt and so on. The condition may be transient or prolonged and, once again, is considered 'organic' when there is a relationship with a likely physical cause. For example, one patient aged in her fifties who received radioactive iodine treatment for thyrotoxicosis was not seen in the follow-up endocrine clinic until several months later, when she attended for an urgent consultation because of the development of acute mental illness. She was quickly admitted to inpatient psychiatric care because she was experiencing a great many delusions centred upon persecution of members of her family. Thyroid function tests, when the results became available, revealed that she had no recordable thyroid function.

Epilepsy (particularly with a temporal lobe focus), brain injury, brain infection (for example, AIDS or neurosyphilis), hypothyroidism, systemic lupus erythematosis, porphyria, corticosteroid therapy and amphetamine ingestion are just examples of the multitude of physical conditions which are associated with delusional disorders of this kind.

Organic mood disorder

As with organic delusional disorder, cerebral dysfunction due to physical illness may lead to depression, mania or a mixed affective state. The possible causes are again very numerous; the list in the above section contains many of the known associations.

The management of these organically caused states of hallucinosis, delusion and mood disorder has two main components. First, it is important to identify and deal with any underlying medical condition, or implicated substance, or any drug treatments which may be involved. Second, these conditions tend to respond symptomatically to standard psychiatric drug treatment. In the case example above, the lady without thyroid function improved markedly with a neuroleptic drug before it could be proven that she needed thyroxine replacement and the specific treatment began. Neuroleptic and antidepressant drugs may have an important place in management.

Organic personality change

Cerebral insult may produce enduring change in attitudes, emotion and behaviour. The most obvious example is where such change occurs as part of dementia, when it is one of the features of the condition most upsetting to the patient's relatives. However, change of this kind may take place in states other than dementia, and in the absence of intellectual decline. For example, patients who have been subject to brain trauma or infection may become listless and apathetic; develop emotionalism or other lability of mood; lose concern for social conventions or for other people; become seriously disinhibited in behaviour (perhaps including sexual conduct); become suspicious or aggressive; become ritualistic, pedantic or circumstantial; or take on any of a number of other attributes. Not only traumatic and infective damage but also vascular, space-occupying and other lesions can be implicated. It has long been accepted that frontal lobe damage is particularly associated with changes of this kind. However, more widespread cerebral damage and lesions in other brain areas may also produce changes of this kind.

Further reading

Lishman, W.A. (1987) *Organic Psychiatry: The Psychological Consequences of Cerebral Disorder*, 2nd edn, Oxford: Blackwell Scientific Publications.
Lloyd, G.G. (1991) *Textbook of General Hospital Psychiatry*, Edinburgh: Churchill Livingstone.

8

Misuse of alcohol and other substances

A great many substances are taken purposely in order to derive some psychological or physiological effect. Most of these, if not all, may affect mental state adversely. This chapter will describe the general pattern of such problems and describe some of the more common and important syndromes which arise. Alcohol misuse is much the commonest problem. Many of the difficulties with other drugs are similar to those seen with alcohol; for that reason alcohol is dealt with first and in the most detail.

There is no ideal psychiatric classification of substances used. Any list of practical value will comprise, first, drugs which are in common use – whether single drugs or categories of drugs with similar effects – and, second, those for which there is an established association with abnormal mental states. The latest version of the International Classification of Diseases (ICD-10) sets out such a list. Psychiatric disorders are classified by the substance involved (Table 8.1a), and by the clinical state (Table 8.1b).

Use of a substance shown in Table 8.1a may result in a clinical state shown in Table 8.1b. Some drugs seem to lead only to one or two of these states. In the case of tobacco, for example, although dependence is readily apparent, there is little evidence that it causes clinically important states of withdrawal, intoxication or precipitation of psychotic mental illness. All of the other substance categories in the list, however, are associated with one or more of these phenomena. Cocaine, for example, is

Table 8.1a *Substances whose use may result in mental or behavioural disorders*

- Alcohol
- Opioids
- Cannabinoids
- Sedatives or hypnotics
- Cocaine
- Other stimulants
- Hallucinogens
- Tobacco
- Volatile solvents
- Multiple drugs
- Other and unidentified substances

Table 8.1b *Clinical states associated with substance misuse*

- Acute intoxication
- Harmful use
- Dependence syndrome
- Withdrawal state
- Withdrawal state with delirium
- Psychotic disorder
- Amnesic syndrome
- Residual or late-onset psychotic disorder

associated with at least five of the eight categories of clinical state presented in Table 8.1b (see later in this chapter). The nature of the clinical states set out in the table will be described when dealing with specific substances.

Alcohol

Excessive drinking

Many circumstances may contribute to a shift from modest to excessive alcohol consumption. Some of these are obvious: when young people become old enough to buy and consume alcohol in public, when they leave home and forsake parental constraint, when they experience a rise in income; when life is affected by chronic difficulties or untoward events; when loneliness becomes intolerable; when occupation results in regular close contact with alcohol; and many others. Often, many such influences are brought to bear – added to which, alcohol also holds inherent attractions for the consumer. Why is it so widely used? What are its physiological and psychological effects?

It is widely recognized that alcohol can induce feelings of warmth, well-being and general exhilaration. It is not, however, a stimulant but a cerebral depressant. Such relief as it may bring results from stifling self-criticism and the nagging voice of conscience, from suppressing worry about problems, from damping down anxieties and inhibitions. However, even when alcohol consumption improves outlook on life, such dubious benefit is short-lived and is likely to be achieved only at a level of intake which is excessive and repeated. Its depressant powers on the other hand are, unfortunately, all too evident in common experience: gloom and despondency are often accentuated by drink.

One important result of repeated alcohol consumption is *tolerance* – more is needed for the same effect. Tolerance is a powerful factor in the cycle of deleterious effects: life's problems lead to heavy drinking, some transient 'benefit' seems to occur, further but increasing alcohol

ingestion takes place, and the many adverse consequences of such harmful use of alcohol merely add to the person's original problems.

Alcohol dependence syndrome

Dependence on alcohol (or any other substance for that matter) is a state beyond excessive intake. It exists when the pattern of consumption has taken precedence over the original reasons for the excess intake. It cannot be defined simply, but results from a combination of phenomena (Table 8.2).

Those who drink heavily are often aware of a strong, indeed compelling, *desire to drink*. Where alcohol was once consumed only in certain settings, it is now avidly sought. This urge may be described by a spouse or other informant but may also be reported by the subject, especially when he is also aware that his *control of drinking is impaired*. He may say that he can no longer refuse a drink if offered, or cannot pass an open public house. He may not be able to have only one drink but always progresses to intoxication. There is an old adage which is sometimes apt: 'When one drink is too many and twenty isn't enough.' It should

Table 8.2 *Features of alcohol dependence syndrome (derived from ICD-10)*

- Strong desire to drink
- Awareness of impaired control over drinking
- Narrowing of personal drinking repertoire
- Progressive neglect of alternative activities
- Persistent drinking despite clear evidence of harmful consequences (physical, social, psychological)
- Evidence of tolerance
- Evidence of physiological withdrawal
- Drinking, with the intention of alleviating withdrawal symptoms
- Reappearance of the dependence syndrome after abstinence

be emphasized, though, that dependence syndrome may be present without such severe loss of control.

Where alcohol consumption remains at an acceptable level, the desire to drink is only one element of lifestyle, but in dependence syndrome drinking becomes the pre-eminent activity and the pattern of its use becomes stereotyped. The daily activity *repertoire is narrowed* and drinking takes place almost regardless of circumstances and despite other important considerations. For example, heavy intake or daytime drinking, hitherto restricted to weekends, may become the norm on workdays as well. In severe dependence, the daily timetable may have resulted from a need to maintain adequate blood levels of alcohol. As the repertoire narrows, other aspects of life are relegated to a less important role. It is in self-care, attendance and capability at work, family role, and interests and pastimes that this *progressive neglect of alternative activities* is evident.

Unfortunately, dependent drinkers will often persist in *drinking despite clear evidence of harmful consequences*. Patients who, for example, have developed duodenal ulcers or alcoholic hepatitis, those who have been warned by their employers or spouses about serious social consequences if they drink again, those who know that their low mood is exacerbated and not helped by alcohol – all of these and many others may yet continue with excess consumption. The reason, it seems, is due to the changes in lifestyle which have already developed, and the physical dependence factors described below.

The physiological phenomenon of *tolerance* which was described above may become particularly evident in dependent patients, who may tolerate very high doses of alcohol. In such cases, repeated high intake and almost permanently high blood levels may seem to have remarkably little deleterious effects on performance. In fact, there are often serious deficits in subtle aspects of behaviour, such as poor judgement and disinhibition, even when speech and motor functioning seems little impaired. Later, when liver function and drug metabolism have declined, an opposite effect

may be noticed – that only small amounts of alcohol have intoxicating effects.

Among the most striking clinical aspects of dependence upon any drug are the symptoms and signs of *physiological withdrawal*. Withdrawal symptoms occur when prolonged high intake is followed by a reduction. Alcohol withdrawal symptoms may occur after as little as three or four hours of abstinence, and are therefore often apparent in the morning when no alcohol has been taken since the night before. Edwards describes four core symptoms. *Tremor* may range from a single episode where the hands are shaky, to recurrent severe shaking of the whole body. *Nausea* may exacerbate poor nutritional intake and in many instances is accompanied by retching and vomiting. *Sweating* results in a clammy feeling, but when severe, patients may report that they become soaking wet. *Mood disturbance* ranges from a typical edginess, restlessness and subjective agitation to a more profound fearfulness which is most obvious when severe withdrawal symptoms are accompanied by delirium (see below). Over-sensitivity to noise, tinnitus and muscle cramps are also well-recognized symptoms. Alcohol withdrawal seizures are a risk and may take less than 12 hours to arise, although they are more common after one or two days of abstinence.

In milder cases, symptoms may emerge only occasionally. As severity of dependence increases, they may occur each morning but settle with the first drink. Later, symptoms may break through decreasing blood levels and waken the patient in the night, perhaps even affect him in the daytime despite recent drinking. The serious state of *withdrawal with delirium* (delirium tremens) usually develops its full clinical picture within a few days and lasts for several days or longer (see Chapter 7). Dependent patients know how to seek temporary relief and, consequently, *drink with the intention of relieving withdrawal symptoms*.

One of the most unfortunate features of the syndrome is that when alcohol is taken again after a period of abstinence, *reappearance of dependence* may occur much more rapidly than among other persons drinking similar amounts.

Consequences of excessive drinking and dependence

Acute intoxication, even on a rare occasion, holds a number of risks. Involvement in accidents, and becoming a victim or perpetrator of violence are perhaps the most frequent untoward consequences. Repeated excessive intake and dependence have many adverse *physical*, *social* and *psychological* outcomes.

1 Physical

The physical effects of excess alcohol are too numerous and complex to describe in detail here. Table 8.3 sets out some of the important alcohol-related disorders; they will not be further discussed here. The reader should consult textbooks of medicine, or the excellent book about drinking problems by Edwards (see Further reading, page 79).

2 Social

The social effects of heavy drinking are responsible for much of the suffering by patients and their families, and for a high proportion of the overall cost of alcohol abuse. At *home*, there is a long catalogue of unhappy outcomes: loss of mutual support in the marriage; impaired parenting; conflict with and violence towards spouses and children; deterioration in sexual relationships; loss of income due to absenteeism from work and unemployment; high expenditure on alcohol; and many others.

At *work*, poor time-keeping and attendance, together with decreased efficiency, jeopardize employment. Physical risk to self and others is not infrequent, whether it be from machinery or driving vehicles or from more subtle matters of safety; for example, medical practitioners may constitute a risk to others when dependent on alcohol. *Training and education* also fall victim to alcohol problems. Students or trainees are sometimes barred from courses, resulting from one or more untoward incidents when drunk; frequently, such episodes reflect more chronic excessive drinking.

Sadly, the outcome of heavy drinking for some includes no home, no spouse and no job. There are many reasons for *homelessness*, but alcohol problems are prevalent among those who are homeless and especially in those who are also destitute and itinerant. *Crime* – from driving offences or stealing from the gas meter to violent offences, even homicide – has a marked association with both acute and chronic alcohol excess. In public disorder offences, from brawls to riots, alcohol is very often implicated.

Table 8.3 *Alcohol-related physical disorders*

Gastro-intestinal disorders	Oesophagitis, gastritis, Mallory-Weiss lesions, peptic ulcers, pancreatitis, hepatitis, cirrhosis, portal hypertension and varices, liver failure, malignant neoplasms
Neurological disorders	Peripheral neuropathy, seizures, cerebellar degeneration, Wernicke's encephalopathy, sub-dural haematoma, erectile failure (impotence)
Cardiovascular disorders	Arrhythmias, cardiomyopathy, coronary artery disease, hypertension, stroke
Respiratory disorders	Respiratory depression or inhalation in acute intoxication, increased incidence of tuberculosis and smoking-related disease
Haematological disorders	Anaemia (iron deficiency, megaloblastic or haemolytic), thrombocytopenia
Locomotor disorders	Myopathy

3   Psychiatric

Alcohol excess may lead to depression of mood and *depressive illness*. This may result from a combination of the direct depressant effect of the drug, the guilt and self-recrimination of the drinker, and the impact of the adverse events and difficulties due to chronic excess. Fairly mild withdrawal states produce anxiety symptoms, and *anxiety states* may arise in this secondary way. Prolonged alcohol misuse in some subjects seems to accentuate a suspicious attitude towards others. In severe cases this suspiciousness becomes morbid and may be manifest in maladaptive behaviour. The most typical clinical picture is one of *morbid jealousy* towards the partner (see Chapter 6).

There are several neuropsychiatric complications of alcohol excess. *Withdrawal state with delirium* (delirium tremens) has been mentioned and is described in Chapter 7. Another disorder which emerges particularly in association with cessation or reduction in alcohol intake is the *alcohol-induced psychotic disorder* widely known as '*alcoholic hallucinosis*'. The patient typically experiences auditory hallucinations, often persecutory in quality, in the absence of delirium. They may take the form of third-person voices discussing the patient or commenting on his actions, and they are often accompanied by delusions of being watched or followed. When transient, perhaps lasting only a few weeks, the condition is distinguishable from schizophrenia – especially if the alcohol consumption history is typical. However, when psychotic symptoms persist the clinical state may be comparable with that seen in chronic schizophrenia.

Wernicke's encephalopathy is due to thiamine (vitamin B1) deficiency. Alcohol dependence is the most frequent cause of clinically evident deficiency; it leads to poor nutritional intake and impaired thiamine absorption and storage. To make matters worse, the need to metabolize alcohol increases requirements. The condition is manifest by a triad of signs: delirium; ataxia; and eye signs, including ophthalmoplegias and nystagmus. In a substantial proportion of cases, although the acute signs may disappear with treatment, the patient is left with a persisting intellectual impairment.

Although this process is sometimes sub-acute and the chronic impairment may be global, typically there develops a specific disorder of recent memory. In its florid form this condition, known as the *amnesic syndrome* (synonyms: dysmnesic syndrome, Korsakov's psychosis), is a curious disorder. Whereas attention, language function and spatial function may be unaffected, and the patient retains the capacity for both immediate recall and remote memory of events long ago, the striking feature is the inability to recall events between a few moments before and years past. The result is someone who may retain all the social graces and a good vocabulary and at first sight may seem normal, but who is quite unable to function independently. For example, the patient will often have no idea of time, place or the role played by other people. Retained verbal ability may lead some patients to attempt to fill the gap in memory with a semi-appropriate answer, the content of which may be entirely imaginary; this process is known as *confabulation*.

Detecting and assessing alcohol problems

All doctors need to be aware that alcohol-related health and social problems are common in the community, and especially so among those who visit a general practice surgery or accident and emergency department, and among hospital inpatients. It is therefore important to recognize early evidence of the signs and symptoms described above, and to be alert to the social aspects of heavy drinking. The doctor may also be presented with obvious signs such as acute intoxication, empty bottles or unexplained trauma or may be offered strong clues by a concerned relative.

High risk groups

In addition to these clinical clues, it should be remembered that some *occupations* have particular associations with alcohol problems. These include those who deal directly with alcohol, such as bar or catering staff and brewers' draymen; those whose jobs involve expense-account entertaining, such as journalists, sales executives and the like; and those who work long or antisocial hours or who may be segregated by occupation and unusual responsibilities and stresses, such as doctors, police officers, seamen or members of the armed forces. The *unemployed* have higher than average risk too. Social standing confers no immunity – alcohol is a great leveller. *Family history* is also relevant. Whether by genetic or environmental influence, or both, alcohol problems are more likely in families where one member, particularly a parent, has been affected previously. Some patients may be *evasive* about their activities and their alcohol intake, which should lead the doctor to consider its role more seriously.

Questions to ask when trying to detect those affected

Some questionnaires used for research purposes have been recommended for clinical use in screening patients – for instance, in general practice – for serious alcohol problems. One of these, the *CAGE*, is very short and has some useful questions about attitudes to drinking which are worth asking in any case where excess intake is suspected (Table 8.4). Positive response to any two of these questions indicates high likelihood of established and moderately severe alcohol problems.

Taking a case history

As in all interviews, taking a history is an important part of the therapeutic process. Patients with established alcohol problems are particularly likely to be defensive or reticent about some matters. In such cases the following aspects of the history need to be covered:

- when alcohol consumption began, when it became regular, when further symptoms such as withdrawal phenomena started, when the patient became aware of a problem;
- a detailed account of current drinking, with close questioning as to timing and circum-

Table 8.4 *The CAGE questionnaire*

C	Have you ever felt you should Cut down on your drinking?
A	Have people Annoyed you by criticizing your drinking?
G	Have you ever felt bad or Guilty about your drinking?
E	Have you ever had a drink first thing in the morning to steady your nerves or get rid of a hangover (Eye-opener)?

stances, nature of beverages taken and quantities – particularly on days when drinking is heavy;
- the effect of drink on the patient – asking about drunkenness, conduct, falls, memory blackouts, trouble with the law;
- attitude towards reduction or abstinence, and history of past help-seeking;
- whether, as described above, the person is dependent and if he has experienced any adverse physical, social or psychological outcomes.

It is important to record quantities of alcohol consumed, ideally in grams of absolute alcohol. However, a rough approximation of equivalence can be made in 'units', where each unit is roughly 10 g of absolute alcohol and can be simply estimated: half a pint of normal-strength beer, lager or cider; a standard measure of wine; a single pub measure of spirits (not the more generous drams often provided elsewhere); a pub measure of sherry.

Management

Physical investigations

Occasionally, abnormal blood tests may suggest, or help to confirm, that the patient is drinking excessively. More often, such serum measures help to quantify the physical damage related to established heavy drinking. Two common batteries of blood tests are helpful. In the full blood count, the mean corpuscular volume (MCV) may be raised. In the liver function tests, several enzymes may show raised values: gamma-glutamyl-transpeptidase (γ-GT) is the most sensitive indicator.

Talking with an informant

Meeting and talking with a spouse or other key informant should be standard practice in psychiatric care (see Chapter 3). It is particularly important in alcohol problems because of the reticence and understatement of many patients concerning the degree of the problem and its widespread effects. If the assessment is inaccurate the treatment is likely to fail. The key informant will often be an important part of that treatment.

Objectives of treatment

Treatment has immediate and longer-term objectives, outlined in Table 8.5. Some dependent patients and non-dependent alcohol abusers can stop alcohol intake without ill effect; others, especially the more severely dependent, cannot. Where withdrawal symptoms are likely, or already present, therapeutic drugs are required to reduce the physiological and psychological consequences of a withdrawal state. Care in hospital is necessary in some

Table 8.5   *Objectives of treatment*

Immediate management of dependence

- Eliminate alcohol without severe withdrawal symptoms
- Avoid delirium tremens
- Anticipate thiamine deficiency and prevent serious sequelae

Long-term management

- Agree on whether reduction or abstinence is appropriate
- Support this decision with:
  supportive therapy
  alcohol unit
  Alcoholics Anonymous
  deterrent drugs

---

cases. In this process of *detoxification* the most widely used drugs are benzodiazepines such as chlordiazepoxide. Initial doses are much higher than those used in the treatment of anxiety states, and may range from 5–10 mg three or four times a day in the case of prophylaxis or mild withdrawal symptoms, up to 30–40 mg four times a day, or even more in patients with established and severe withdrawal symptoms.

The aims of medication are to reduce autonomic over-activity, prevent perceptual abnormalities and protect against withdrawal fits. Delirium tremens, which may otherwise occur, is a serious psychiatric and medical disorder with appreciable mortality as well as morbidity (see Chapter 7). In severely dependent and malnourished patients being detoxified in hospital, glucose intake may precipitate the development of Wernicke's encephalopathy and possibly result in a permanent amnesic syndrome. It is therefore important to protect against such an event by administration of parenteral B vitamins; administration of 'Parenterovite' is recommended by the intramuscular route.

In the long term many, perhaps almost all, chronically dependent patients are unable to return to reasonable levels of drinking; for them it is either abstinence or dependence. For many people who have had alcohol related problems and for some with less severe or less chronic dependence, controlled drinking is an achievable target. In some patients who are strongly opposed to a life of abstinence, controlled drinking is worth trying, at least for a trial period.

Whatever the decision, those who have alcohol problems will need support in the battle to free themselves from maladaptive drinking. As well as family and friends, professional staff can have an important role. Specialist alcohol units may provide inpatient or day-patient care, sometimes using group therapy. Specialist teams may have Community Nurses or other staff who can offer support at the patient's home. Some patients find the meetings of the self-help organization Alcoholics Anonymous invaluable. AA have a distinctive brand of group therapy and individual support built around an ethos of strict abstinence.

Some patients are helped to remain abstinent by prescription of drugs which, once taken, act as a deterrent from alcohol intake. Disulfiram ('Antabuse') blocks the metabolism of alcohol at the acetaldehyde stage. This has the effect of causing unpleasant symptoms which occur shortly after ingestion of a small amount of alcohol: congestion of the face and conjunctivae, tachycardia, giddiness, headache and a feeling of general distress. The hope is that the patient will take the drug in the morning when resolve is high and then be deterred from alcohol intake throughout the day. Unfortunately, concurrent alcohol consumption is not without real risk. While some patients certainly benefit, deterrent drugs have a limited place in therapy.

Other substances

Opioids

Opioids (synonyms: opiates, narcotics) occur naturally as opium, derived from the poppy *papaver somniferum*. Opium contains alkaloids such as *morphine* and *codeine*; these alkaloids can be altered slightly to produce other compounds such as *heroin*. Many synthetic opioids have also been synthesized. In addition to their analgesic effects, all these drugs bring about euphoria – their main attraction in non-therapeutic use. Tolerance is common and holds great danger because doses which may be taken regularly by one person may be lethal to another, or to the same person after a period of abstinence. Respiratory depression and respiratory arrest are the most dangerous physical effects. *Dependence* is common in regular use and develops most rapidly when drugs are taken intravenously ('mainlining') or, in the case of heroin, burned and inhaled ('chasing the dragon').

Withdrawal symptoms and signs include:

- misery, craving and drug-seeking
- yawning and sweating
- coryza with running nose and salivation
- restlessness and insomnia
- dilated pupils

- piloerection ('gooseflesh' or 'cold turkey') and shivering
- vomiting, diarrhoea and abdominal colic
- hyperaesthesia, paraesthesia and muscular cramps

The withdrawal syndrome is worse with rapidly acting drugs and with high doses. Marked withdrawal is profoundly distressing but rarely life-threatening. Neither delirium nor psychotic disorders are prevalent in withdrawal or dependence. Morbidity and mortality of opioid use are high, resulting from: depression and arrest of respiration; secondary effects of injection, such as septicaemia, endocarditis, hepatitis, AIDS, pulmonary microemboli (from crushing and injecting poorly soluble tablets); and suicide.

Medical management of opioid use or dependence is a difficult task. Because some patients are prescribed a maintenance opioid – *methadone* – there is considerable demand for such treatment. There are legal restrictions on prescription of opioids in drug dependence, and there are requirements for doctors to notify the Chief Medical Officer at the Home Office of persons they believe to be addicted to certain controlled drugs. Much of the medical management of opioid dependence is carried out in specialist clinics and units.

Cannabis

Cannabis is much more widely used than opioids and has very different characteristics. It too is derived from a plant – from *Cannabis indica* or, more commonly, from *Cannabis sativa*. Different parts of the plant and different preparations lead to an array of substances with different names: cannabis resin, ganja, marijuana and others. All contain the active compounds: cannabinoids, particularly *tetrahydro-cannabinol* (THC). The drug is most often smoked and imparts a relaxed feeling, even euphoria, within a few minutes. Elimination of even a single dose takes several weeks and it seems likely that repeated doses may accumulate in the body.

There are multiple controversies about the ill effects of cannabis. Tolerance is not clear-cut, as it is with opioids. It is reported amongst those who are users of very large quantities, but may not be clinically important in the majority of users in European countries, where total doses are relatively low. So it is also with withdrawal, which is not conspicuous even in regular users in the United Kingdom. There have been many reports of psychotic disorder developing. Whether such a state is caused directly by cannabis remains uncertain; evidence for a brief state of confusion, delusion and hallucination is more convincing than that for the existence of a more chronic disorder.

Sedatives and hypnotics

Barbiturates were, until quite recently, widely prescribed for insomnia and anxiety. Dependence was common, and responsible for a number of clinical conditions similar to those encountered with alcohol dependence. Fortunately they are rarely prescribed nowadays. Unfortunately, the sedative drugs which replaced them, and which became even more popular, have also been found to be responsible for adverse effects.

The *benzodiazepine* drugs now account for the great majority of prescriptions for hypnotics and sedatives. Their relaxing effect is very marked and they are traded illicitly by multiple-drug users. It has gradually become clear that, although less addictive and much less toxic than barbiturates, they do produce *tolerance, dependence* and *withdrawal* symptoms in a substantial proportion of patients. For these reasons they should be prescribed with caution, in low doses and for short periods only (see Chapters 21 and 23). Unfortunately, short-term effectiveness of the drugs in both anxiety and insomnia often renders the intention to stop a difficult task, even after only a few weeks. The withdrawal syndrome can include severe symptoms such as epileptic seizures and psychotic states; more common are return of anxiety and insomnia, tremor, restlessness, craving for the drug and mild perceptual disturbance. It seems that shorter-acting benzodiazepines are often more difficult to stop than the longer-acting compounds.

Cocaine

Over recent years cocaine has become, in some countries, very widely available. At the time of writing, the widespread use predicted for the United Kingdom in the late 1980s has not fully materialized. This is fortunate not least because of the close association between the drug and serious psychotic illness. The drug is a *stimulant* alkaloid derived from the coca leaf of Central and South America. It may be smoked, taken intravenously, or delivered by almost any route. Sniffing it through a straw ('snorting') is perhaps the most popular method, although purified crystalline cocaine ('crack') is usually smoked.

The rapid stimulating and euphoric effect can be intense and lead very quickly to craving for more. This *craving* and the accompanying drug-seeking behaviour are amongst the most prominent effects of repeated cocaine use. Tolerance, physical dependence and withdrawal symptoms also occur. Repeated use may be associated with agitation and suspicious mood. Persecutory delusions, hallucinations – auditory and tactile ('formication' or 'cocaine bugs') – and motor stereotypies are the main features of *psychotic episodes*.

Other stimulants

Amphetamines are the other important stimulants encountered in psychiatric practice. They are often ingested and they bring about alertness and elevation of mood; many effects are directly related to their sympathomimetic properties. Effects are, however, short-lived and repeated use can quickly lead to marked tolerance. Physical dependence is not a conspicuous finding. The most striking clinical condition related to amphetamines is serious *psychotic illness*. The typical case occurs during a period of high intake, although it can arise in a first-time user. The clinical state may be indistinguishable from schizophrenia, with auditory hallucinations and persecutory delusions in clear consciousness the main features. The course of such episodes is usually relatively short – measured in days rather than weeks – although more prolonged illnesses do occur.

Another stimulant deserves a brief mention: *caffeine*. Present in tea, coffee and some cola drinks in appreciable quantities, there are many reports that the stimulant effect may have an association with anxiety symptoms and insomnia. Some psychiatrists suggest a trial of caffeine reduction or elimination in patients with anxiety and panic symptoms (see Chapter 10).

Hallucinogens

Lysergic acid diethylamide (LSD, colloquially 'acid') was first synthesized from the fungus ergot about fifty years ago. It remains the best known and most widely used hallucinogenic drug. Many others have been synthesized since, such as *phencyclidine* (PCP, colloquially 'angel dust') or *dimethyltryptamine* (DMT). They produce, in minute quantities, heightened visual imagery, illusions and hallucinations. Many users have also described transient elevation of experience to levels not otherwise encountered. Unfortunately, so-called '*bad trips*' are not uncommon. Euphoria can be replaced by profound fear and distress which, together with false beliefs and perceptions, may lead to disastrous consequences; for example, jumping from high places either in fear or with confidence in the ability to fly.

The other disturbing outcome for many who have taken hallucinogenic drugs is recurrent '*flash-back*' experiences in which the person has a return of sensations, often unpleasant ones, which occurred during intoxication. Hallucinogens are subject to marked tolerance but are not apt to induce dependence, although PCP may be more likely to do so than LSD. Psychotic symptoms are evident most often in acutely disturbed states but may occur in more chronic form.

Volatile solvents

A large number of volatile organic chemicals have, in recent years, become prevalent drugs of abuse. These substances are readily available glues and solvents and are usually inhaled from a plastic bag by adolescents and young adults. Episodes of psychosis, usually short-lived, are described in solvent users. Some of the solvent is excreted through the lungs and a characteristic smell therefore occurs for a few hours. Some users develop a perioral and perinasal rash from the method of inhalation. The fumes produce many serious effects and appreciable physical morbidity and mortality. The effect on the mental state is one of rapid intoxication with a sense of euphoria – similar to that obtained from alcohol but quicker and often cheaper. Impulsive behaviour while intoxicated is common and there have been many serious accidents, as well as incidents of crime, including violent offences.

Further reading

Edwards, G. (1987) *The Treatment of Drinking Problems: A Guide for the Helping Professions*, Oxford: Blackwell Scientific Publications.

Ghodse, H. (1989) *Drugs and Addictive Behaviour: A Guide to Treatment*, Oxford: Blackwell Scientific Publications.

Raistrick, D. and Davidson, R. (1985) *Alcoholism and Drug Addiction*, Edinburgh: Churchill Livingstone.

Royal College of Psychiatrists (1987) *Drug scenes: A Report on Drugs and Drug Dependence by the Royal College of Psychiatrists*, London: Royal College of Psychiatrists.

9

Neurotic disorders

The classification of those conditions for which the generic term *neurotic* is used, is controversial. William Cullen, in 1769, introduced 'neurosis' to medical terminology to describe disturbances of feeling and behaviour without organic cause. Most people, although not all, manifesting neurotic behaviour also show abnormality of personality, and conversely most of those whose personality shows evidence of disorder will at times produce neurotic symptoms. Disorder of mood is a feature of neurotic disorder and the two often concur. Most patients with severe neurosis will describe some degree of depression; the vast majority of those with depressive episodes, recurrent or persistent depression will also show considerable neurotic psychopathology.

Definitions

Neurosis is a psychological reaction to perceived stress, expressed in emotion or behaviour which is ultimately inappropriate in dealing with that stress. Such a definition, of course, includes all of us at some time or other, and it is difficult to define what is neurosis and what is a normal emotional reaction. This depends upon individual perception of what is an unacceptable symptom. This, in its turn, depends upon social and cultural factors, such as what help is available for the treatment of symptoms, and where or from whom this help comes: doctor, social worker, personnel officer or priest. The difference between normality and neurosis lies partly in whether the reaction is appropriate in degree, and partly in whether the type of behaviour in response to what the sufferer perceives as stress helps to lessen that source of conflict. Patients with neurotic disorder experience and complain of symptoms continuously and severely for some time, whilst for the normal person such experience is transient even in response to considerable stress. The neurotic patient does not achieve a successful adaptation to his symptoms, nor does he manage to prevent further stressful situations, unlike a healthy person.

Neurosis is not a comprehensive description of a condition like *pneumonia* which one either has or does not have; it is possible to be minimally neurotic, and the border between normality and abnormality is not a clear one. Neurosis is often contrasted with psychosis, in which there is gross impairment of mental functioning to such a degree that insight and judgement of reality are affected. In neurosis the subject's personality structure is preserved, so that he does not strike those around him as completely irrational or out of contact with reality. His condition can, in fact, be 'understood'; his anxiety or other neurotic state, despite seeming unjustified by causal circumstances, is an experience which is familiar and understandable to the observer. Indeed, there appears to be no qualitative difference between *normal* and *morbid* anxiety, only in the circumstances which occasion them. The quality of experience of the psychotic patient is, in contrast, completely strange and unfamiliar, or in Jaspers' terminology, *un-understandable*.

It is often difficult to make a clear-cut distinction between psychosis and neurosis. It is a mistake to contrast psychoses as serious and causing permanent disability with neuroses as minor mental disturbances. For example, a severe obsessional disorder may be so intractable as to be lifelong and far more crippling than several bouts of relatively short-lived psychotic depression. Similarly, some sufferers from neurosis kill themselves. Much depends on the criteria of illness applied.

The neurotic disorders are extremely common; anxiety and depression, separately or together, are much the most frequent psychological symptoms in primary care, accounting for over 90 per cent of psychiatric morbidity in that setting. The different neurotic syndromes should not be thought of as discrete disease entities; cases cross over from one neurotic diagnosis to another over time and they share a common prognosis. There are many intermediate and mixed cases, sometimes all the differing neurotic syndromes will occur in the same patient at the same time. The methods of treatment and the services for management have some similarities for the various neurotic disorders.

Psychopathology

Should neurotic disorders be regarded as illness at all? This, of course, entirely depends upon how one defines illness. Certainly, patients with neurotic disorders regularly present to doctors with physical symptoms, and there is also biological disadvantage in that those with severe neurotic disorders have a higher mortality than expected. Such people suffer a great deal because of their symptoms and disturbed social relationships. Neurosis often overlaps with physical disease: it may occur in association with and result in physical illness; it may mimic physical disease causing diagnostic confusion; and it may complicate the symptoms and course of established disease.

The psychopathology of neurotic disorder is listed in Table 9.1. Neurotic thinking and behaviour, however inappropriate and unacceptable, is usually understandable when the doctor talks with his patient in detail. The doctor may be able to say, 'If I had been in that situation with those experiences, I can understand how I could have done or could have felt that'. Often such people describe the tyranny of inevitability. They understand what is going wrong but feel themselves to be completely powerless to put it right.

The self-experience of people with neurotic disorder always shows some degree of disturbance. Chronic low self-esteem often results in indecision and an inability to initiate effective action. Anxious deprecatory over-involvement with self results in a cycle of demoralization (represented graphically in Figure 9.1). There may also be distortion of body image. The neurotic patient, unlike the psychotic one, always recognizes his actions as his own but feels that they are constrained by external circumstances: there is no freedom of action. He may polarize different parts of himself – 'myself as I know myself to be, incompetent, an abject failure', and 'myself as I would like to be, successful, popular and happy'. He may feel himself to be irretrievably deteriorated because of circumstances outside his control. He knows precisely what are the boundaries of self but feels a loss of capacity to influence the outside world.

Disturbance of mood is an invariable part of the psychopathology of neurotic disorder:

- *Anxiety* is variable in severity. It may be *generalized* and diffuse;

Table 9.1 *The psychopathology of neurosis*

1 Disturbance of self-experience
2 Disturbance of the experience of relationships
3 Disturbance of mood
4 Bodily symptoms

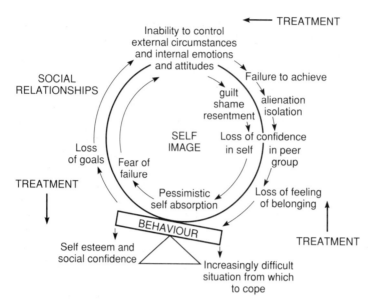

Figure 9.1   Cycle of demoralization

situational in response either to external stimuli, as in agoraphobia, or internal stimuli as in illness phobia;

episodic in panic attacks; or,

precipitated by external events, as in post-traumatic anxiety.

- *Depression* also is a very frequent mood state associated with feelings of loss, low self-esteem, feelings of learned helplessness and difficulties with coping.
- *Irritability* implies reduced control over temper usually with verbal or behavioural out-bursts, and experienced by the individual as unpleasant.
- *Depersonalization* is a common symptom, often overlooked because not enquired for, in which the subject *feels* himself or his surroundings to be unreal or altered in some way (see page 106).
- *Feelings of self-reference* may also occur in neurotic disorder in which the person feels himself to be the object of others' adverse attention.

Bodily symptoms include the various features of the somatoform disorders (see page 103). There are also bodily symptoms commonly associated with the abnormal mood of both anxiety and depression. Disorder of self-image may manifest in bodily symptoms such as *dysmorphophobia*, in which the person complains persistently that a

bodily organ – for example, the nose or the breasts – is deformed and very unattractive (see page 107). *Sleep disorder* is a frequent complaint with neurotic patients, especially increased wakefulness in the first third of the night, with more time awake, and awakenings during the night, and decreased time in deep sleep.

Disturbance of relationships is invariable in neurotic disorder. Individuals describe real or perceived deficiency in relationships, failing to receive care, concern, comfort, interest and support from others. They describe problems with work, or obtaining work, with family and marital relationships, and with the people they come into contact with. Because of previous bad experiences in relationships, they tend to lack confidence and be suspicious in subsequent social contact and this sets the scene for further failure. The many difficulties in the background of the person with severe neurotic disorder tend to be self-perpetuating. This again is the tyranny of inevitability in which failure of relationships produces a reinforcing vicious circle of low self-esteem and further difficulties with others.

Aetiology

Both hereditary predispositions and adverse environmental circumstances contribute to the formation of neurotic disorders, although most authorities would agree that, here, nurture is of much greater importance than nature. There is some evidence that personality type is at least in part inherited and that there may be genetic influence upon the type of abnormal emotional reaction manifested. The environmental influences which appear to foster adverse emotional reactions can be summarized into those associated with early life experiences and those developing later in response to adverse life events or current stresses.

As other behaviour patterns are acquired in the family, neurotic reaction can be learnt from parents as a way of responding to stress. It can also be provoked by the conflicts which may arise within a family; quarrels and arguments between the parents causing split loyalties in the child, adjusting to an absent or delinquent parent, coping with the rivalries and competing claims of brothers and sisters. The importance of developing a secure emotional bond between mother and child in the first year of life has been stressed for subsequent normal emotional responses. However, not only is this earliest period of relationship with mother crucial, but also how child and mother relate later; the relationship with father is also important for subsequent development. Continuing conflict and family disturbance is generally more damaging than complete loss of a parent – for instance, through bereavement. Family atmosphere and the quality of relationships are highly influential upon the developing children in determining future emotional reactions; they also create the pattern for the home atmosphere and relationships the children will establish when they themselves become parents.

Psychodynamic theory as originally propounded by Sigmund Freud claims that neurotic behaviour arises from personal conflicts that have remained repressed at an unconscious level since early childhood and can now only find expression in this inappropriate and censored way. Freud considered all such conflicts ultimately to be sexual in nature, and to be established in early childhood, usually by the age of 3 or 4. The intolerable emotion, usually of guilt, could not be faced and might therefore be converted into a physical symptom – *conversion* *hysteria*. Such theories are useful when looking for underlying causes of problems, but evidence for the universal validity of Freudian theory is absent.

The immediate cause of a neurotic reaction is stress (see page 31). What is stressful to one person may be regarded as stimulating and exciting to another; what one regards as a satisfactory, calm way of life may by another be perceived as boring and hence stressful. Stress may refer to the response to a noxious stimulus, or it may be considered to be the circumstances that provoke such a reaction, stressors or adverse life events. It is best to see stress as existing in the relationship between the person and the way he perceives his environment; at work and at home.

It is part of common human experience that unfortunate circumstances or *adverse life events* cause misery and fear, and such emotions may transcend what could be considered an appropriate reaction, and become abnormal. The particular categories of life event which are associated with a depressive reaction are those that are undesirable, those that represent *loss*, or 'exits from the social field', such as death of a relative or leaving home for the first time, and events which reveal 'interpersonal difficulties' such as family arguments. *Threat* is particularly conspicuous in causing anxiety. Adverse life events are prominent at the beginning of many neurotic illnesses.

Abnormal emotional reactions may be seen as *learned behaviour*. One account of how this occurs is the hypothesis of *learned helplessness*, originally described in experimental work carried out with dogs, but subsequently applied to humans in social conditions. The theory is that recurrent exposure to unpleasant situations of suffering or personal failure where the subject is incapable of escape eventually produces a response where no attempt to escape is made even though it is now possible. The victim assumes that activity is hopeless, that everything will inevitably go wrong and accepts this with resignation.

Possible social causes of neurosis could include deficiencies in the individual's social network, especially social interaction and attachment, and also lack of perceived adequacy of those who are available. These may both contribute to poverty of relationships and the development of neurotic disorder. This failure of emotional bonding may result from deficiency established very early in life.

Classification

The neurotic syndromes are not discrete entities but overlap with one another; many neurotic symptoms may occur in the same individual, resulting in mixed and intermediate cases. The distinction from both depression and personality disorder may be difficult or impossible, as

neurosis, depression and personality disorder may occur in any combination. The classification used here is that of the International Classification of Diseases, 10th edition (ICD-10), and is listed in Table 9.2. This is complex and is given here for guidance; it should not be learnt in detail!

The major categories of this classification are dealt with in Chapters 10 to 12. These diagnostic divisions are by no means watertight, as many people may show two or more features of neurosis concurrently. Although it is customary to include phobic reactions under the heading of anxiety states, many such reactions are similar to certain obsessional disorders. Anxiety itself may also be prominent in many cases of

Table 9.2   *Neurotic, stress-related and somatoform disorders in ICD-10 (1992)*

Neurotic	
Phobic	Agoraphobia
	Social phobia
	Specific or isolated
Other anxiety	Panic
	Generalized
	Mixed anxiety/depressive
Obsessive-compulsive	Obsessional thought
	Compulsive acts
	Mixed
Dissociative	Psychogenic amnesia, psychogenic fugue
	Psychogenic stupor, trance/possession
	Multiple personality
	Psychogenic motor disorder, psychogenic convulsions
	Psychogenic anaesthesia or sensory loss
	Other dissociative, unspecified dissociation or conversion disorder
Other	Neurasthenia
	Depersonalization
	Derealization
Unspecified	
Stress/adjustment	Acute stress reaction
	Post-traumatic stress disorder
	Adjustment disorder
Somatoform disorders	Multiple somatoform disorder
	Undifferentiated somatoform disorder
	Hypochondriacal syndrome
	Psychogenic autonomic dysfunction
	Pain syndrome without organic cause
	Other

obsessional disorder, while mixtures of obsessional and dissociative symptoms are not uncommon.

Acute emotional crisis (acute stress reaction)

Acute emotional crisis is a short-lived disturbance in behaviour which can be severe enough to justify the attention of a doctor and is usually quite clearly caused by an emotionally disturbing experience or trauma. Bereavement reaction provides a good example. Anyone will react with grief to the loss of a near relative, or with anger to an unprovoked insult. Such emotional reactions are entirely normal, although, when severe, may still bring a patient to the doctor for sympathetic counsel or to ask if it is normal. There are, however, emotional responses to bereavement which are clearly outside the normal range leading to an over-prolonged reaction which fails to resolve as expected. In such cases there is frequently, but not always, an ambivalent relationship between the deceased and the bereaved.

Psychogenic (reactive, neurotic) depression

Although depression is not classified with the neurotic disorders in ICD-10, it is generally found that neurotic or reactive depression is the commonest form of abnormal reaction. Psychogenic depression bears a certain resemblance to more severe forms of depression (described in Chapter 5) as regards the actual mood change and other psychological features, but does not as a rule show such symptoms as early morning waking, the characteristic diurnal variation of mood, loss of weight, or other somatic or so-called biological symptoms. This type of depression includes reactions such as those which occur in those facing any major life crisis or loss. Much of the confusion which surrounds this matter is of semantic origin, bound up with the meaning of the term 'depression'.

On all occasions when a diagnosis of a neurotic disorder is made, the possibility of depression also being present should be considered. If depression is present, both diagnoses should be accepted; if possible, it should be stated which of the two diagnoses is more significant.

Mental mechanisms

A considerable part of the terminology used traditionally by psychiatrists to describe the presumed processes occurring in those who show abnormal emotional reactions was derived from psychoanalysis. Such terms should be regarded not as factual entities but as hypothetical working concepts. They are included here not because they are regarded as essential for undergraduates but because of their historical interest and the illumination they may give into understanding an individual's predicament.

Mental mechanisms are modes of irrational, emotionally determined thinking and action; they assume the influence of unconscious parts of the mind. They provide an escape from having to face unpleasant reality which would otherwise occasion anxiety or some other disagreeable mood. They play some part in everyday mental activity, but when they predominate in certain areas of the patient's mental life and modify behaviour to any degree, they may in themselves be regarded as abnormal. The difference between ordinary evasion of difficulties and pathological reactions to situations or psychological stresses is one of degree rather than kind.

Compensation is the development of a personal quality to offset a defect or sense of inferiority; for instance, exaggerated tidiness. Within certain limits this is a normal, useful process but may be excessive, becoming a matter of *over-compensation*, when it is a reaction to repressed and therefore unconscious drives. The excessively conscientious and scrupulous individual may be over-compensating for opposite and contrary tendencies.

Conversion is the manifestation of repressed ideas in the form of bodily symptoms. Thus an hysterical paralysis of the legs may represent a crude form of escape from anxiety that might be occasioned if the sufferer were not prevented by his disability from having to go out and about.

Displacement is the shifting of emotion from one subject or situation which occasions it to another. This serves as a means of disguising or avoiding unacceptable ideas and tendencies. This is the psychodynamic explanation to account for irrational and apparently meaningless fears and phobias, though the hypothesis derived from experimental psychology would regard conditioning as likely to play a greater part, particularly in phobia formation.

Dissociation is a splitting of consciousness whereby inconsistencies in thought and conduct are overlooked; for example, the aggressive individual who asks for the doctor's assistance 10 minutes after threatening him with violence. It is also a mechanism which is thought to be operative in hypnosis, in sleep-walking and in hysterical trance states.

Fixation is arrest of development of personality at a state short of emotional maturity, even though general intelligence may measure up to average or above average on rating scales. Childish ways of reacting to difficulties, excessive dependence on others and marked egotism are all manifestions of fixation. The Freudian school stresses arrest of psychosexual development as a basis for pathological mental states and in fact all neurotic adaptations to life situations.

Identification is the conscious or unconscious placing of oneself in the situation of another person and may include the assumption of the characteristics of that person. It is normal for young people to imitate the attitude and behaviour of older persons whom they hold in high esteem. However, it is also normal, particularly in the case of adolescents, to try and escape from identification as part of their own search for self-identity. Persons drawn together by a common bond of empathy may also identify strongly with each other; hence the often observed phenomenon of the registrar 'catching' the consultant's mannerisms.

Introjection is the turning inwards of aggressive feelings and attitudes towards others which might otherwise give rise to conflict.

Thus, hostility towards others may be repressed and introjected in the form of suicidal impulses.

Projection is the displacement of personal attitudes onto the environment, and thus is the opposite of introjection. It is a way of avoiding self-blame and feelings of guilt. Personal shortcomings and failures are ascribed to 'bad luck' or an unfavourable material or psychological environment; for instance, the cruel father who blames his own parents for his current behaviour.

Rationalization is another means of self-deception by finding satisfactory socially acceptable reasons for conduct which is really prompted by less worthy or unethical motives.

Regression is a reversion to modes of thought, feeling and behaviour which are more appropriate to an earlier stage of development. Thus an adult may be said to regress to childish petulance and temper tantrums, while a physically or mentally handicapped person may regress to a child–mother dependent attitude towards a nurse.

Repression is the thrusting out of consciousness of ideas and urges to action which are incompatible with ideals, conscience or ethical standards. It is regarded as an unconscious, involuntary process in contrast to suppression, which is a conscious, willed checking or inhibition of thoughts, feelings and actions which conflict with moral standards.

Resistance is the barrier between the unconscious and the conscious, preventing resolution of incompatible elements in mental activity. The patient resists mental exploration, clings to his symptoms and in various ways fails to cooperate in treatment although he does so unconsciously and not wilfully.

Sublimation is the direction of undesirable or forbidden tendencies into more socially acceptable channels. Childish, egocentric conduct should, as a result of increasing maturity, be sublimated into more altruistic social behaviour. Surplus energies may be sublimated into useful channels.

Transference refers to the expression of emotions towards one person which are derived from experience with another. Thus a patient may transfer anxious or hostile feelings which he previously experienced in relation to a harsh dominating parent towards all those whom he later regards as authority figures. This mechanism plays an important part in psychotherapy, where the patient expresses feelings towards the therapist which he has transferred from elsewhere, but it is equally operative in all other doctor–patient relationships, such as that between the general practitioner and an adolescent patient.

Further reading

Henderson, A.S. (1988) *An Introduction to Social Psychiatry*, Oxford: Oxford University Press.
Sims, A.C.P. (1983) *Neurosis in Society*, Basingstoke: Macmillan.
Snaith, R.P. (1991) *Clinical Neurosis*, 2nd edn, Oxford: Oxford University Press.

10

Anxiety disorders

Anxiety, and the various disorders in which it is manifested, have been neglected by general physicians, general practitioners and psychiatrists. This is probably because they are so common that they are often thought to be a normal part of human experience and not requiring treatment. This, however, is a fallacy, and it is important to make the distinction between *normal* and *abnormal* anxiety, and between anxiety *trait* and an anxiety *state*.

Normal anxiety is a usual, even necessary, if unpleasant, response to threatening circumstances and is adaptive and of biological advantage. In abnormal anxiety the mood state is either an inappropriate response to the stimulus, or out of proportion to its severity, or prolonged when the stimulus has been removed, or associated with other maladaptive behaviour. It does not assist the individual in dealing with a threatening situation. *Anxiety state* is temporary, whilst *anxiety trait* is a lifelong tendency of the individual always to experience a high level of anxiety; this is considerably exacerbated by any additional external stress.

Normal and abnormal anxiety

Although the emotional response of anxiety is essential for survival, the consequences of abnormal anxiety can be disastrous. Anxiety may pervade every aspect of life and prevent the individual from coping with ordinary demands. It may impair ability to carry out responsibilities at work, resulting in unemployment and economic hardship. It may exacerbate the distress and discomfort of, and hinder recovery from, physical disease. It may lead to alcohol or drug abuse in an attempt, by self-medication, to alleviate the misery of anxiety. It may result in deteriorated performance in personal relationships, or in public activities such as examinations. The methods used to treat anxiety both by doctors and by the sufferers themselves have their own risks and hazards. The damaging consequences of abnormal anxiety have been much underrated in the past.

Anxiety is both a mood and a drive. When a healthy person is faced with a challenge, he may experience both the somatic symptoms and the mood of anxiety, and this constitutes the driving force resulting in successful accomplishment. Anxiety occurs with arousal; with increasing levels there is improved performance until a plateau is reached, as shown in Figure 10.1. Beyond this, increasing arousal is associated with anxiety *symptoms* and a decreased level of performance. So an optimum level of the mood and drive of anxiety results in appropriate behaviour, but if this is exceeded abnormal anxiety occurs. This is out of proportion to the stimulus, persists after the stimulus has been removed, and does not help in dealing with that stimulus.

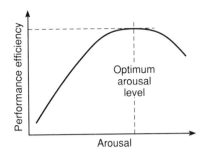

Figure 10.1 Yerkes–Dodson curve for anxiety from Sims and Hume 1984

'Mood (affective) disorders'. Although it is helpful to evaluate anxiety symptoms separately from other conditions, very frequently in the patients we see with anxiety disorders there are also prominent symptoms of depression present, and so both diagnoses will be required; there may also be other neurotic symptoms.

Anxiety is the description of the subjective state as made by the patient, whilst *stress* is the explanation by the outside observer of what he sees happening to the person who feels anxious (Chapter 4).

If the source of morbid anxiety is specific, it is designated *phobic disorder*, whilst *generalized anxiety disorder* arises with no single cause of stress. When anxiety, with other psychological symptoms, occurs following individual catastrophe or mass disaster, the condition is described as *post-traumatic stress disorder*. Anxiety is also the emotion associated with *threat* or *anticipation* of an unpleasant event involving severe discomfort, or loss, or both. In the 10th revision of the International Classification of Diseases, chapter V (ICD-10), the different anxiety disorders are classified under 'Neurotic, stress-related and somatoform disorders' whilst depression is classified under

Classification of anxiety disorders

A schematized representation of the commonly occurring anxiety disorders is shown in Figure 10.2. The anxiety disorders listed in ICD-10 are shown in Table 10.1.

Epidemiology

A major difficulty in carrying out epidemiological studies in this area is to decide who is a *case*; that is, the distinction between a normal and appropriate level of anxiety and what

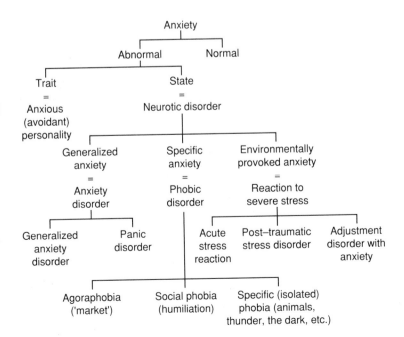

Figure 10.2 The anxiety disorders

Table 10.1   *Anxiety disorders in ICD-10*

F40   Phobic disorder
        Agoraphobia, with or without panic
            disorder
        Social phobia
        Specific (isolated) phobia

F41   Other anxiety disorders
        Panic disorder (episodic paroxysmal anxiety)
        Generalized anxiety disorder
        Mixed anxiety and depressive disorder

would be regarded as morbid and pathological. Another problem is the distinction between prevalence and incidence. Phobic disorders are generally of shorter duration and therefore have higher incidence and lower prevalence, whilst generalized anxiety is often long-lasting and so conversely has high prevalence and lower incidence. This means that the figures obtained are very dependent upon the manner of their collection.

In a community survey, a questionnaire study of the population found the one-year prevalence for agoraphobia with panic to be 1.2 per cent, all other phobias 2.3 per cent, and generalized anxiety 6.4 per cent. The female:male sex ratio has been found for phobias to be 2:1, and for generalized anxiety disorder 3.5:1.

Point prevalence data – that is, the number of cases at any moment in time – is summarized in Figure 10.3. At any particular time it is likely

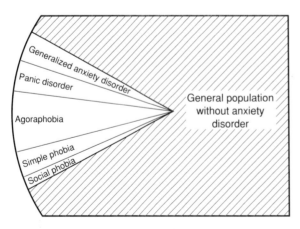

Figure 10.3 Prevalence of anxiety disorders in a general population

that about 3 per cent of the population will be suffering from panic disorder, 6 per cent from agoraphobia, 3 per cent from generalized anxiety disorder, 2.5 per cent from specific phobias and 1.5 per cent from social phobia; totalling 16 per cent from all anxiety disorders. There are no known differences quantitatively between different societies; however, there are marked cultural differences in presentation of symptoms and in their manifestation. This is an important area for transcultural research.

Disease concept of anxiety

Anxiety has changed surprisingly little in meaning since its derivation from the Latin word *'anxietas'*, meaning troubled in mind. Phobia and panic both originated as the personification of an emotion in the Greek gods, Phobos and Pan. Anxiety was linked in medicine in earlier centuries with somatic symptoms, especially cardiac disease, and also with constriction ('straits'). In psychiatry it was used to describe agitation in depressive psychosis, and then from about 1920 as anxiety neurosis. Phobias have been seen as morbid mental states since a description by Hippocrates, but agoraphobia as a separate syndrome was described in the mid-nineteenth century. Panic state was recognized by Freud as psychiatric disorder at the end of the nineteenth century but only formulated as a discrete diagnostic category in 1980.

An emotion which is regarded as an entirely appropriate response in the anticipation of threat and challenge in one situation may be regarded as pathological in another. There is a tendency for anxiety to become chronic, especially as avoidance of the provoking stimuli tends to perpetuate the emotion. There are a number of different overlapping anxiety disorders. Anxiety state is commonly found in all areas of medicine, in primary care as one of the commonest responses to the stresses of everyday life, amongst general hospital inpatients especially as a response to their experience of a severe illness, and also in psychiatric practice.

Symptoms

Anxiety state is manifested by symptoms of *mood*, of *cognition* (that is, thought and attitudes), and of *somatic* disturbance. These are not necessarily all present at the same time and there is considerable individual variation. In anxious mood there is a feeling of fear for an unknown disaster which in panic disorder amounts to terror. *Generalized anxiety* is characterized by motor tension, autonomic over-activity, apprehensive expectation of an unpleasant event and increased vigilance; it is persistent and free-floating. *Free-floating anxiety* – that is, without specific provocation – is associated with over-arousal, abnormal vigilance and sleep disorder, especially difficulty getting off to sleep.

Somatic symptoms are of two main types, increased muscular tension and autonomic over-arousal. Typical of the muscular symptoms are tension headache from the scalp muscles, restlessness, especially of the limbs, from an inability to relax, and tremor of the hands. Autonomic stimulation produces a number of symptoms, including palpitations, sweating, dryness of the mouth, loss of appetite, bowel over-activity, and frequency of micturition. A sense of suffocation may result in hyperventilation, causing decrease in arteriolar carbon dioxide and consequent paraesthesiae, tetany and even, rarely, convulsions. The characteristic cognition of anxiety is a feeling of insecurity. The individual is limited in what he can do by fear, and there are worrying thoughts which may be pervasive or focused on particular situations (phobias).

Trait anxiety is described by the sufferer as: 'I've been anxious all my life, a born worrier'. It is partly constitutional, and partly that anxious people tend to have been brought up in anxious families where the parents have responded with anxiety to all the situations in their environment. A person with trait anxiety will respond to minimal increase of stress with more marked anxiety symptoms. Generalized anxiety disorder arises gradually as a response to increasing levels of stress or conflict. The individual often has background proneness, with trait anxiety

symptoms occurring in variable degree. There is a general feeling of insecurity with a number of different situations avoided. Once established, anxiety states tend to persist unless they are treated adequately.

Panic disorder characteristically occurs first in young adult life and is commoner in women than men. There may have been no previous experience of pathological anxiety. The panic attack may first occur without any comprehensible provocation but quickly becomes associated with particular situations such as being in a public place or on a bus. The panic attack usually lasts for about 20 minutes and results often in the person rushing out of the place where it has occurred, or, alternatively, collapsing into a convenient armchair. The acute symptoms include tachycardia, a choking sensation, paraesthesiae, dizziness and faintness; they are often associated with a fear of dying, especially from a heart attack, or fear of going mad. The patient describes his mood as terrifying. Attacks tend to recur, and when they occur again in particular circumstances, this results in avoidance of those situations (panic disorder with agoraphobia).

Social anxiety is the emotion which is common to both agoraphobia, fear of being in a public place, and social phobia where there is fear of humiliation. In *agoraphobia* – literally, fear of the market place – the individual feels himself to be trapped in a situation from which he cannot easily escape without becoming the object of curiosity or contempt. Such an individual may make sure that if he goes to the theatre at all he will sit at the end of a row near the back. *Social phobia*, fear of being socially conspicuous, is associated with feelings of personal insecurity and sensitivity to others' criticism. It may manifest as anxiety about eating in public or public speaking. It usually starts in childhood and is associated with a need to conform. There is a general lack of self-confidence.

Illness anxiety may occur in which there is fear of illness amounting to phobia. The sufferer may describe extreme fear of developing a condition such as cancer or AIDS, even when it is extremely unlikely. Alternatively, the patient may present with physical symptoms that elude diagnosis despite referral from specialist to specialist. In the latter situation anxiety symptoms are only elucidated on careful enquiry. A patient with an intense dread of cancer said she would drive for miles to avoid a suburb of the city where there was a hospital with a radiotherapy unit. *Sexual anxiety* is one of the commonest reasons for sexual dysfunction: one partner has what has been called 'performance anxiety' which inhibits sexual intercourse and therefore increases subsequent anxiety in this situation.

A *specific phobia* may occur in response to any number of objects or situations that come to have great and fearful significance for the individual. Phobias are frequent for insects, snakes, worms, cats, dogs, thunderstorms, high winds, aeroplanes, lifts and so on. It is the accompanying behaviour of avoidance that so disables the patient; for example, a woman with a cat phobia was unable to make any social visits in case her hosts kept a cat. Another woman with a phobia for thunderstorms was virtually unable to leave her home during the summer in case there was a storm whilst she was out. In the past, each frightening object was designated by a different Greek word, such as 'claustrophobia' (fear of enclosed spaces) or 'arachnophobia' (fear of spiders).

Acute stress reaction is a transient disturbance lasting for a few hours or days. The individual feels dazed, and there is a narrowing of attention and difficulty in grasping what is going on around him. It occurs in response to exceptional stress for the individual, such as involvement in natural catastrophe or sudden bereavement. Panic and agitation often follow initial numbness. *Post-traumatic stress disorder* is a much longer-lasting response to an extremely stressful event. Provoking situations may be *mass* disaster, either *natural*, such as an earthquake or a bush fire, or *man-made*, for instance, a bomb exploded in a public place; or *individual* disaster, which also may be *natural*, such as involvement in a serious accident or *man-made*, such as being a victim of rape or torture. Symptoms may include repeated visual images of the disaster, avoidance of anything that recalls the trauma such as travelling near it, and persistent high arousal with feelings of anxiety. *Adjustment disorder* may follow a significant life change,

especially one that involves loss such as bereavement, emigrating under duress, and so on. Symptoms usually occur for between 1 and 6 months, and include depressed mood and anxiety, with difficulty in dealing with everyday social circumstances.

Sometimes the symptoms of an individual patient are relatively clear-cut examples of one of the above anxiety disorders. However, a much more common state of affairs is to find a mixture of various anxiety disorders, and also other neurotic symptoms. The different neurotic syndromes are not discrete but merge with one another. The same patient may present with a different mixture of symptoms on different occasions.

Differential diagnosis of anxiety disorder

Anxiety symptoms may occur as part of another psychiatric disorder and thus obscure its diagnosis. Much the most frequent overlap of symptoms is between depressive illness and anxiety state, and, in fact, panic disorder and some phobic conditions frequently respond to treatment with drugs that are normally regarded as antidepressant in their activity. Symptomatic discrimination between depression and anxiety may be made by looking for the characteristic symptoms of depressive illness such as *anhedonia* – the loss of the ability to feel feelings, and especially to experience pleasure. Individuals with learning difficulty are very prone to anxiety symptoms especially in novel situations, and they may express their anxiety in agitation and avoidant behaviour rather than in words. Anxiety and apprehensiveness may be early symptoms in developing organic psychosyndromes – for example, in early dementia. Anxiety may also be the most prominent symptom in substance misuse or its withdrawal. Especially important, because it is common and readily dealt with, is the association between excess caffeine intake in coffee-drinking and the occurrence of anxiety symptoms. In schizophrenia there may be prominent complaints of anxiety, especially when delusional atmosphere is the symptom which precedes the fully developed condition.

Depersonalization and derealization commonly occur with anxiety.

Symptomatic anxiety is a common response to the experience of severe physical illness. In some conditions anxiety is a symptom and indeed a sign of the condition itself. Such conditions would include hypoglycaemia from insulin excess, or rarely an insulinoma. In hyperthyroidism, phaeochromocytoma, carcinoid syndrome and also in some types of acute cardiac disease, and in epileptic illnesses, especially temporal lobe epilepsy, anxiety symptoms may occur. Anxiety is a prominent symptom in the acute stages of withdrawal from alcohol, benzodiazepines and opiates.

Not only do an individual's anxiety symptoms comprehensively affect his own behaviour and capacity to cope, but they also have an effect on other people. When symptoms are so disruptive that he regards himself and others regard him as sick, then this assumption of the sick role may add to his disabilities. Anxiety symptoms, especially somatic symptoms, have often been misinterpreted, and fruitless prolonged physical investigation has reinforced the individual's belief that he is suffering from a serious, rare and potentially lethal physical illness. He may respond to this by ceasing from all physical activity and stopping work. In the past such conditions have been described as 'disorderly action of the heart', 'effort syndrome', or 'soldier's heart'. There has been a close association between anxiety and presumed cardiac disease because of the similarity of symptoms.

Aetiology

The causes of anxiety state are described here for convenience as biological and psychosocial factors. However, it is important to realize that these overlap and in practice cannot be separated from each other. At present, the biological evidence is fragmentary, not necessarily applicable in all cases, and may be secondary to anxiety, whilst the psychosocial factors probably have more general relevance but are also subject to greater potential for methodological error. Thus knowledge of the aetiology of anxiety disorders is still highly tentative.

Biological factors

Genetic studies of aetiology in anxiety disorders have been of two main types, familial and twin studies. Anxiety has certainly been shown to be familial, but it is not always possible to distinguish in the family between biological factors and the initiation of other members. Twin studies have looked at concordance in monozygotic and dizygotic twins. There is still, of course, the problem that identical twins are likely to be reared similarly to each other and somewhat differently from other siblings. However, in general, studies have shown that there is no greater concordance for generalized anxiety disorder in monozygotic than dizygotic twins but there is weak increase of concordance where the individual suffers from panic disorder.

The James–Lange hypothesis of emotion proposes that a startling experience causes the heart to beat rapidly and the awareness of this physiological state results in the emotion of anxiety. Cannon considered the opposite sequence to occur; that is, the emotional experience was primary and bodily changes occurred in consequence. This theory proposes that the response to threat is conveyed in the beta-adrenergic fibres of the autonomic nervous system, and the thalamus processes the information; this circuit comprises the mammillary bodies, the fornix, anterior-thalamic nuclei, parahippocampal and cingulate gyri connecting with the temporal lobes. The septohippocampal system may be associated with vigilance especially involving the locus coeruleus. There has been some supporting evidence from positron emission tomography (PET) studies.

Further investigations for the localization of anxiety have involved the demonstration of benzodiazepine receptors. When benzodiazepine antagonists bind at these sites, anxiety is the resultant emotion. Pharmacological studies have demonstrated panic occurring from beta-adrenergic activation. This may occur with excess intake of caffeine, carbon dioxide inhalation, or sodium lactate infusion.

Panic disorder has been treated with imipramine and other related drugs.

Psychosocial factors

In Freudian *psychoanalytic theory* (see Chapters 4 and 9), adult anxiety is considered to have started with the repression of unacceptable ideas into the unconscious in early childhood. When this emotion returns to consciousness, it is expressed as anxiety. Repression allows different unpleasant experiences to become associated unconsciously, and hence phobia may arise from what would be considered a relatively minor immediate provocation. Panic has been explained as resulting from a repressed memory of sexual trauma.

In *attachment theory*, bonds between the infant and its mother are formed at a crucial stage of development. If there is maternal deprivation at this age – for instance, because the child has to go into hospital – the child develops anxiety about the reliability of attachment figures. This may subsequently develop through separation and threat of loss into chronic, all-pervasive anxiety.

Learning theory has been used to explain the occurrence of anxiety state. In *classical conditioning* as described by Pavlov, if a conditional stimulus is repeatedly presented just before the unconditional stimulus, eventually the response of the unconditional stimulus will be produced for the conditional stimulus. In Pavlov's experience with dogs in St Petersburg, water became a conditional stimulus, resulting in acute terror and panic. Normally, if the conditional stimulus occurs without the unconditional stimulus, it will eventually become extinguished. Thus, to be an adequate explanation for continuing anxiety, it has to take on drive properties. In this theory phobia has been explained as avoidance resulting in diminution of anxiety.

In *operant conditioning* behaviour is considered to occur in response to rewards, thus working on the principle of reinforcement. Phobic behaviour can then be seen as avoidance acting as a reinforcer in a situation where anxiety has become associated with certain specific circumstances. Avoidance results in

relief of anxiety, thus strengthening the association of anxiety with the situation avoided.

With *cognitive theory* the individual's mood and behaviour is considered to be largely determined by his cognitions; that is, the thoughts and attitudes with which he structures his own place in the world. These cognitions are based upon previous experience. If his cognition is associated with a particular situation, of failure and humiliation, then the resultant emotion when he is faced with this situation once again will be anxiety. Anxiety readily becomes associated with that particular situation and may spread to other areas of life.

The *social conditions* under which an individual lives are potent cause of stress and hence the subjective emotion of anxiety. For instance, work conditions may provoke so-called 'executive stress' or 'burn-out'. Unemployment and, even more, the threat of unemployment are potent causes of anxiety which may amount to pathological anxiety disorder and require treatment. Marital disharmony and sexual dysfunction both result from and cause anxiety. Agoraphobia and social phobias may occur, for social reasons, in young married women (the housebound housewife). It may to some extent be associated with the change of social role in leaving the parental home and area of the town to live in a new area where people outside are seen as hostile and competitive. Anxiety may result from disturbed relationships with other family members such as parents-in-law. Problems in relationships in the family – for example, between parents – are potent causes of anxiety in the children. It is also common for a specific phobia of one or other parent to be communicated to a child.

Major disaster may be a provocation for anxiety, and those in such a situation who develop anxiety disorder are likely to manifest anxiety amongst other symptoms. Anxiety may be communicated to others in epidemic form. Close contact with an individual who is already very anxious may result in transmission of anxiety to those around who were previously unaffected. Such epidemics have been described throughout history and have tended to be reported in communities of young females – for instance, in a girls' school. Symptoms most typically are of over-breathing, dizziness, faint-ness, headache, shivering, pins and needles, nausea, pain in the back or abdomen, hot feelings and general weakness, with the emotion of anxiety.

Outcome

When symptoms have occurred for a long time, in any of the anxiety disorders, there is likely to be continuing long-term disturbance both symptomatically and in social relationships. When those who suffered from severe anxiety disorders are followed up, they have been found to have a considerably raised rate of both alcohol and drug misuse even though there was no evidence of excess intake at the time of initial treatment. Dependence upon benzodiazepines is a problem with those suffering from anxiety disorders.

Generalized anxiety disorder, in particular, is likely to be prolonged and to persist over many years or decades. Phobic disorders, especially specific phobias, are often of shorter duration, but may recur at times of increased stress. Panic disorder is variable in outcome; it may be of short duration, or may persist over many years. Although post-traumatic stress disorder neces-sarily starts after a major precipitant, in a small proportion of cases onset is delayed by more than six months after the traumatic event. Most frequently symptoms have substantially diminished after about 18 months. Sometimes, however, especially where the stress was prolonged over a long time – for example, when prisoners of war are held under conditions of torture – symptoms may persist for years or decades, or even for the rest of the individual's life. One disturbing feature of such severely traumatized individuals is that the symptoms may not diminish as the years go by but even increase, so that a man held as a prisoner of war in his twenties occasionally becomes even more emotionally disturbed in his sixties.

An unexpected finding in the long-term out-come of anxiety disorders is the demonstration of an increased premature mortality; for example, sufferers from panic disorder were found at follow-up to have an unexpectedly high death-rate both from suicide and from cardiovascular disease. This has been demonstrated for other types of anxiety disorder. There is a marked increase of suicide above the expected rate; this is in many studies found to be as high as for depressive disorder. There is also a persistent increase in the mortality from natural causes, particularly arteriosclerotic disorders.

Treatment

Accurate diagnosis is essential for the effective management of anxiety; that is, the type of anxiety must be elucidated, the relative import-ance of biological and psychosocial factors assessed, and the presence of any other causa-tive factors such as other mental or physical illnesses taken into consideration. Caffeine intake is a particularly important factor. On occasions, advice to decrease or cease altogether drinking coffee and tea may result in relief of symptoms.

Drug and psychological treatments both have some disadvantages. It is a forlorn hope to seek a pharmacological solution to psychogenic anxiety, but on the other hand, psychotherapy is extremely time-consuming of highly skilled personnel, and hence a scarce resource. Treat-ment is discussed briefly here and reference is made also in Chapters 21 to 23.

Amongst the psychotherapies used in the treatment of anxiety are exploratory, behavioural, cognitive and group methods. *Exploratory methods* have most frequently been based upon the work of Freud, and involve making conscious the underlying conflicts, especially of a sexual nature, that have manifested in altered form as anxiety in adult life. Such methods are highly time-consuming and not necessarily effective. Briefer methods have been described by workers such as Carl Rogers in his 'client-centred psychotherapy'. This deals more with factors going on now in the patient's present experience rather than with past conflicts.

Behaviour therapy was developed by Wolpe, and the *classical* and *operant conditioning theories* have been applied to give methods of treatment. Such treatments, which can take place in a relatively small number of sessions, have been shown to be at least as effective as the more prolonged psychoanalytic treatments. *Cognitive therapy* is based upon the view that anxiety results from poor self-esteem, rather than vice versa. In essence, the method of dealing with these adversive cognitions is to set up a situation in which the individual produces his own arguments in a debate within himself against his negative cognitions, thus producing a change of attitude. *Group methods* have proved effective where there is social anxiety and difficulty in relationships.

Drug treatment has chiefly involved the sedative-hynotic groups of drugs, the beta-blockers, and those drugs normally considered to be antidepressant. The most commonly used drugs for the treatment of anxiety have undoubtedly been the benzodiazepines. Initially these were thought to be the ideal anxiolytic, but it is now realized that there are considerable problems with drug dependence and relatively severe withdrawal states. If used at all, these drugs should only be used in the short term for the management of acute anxiety, and the individual should be warned of the risk of dependence.

Beta-blocking drugs, such as propanolol, diminish the somatic components of anxiety. They have been used in the treatment of anxiety disorder but have not, in general, proved to be very effective.

The chief uses of the antidepressant group of drugs, such as imipramine, in the treatment of anxiety disorders is in those circumstances where there is 'masked depression' in addition to anxiety, in panic disorder, and in some cases of resistant phobic disorder. In Figure 10.4, the Hospital Anxiety and Depression Scale chart is shown for a patient with marked anxiety, who also had some depressive symptoms. Treatment for anxiety by psychological methods did not produce diminution of symptoms until the depressive symptoms were also treated with imipramine. It has been shown that panic disorder frequently responds to treatment with imipramine, and this in lower dose than is necessary for depressive illness. Phobic illnesses

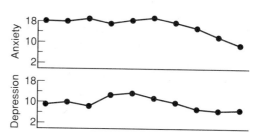

Figure 10.4 Hospital Anxiety and Depression Scale chart for a patient with mixed depression and anxiety

have frequently responded to treatment with tricyclic antidepressants, especially with the drug clomipramine.

In considering pharmacological agents in treatment, it is also important to mention drugs that may precipitate or exacerbate anxiety. Alcohol is frequently used as self-medication for anxiety and it is, of course, to some extent effective in the short term. However, the risk of dependence and addiction should discourage its use for this purpose. Caffeine, which is present in tea, coffee and cola drinks, is a potent cause of anxiety symptoms, and patients with anxiety disorder should be recommended to refrain from such drinks altogether, at least for a therapeutic trial.

Brief anxiety management techniques (Chapter 21) usually include both cognitive and behavioural elements. They combine the different components listed in Table 10.2. Explanation of why the treatment is effective, perhaps to relatives as well as to the patient, is important in ensuring the patient's motivation for involvement in what will require hard work and cooperation to achieve freedom from anxiety. Relaxation is induced through a series of exercises, and it is important for the subject to

Table 10.2 *Components in anxiety management*

1	Exploration and motivation for change
2	Relaxation or meditation
3	Exposure to anxiety
4	Restructuring of attitudes
5	Self-control

develop self-mastery of this process so that it can be used subsequently as a self-administered 'panic button'. Once the stage of relaxation has been achieved, exposure to anxiety, as a further stage in treatment, is essential so that the patient knows that production of and relief from anxiety is under his own control. In restructuring of attitudes the sufferer comes to realize that anxiety is not inevitable and is under his control through the procedures that have already been learned and an 'internal dialogue' within himself. Finally, it is important that the patient realizes that the technique is entirely under his own control and this is learned by practice between sessions with the therapist, with self-monitoring and achieving goals that have already been established.

Further reading

Sims, A. and Snaith, P. (1988) *Anxiety in Clinical Practice*, Chichester: Wiley.

Snaith, P. (1991) *Clinical Neurosis*, 2nd edn, Oxford: Oxford University Press.

Weismann, M.M., Myers, J.K. and Harding, P.S. (1978), 'Psychiatric disorders in a US urban community: 1975–6', *American Journal of Psychiatry* 135: 459–62.

11

Dissociative, somatoform and other neurotic disorders

This chapter is concerned with a motley group of conditions listed in Table 11.1. They all present with somatic symptoms, and the patients usually regard themselves as being physically ill. Often they strenuously resist psychiatric diagnosis and any suggestion that psychosocial factors are acting as precipitants.

Table 11.1 *Dissociative, somatoform and other neurotic disorders, from ICD-10*

Neurotic, stress-related, and somatoform disorders

    Phobic disorders
    Other anxiety disorders
    Obsessive-compulsive disorder
    Reaction to severe stress, and adjustment
      disorders

Dissociative (conversion) disorders

These include dissociative amnesia, fugue, stupor, convulsions, movement disorders, anaesthesia and sensory loss and also trance and possession disorders

Somatoform disorders

These include somatization, hypochondriasis and autonomic dysfunction affecting various bodily systems

Other neurotic disorders

Neurasthenia (fatigue syndrome, Chapter 16)
Depersonalization-derealization syndrome
Dysmorphophobia

Note: Bold type denotes those disorders which are the subject of this chapter.

Other features of neurotic disorders are often present, including disturbance of mood, with anxiety and depression, and marked disturbance in social relationships.

These conditions overlap with one another; mixed states are common. They also overlap with other neurotic disorders, especially depression and anxiety.

In most of medical practice the doctor is used to finding correspondence between the presence of physical disease and the symptoms which are the complaint the patient makes. However, sometimes serious organic disease occurs without any symptoms; for example, carcinoma *in situ* of the cervix. There may also be somatic symptoms without any known organic disease, and these are described in this chapter and represented diagrammatically in Figure 11.1. In *hypochondriasis* there is fear of illness. In *conversion disorder* the patient gains advantage from the presence of physical symptoms; it is presumed that this is mediated unconsciously. With *factitious disorder* physical symptoms are elaborated or intentionally produced. In *malingering* there is no disorder, either psychological or physical, and the apparent illness is simulated for immediate environmental gains.

In the past *dissociation* and *conversion* were included as different forms of *hysteria*; all somatoform disorders were designated *hypochondriasis*. Traditionally, hysteria and hypochondriasis have been considered to be

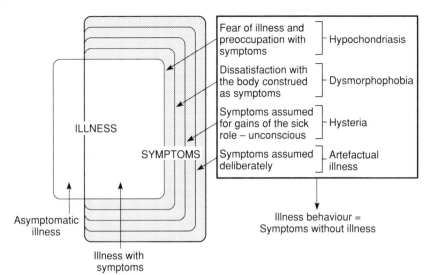

Figure 11.1 Illness behaviour and organic disease

separate conditions but with considerable overlap, often occurring at different times in the same patient, and sometimes even at the same time.

Dissociative (conversion) disorders

What for the last four centuries has been called *hysteria* is given the above rather clumsy designation in ICD-10. There is either a narrowing of the field of consciousness – that is, lack of awareness of most of what is happening, with selective amnesia (*dissociation*) – or limitation of motor or sensory function by transferring an unpleasant mood state into a physical symptom (*conversion*). There are four implications:

1 the symptoms are psychogenic;
2 the cause is not consciously recognized by the patient;
3 the symptoms carry some sort of advantage to the patient;
4 they occur via the psychological mechanisms of conversion or dissociation (as above).

Any or all of the functions of awareness of identity, memory, sensation, and control of motor functioning may be affected. The individual may claim to be wholly unaware of his behaviour. Often an underlying conflict can be demonstrated, and the behaviour is neurotic in that it is an inappropriate way of responding to that conflict and does not resolve the difficulties effectively.

Follow-up studies of patients previously diagnosed as suffering from hysteria have cast doubts on its existence as a distinct condition, as in one study a large proportion of patients developed serious physical illness and in another study, over 60 per cent of patients at follow-up showed definite evidence of affective disorder. Many patients diagnosed as hysterical actually suffered from organic conditions, and a primary depressive illness may sometimes present in hysterical guise. Despite these reservations, there undoubtedly appears to be a small minority of patients for whom the diagnosis of hysteria, or dissociative disorder, is appropriate.

Aetiology

There is no direct evidence of a genetic contribution; as in other forms of emotional disturbance, an account of a disturbed childhood or of unsatisfactory relationships between parents is common amongst those with dissociative disorders.

Loss of self-esteem is usually present either in the short term, such as being charged with a criminal offence, or in the longer term, as in the case of a wife who knows that her husband is having an affair but cannot take steps to resolve this.

Symptoms

The symptoms of dissociation occur at any age in either sex, often influenced by the social group from which the patient comes; thus patients with more sophisticated ideas present more complex symptoms. Suggestibility is frequent, so it is important not to create further symptoms by suggestive questioning or frequent physical re-examination which will reinforce the patient's notion of physical illness. Unwise medical interviewing and examination may on occasions produce such symptoms in vulnerable people. Symptoms may be psychological or physical, often neurological.

Dissociative amnesia

The patient may profess to have forgotten long periods in his life, or alternatively, certain significant episodes. He may appear to have forgotten completely who he is or where he has come from. He usually has nothing on his person which might help to answer these questions. Such amnesia is differentiated from memory loss due to organic cerebral disorder by the preservation of other functions: for example, it may be observed how readily he remembers how to use a knife and fork and how his behaviour is in many other essential respects normal; how he finds his way about the ward; is unperturbed by his situation while at the same time giving an impression of wariness. Such cases not infrequently follow some lapse in conduct – as, for instance, a man who presented in Casualty claiming to have come from America the evening after a criminal charge in a neighbouring borough. Memory may return spontaneously within 24 hours or so but, if prolonged, raises the suspicion of malingering. However, memory of the stressful event itself does not necessarily come back.

Dissociative fugue and stupor

The word '*fugue*' implies flight or wandering, often from a painful or threatening situation. Dissociative amnesia is also present. The individual travels purposefully but beyond the usual range (one patient travelled in a fugue from Birmingham, in the United Kingdom to Montreal, Canada). Whilst in this state the individual is able to interact with others – for example, asking directions – and also to look after himself in terms of eating, avoiding traffic and so on.

Somnambulism, or sleep-walking, most commonly occurs in childhood and is a form of dissociation somewhat similar to fugue. The individual is in a trance and may carry out a complicated routine such as getting out of bed, putting on his shoes, opening the door, going downstairs; he has total amnesia for his behaviour subsequently. *Stupor,* in which dissociation is one antecedent, is profound diminution or absence of voluntary movement and the normal responsiveness to external stimuli such as light, noise or touch.

Dissociative movement disorders and convulsions

There may be total or partial paralysis of a limb with ataxia. In *hysterical astasia-abasia* there is a bizarre gait or total inability to stand up without support. There may be gross tremor of an individual organ or many parts of the body. Almost any motor neurological lesion may be mimicked. Chronic cases may produce contractures and considerable muscular wasting.

Hysterical fits may be confused with those of organic origin and initial full physical investigation will be required. Differential features are not conclusive but include an atypical seizure without normal epileptic features; occurrence only in the presence of others; other evidence of histrionic behaviour; apparently purposive nature of the movements; manifest motivation; absence of injury, tongue-biting or incontinence. During or immediately after the fit the plantar response will not become extensor but this sign also is not wholly reliable. Some patients have both epileptic and hysterical seizures and this causes further confusion.

Dissociative anaesthesia and sensory loss

Typical is the anaesthesia of 'glove and stocking' distribution which does not correspond to known sensory distribution. It demonstrates the patient's *idea* of physical illness rather than what occurs neurologically. Dissociative visual disturbance is not usually total, but more often the complaint is of general blurring of vision or tunnel vision. The patient's movements and coordination often belie the severity of their claimed disability.

A mixture of these various dissociation disorders may occur. Another disturbance of the sense of personal identity is so-called '*multiple personality*', where two or more distinct or independent personalities appear to exist within the same individual at different times. The precise range of symptomatology with dissociation is enormously varied.

Epidemic, communicated or mass hysteria is most likely to occur in closed communities and especially when there is a marked social conflict affecting many members. It spreads by a form of social contagion and is most often reported amongst girls. The first person affected may have a genuine physical illness. Those who transmit the contagion early on in the epidemic are usually of higher social status within their peer group, they are likely to be those who have previously shown instability and are currently going through some personal conflict. From them the epidemic spreads to more normal members of the group. Symptoms may include over-breathing, dizziness, fainting, headache, shivering, pins and needles, nausea, pains in the back and abdomen.

Differential diagnosis

Dissociative disorder is relatively rare in British psychiatric practice but is much more common in developing countries; in general hospital psychiatric units serving other medical and surgical specialties, about 2 per cent of referrals are eventually diagnosed as suffering from hysteria. Hysteria may present to general physicians, surgeons or obstetricians in a manner characteristic for each specialty. Thus hysterical aphonia may present to the ENT

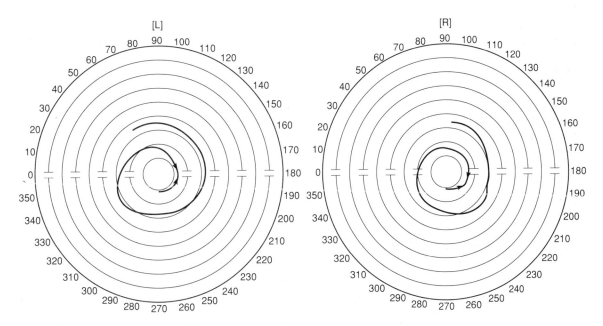

Figure 11.2 Corkscrew visual defect

surgeon; or a corkscrew visual defect to an ophthalmologist (Figure 11.2).

It is important to realize that dissociation is not the only mental mechanism that may result in the appropriation of physical symptoms; indeed, depression with hypochondriacal physical complaints is considerably commoner. Hysterical reactions may also be secondary to other conditions; for instance, amongst known epileptic patients being treated with anticonvulsant drugs, hysterical 'fits' are very common.

There has always been difficulty in separating the concept of *hypochondriasis* from that of hysteria, and, in fact, in the seventeenth century Thomas Sydenham regarded hypochondriasis as the male equivalent of hysteria in the female. Hypochondriasis is described later in this chapter. Some of the important conditions for differential diagnosis are listed in Table 11.2.

Treatment

There is a need for a complete and detailed history, not only from the patient but also from a third party who knows the situation well. Treatment demands a considerable degree of patience and tolerance, with a continuing respect for the patient as a sick person, even though the patient's explanation of his symptoms is unacceptable. Both confrontation and collusion are to be avoided, although there may come a time when confrontation without rejection is necessary. It is important for the patient

Table 11.2 *Differential diagnosis of dissociative disorder*

1 Depressive illness, of any type
2 Epilepsy and other neurological illness
3 Somatization disorder
4 Histrionic personality disorder
5 Deliberate disability
6 Self-poisoning, anorexia nervosa, physiological malfunction
7 Anorexia nervosa
8 Hypochondriasis

to realize that others do not accept sickness behaviour at face value, but still accept him as ill and in need of help.

Common-sense application of relearning is useful, and, to achieve this behavioural modification, biofeedback and physiotherapy may be used; for example, a patient who arrived on the ward on crutches received considerable benefit from walking exercises from a physiotherapist in addition to other, psychological forms of treatment. Treatment has to recommend itself to the patient as being both reasonable and acceptable, and the patient's notion that there is a serious physical symptom may require that the staff use some form of physical treatment. It is very important to build up the patient's feelings of self-respect and esteem. This is achieved by congratulating the patient on successes that occur in the course of treatment and also by encouraging participation in group social activities, and helping the patient to improve in social skills.

It is often very difficult to deal with a hysterical patient's symptoms either as an outpatient or on a general, non-psychiatric ward, and psychiatric admission may be necessary. Instant removal of hysterical symptoms by hypnosis, although sometimes possible, and dramatic and impressive, is unreliable as a form of treatment. It is difficult to predict in which patients it will be effective, the same symptoms or others are likely to recur at a later stage, and dependence on the hypnotist readily develops.

When embarking upon treatment it is worth formulating jointly with the patient what is expected or hoped for, and for how long this should be attempted. Treatment is based upon the acceptance of a patient as a person genuinely needing help, on reassurance that the condition is going to improve, on avoidance of collusion in accepting physical aetiology, and on avoidance of unnecessary confrontation; at the same time work continues with the patient to try to identify and deal with the stresses that have provoked the reaction. It is important for the patient to feel that symptoms are accepted by the doctor as real and worth treating.

There should be a thorough physical examination initially to exclude any organic, neurological or other disorder; any special investigations should be done as early as possible. Having carried out such procedures, and finding them to be negative, the physical symptoms should then largely be ignored. The patient is drawn into cooperation by convincing him that treatment is appropriate and can be effective.

The features of *secondary gain* from the sick role should also be investigated, but not made explicit to the patient. It is important to work out what benefits the patient gains from illness behaviour in order to construct a situation in which the gains from getting better are greater than those in remaining disabled. Such methods of treatment usually involve interdisciplinary cooperation.

Drugs and physical methods of treatment alone can never deal with conversion symptoms. Tricyclic antidepressants and also monoamine oxidase inhibitors have been used, chiefly for dealing with associated depressive symptoms. Electro-convulsive therapy is not indicated in uncomplicated hysterical conversion reactions as it may make them considerably worse.

Prognosis

For a young person with the acute development of a single dissociative symptom in reaction to what he or she perceives to be a severe life stress, the prognosis is generally good. With remission of the stress, and adequate psychotherapeutic treatment, such patients usually make a complete recovery. The prognosis for older patients, for those with chronic disability, and especially where there is evidence of marked personality disorder, is much less favourable. Such symptoms tend to continue. There is also an increased risk of depression, suicide and of death from accident. The condition may recur with similar or different symptoms.

The social setting is important in determining outcome. Where the provoking situation has been removed, the likelihood of complete recovery is very much greater; where there is clear evidence of secondary gain and the provoking situation continues, then improvement is more difficult to achieve. The more disabling and more apparently permanent the

hysterical symptom is, the better the prognosis; for instance, hysterical blindness has a better prognosis than continuing attack disorders, such as 'fits' or vomiting. However, in long-term follow-up, although the initial dissociative symptoms may have completely remitted, many patients show chronic symptoms of anxiety, depression and hypochondriasis.

Somatoform disorders

The patient with somatoform disorder is preoccupied with physical symptoms and fears of illness. There are repeated medical consultations with requests for yet more investigations despite previous negative findings and reassurance often by many doctors in different specialties. The symptoms are out of proportion to and not appropriately explained by any concurrent physical disorder. Neither is the severe distress or preoccupation of the patient so explained. Such patients are very resistant to seeing psychosocial situations as either causing or exacerbating their symptoms, even when this may be obvious. They may be prepared to accept that there are anxiety or depressive symptoms present, in their opinion as a reaction to the physical illness rather than a cause of it. The four somatoform disorders of ICD-10 – *somatization, hypochondriasis, autonomic dysfunction* and *persistent pain* – have some features in common, including the concentration of interest of the patient upon a physical underlying cause; the disorders may occur together. They may also overlap with other neurotic disorders, especially dissociation, anxiety and depression.

Somatization disorder

There is a chronic hypochondriacal neurotic disorder in which there are multiple symptoms, which both recur and change frequently, affecting many different physical systems. Symptoms are usually present for many years before psychiatric referral and continue unabated for many years subsequently. Such patients have had multiple referrals to different hospital specialists, and both their hospital case notes and general practice records are voluminous. There is often a history of many negative investigations and sometimes fruitless operations. Gastro-intestinal and skin complaints are amongst the commonest but virtually every system may be affected. At times the course is chronic and fluctuating, often moving to different systems over subsequent decades. Depression and anxiety are usually present with varying severity.

The condition usually starts in early adult life and continues indefinitely. It is much commoner in women than men. There may be heavy use, amounting to abuse, of a variety of different medications, both prescribed and preparatory.

Diagnosis is based upon the long duration of multiple and variable symptoms, and persistent refusal to accept the advice of many doctors that there is no underlying physical disorder. As is usual with neurotic conditions, there is disturbance in social relationships within the family and outside, and there is also usually some degree of anxiety and depression.

In the past treatment was most often directed at limiting the use of health resources. Reassurance is quite useless as this serves only to reinforce the patient's notion that doctors do not understand the condition. Careful explanation of mechanisms, with reinforcement of positive, healthy behaviour and the application of cognitive behavioural techniques has shown good results, but further studies in this area are required.

Hypochondriasis

In hypochondriasis there is morbid preoccupation with the body or state of health, or with the symptoms of illness. The patient feels the need to express symptoms out of proportion to any disease that may be present. Good health-care provision may have the unfortunate consequence of encouraging over-concern in the predisposed. Hypochondriasis also occurs as a symptom of depressive illness, when it requires pharmacological treatment.

Regarding the social context of illness, the person who considers himself to have symptoms

of illness adopts a 'sick role'. This affects the way he regards himself, and is communicated both to relatives, who are expected to treat him as a sick person, make allowances, be nice to him and not expect too much in return, and also to the doctor, with the implicit message: 'I want both your help and your diagnostic labelling'. In order to come to medical attention the person has to do something, and this activity is called *illness behaviour*. Sometimes hypochondriacal behaviour is an understandable reaction to the misplaced activity of doctors in forcing a sick role upon their patients.

Fear of illness is a prominent part of hypochondriasis. This may show itself as a fear that illness may develop, fear that illness is actually present, anxiety complicating known physical illness, and disease-claiming behaviour as occurs in the *hospital addiction syndrome* (synonym: Munchausen Syndrome).

Psychopathology

The possible disorders of *form* (see page 9) of hypochondriasis are shown in Table 11.3. Not all these occur in hypochondriacal neurosis; for example, a psychotically depressed patient may hear an admonitory voice, an *auditory hallucination*, saying, 'You have cancer.' Such a depressed person may also hold a *delusion*, *secondary* (see page 14) to their depressed mood state, in which they believe, falsely and on delusional evidence, that they have cancer.

Primary delusions occur in schizophrenia and may be hypochondriacal in their content; for instance, a man aged 52 who believed that at the age of 15 an operation had been performed

Table 11.3   *Disorders of form in hypochondriasis*

Disorder of form	Disorder of content
Auditory hallucination Delusion: primary secondary Over-valued idea Obsessional rumination Anxious preoccupation Depressive preoccupation and rumination	Hypochondriasis

upon him, without his knowing it, to insert a golden convolvulus in his abdomen causing him subsequently to become impotent.

An *over-valued idea* is an acceptable and comprehensible idea pursued by the patient beyond the bounds of reason. It is the way that hypochondriacal neurosis commonly presents; for example, a man who spends most of his time worrying about the possibility of his developing cancer from all the various potential carcinogens in his environment. An *obsessional rumination* is recognized by the individual as both 'alien to my nature', but also 'coming from inside myself'. It is resisted yet occurs repetitively; for instance, a person may have a repetitive notion: 'I have cancer'. With *anxious preoccupation* a person, who already has fear of illness, comes to worry that they also have established illness. Normal sensation may be interpreted as symptoms, or symptoms interpreted as serious illness. With *depressive preoccupation* and *rumination* there is an underlying depressed mood.

The symptoms of the hypochondriacal patient may affect virtually any system or function. Most commonly the musculo-skeletal, gastro-intestinal and central nervous systems are involved, with head and neck, abdomen and chest being the parts of the body most frequently concerned. There can also be hypochondriasis for mental symptoms, the two commonest examples of this being hypo-chondriacal concern over sleep and fear of developing madness.

Differential diagnosis of hypochondriasis

It is extremely important to identify *depressive illness* if it is present. Hypochondriasis is a

Table 11.4 *Differential diagnosis of hypochondriasis*

Depressive illness

Neurotic disorder – hypochondriacal neurosis, anxiety state, any other

Schizophrenia

Organic psychosyndromes – dementia

Childhood conditions

frequent presentation of depression, especially in the older, agitated and potentially suicidal patient, who urgently requires and will probably respond to treatment. Hypochondriasis is a frequent symptom of *neurotic disorder* and may occur as a primary condition – hypochondriacal neurosis, but also with any other neurotic condition such as anxiety state, or with depressive neurosis. *Schizophrenic* patients may have bizarre hypochondriacal complaints and will usually show other diagnostic signs. Organic states such as early dementia may be obscured by prominent hypochondriacal complaints. Hypochondriasis and an organic state may coexist, as may hypochondriasis and established, obvious physical illness.

In children the hypochondriasis of the parents may be reflected as over-concern for the child's health; an extreme example of this is the condition described as *Munchausen by proxy* in which the parent manufactures symptoms or signs in the child. The hypochondriasis that parents show may also be communicated to their children, resulting in the latter also showing hypochondriasis.

Treatment

It is essential to make a diagnosis and not fall into the trap of prescribing endless ineffective physical remedies for the various symptoms. It is important to determine whether depression, neurotic disorder, or physical illness or a combination of these explains the symptoms. The hypochondriasis of depression often resolves as the depressive illness improves (Chapter 5).

There is much that the medical profession can do to avoid setting the scene for the emergence of hypochondriasis. Unnecessary repeated consultation and examination should be avoided, as should unnecessary investigations, particularly repeat investigations where the first one proved to be normal. The doctor should come to a decision regarding diagnosis and method of treatment and try not to change his mind.

The treatment of the individual patient is often difficult but may be facilitated by bearing in mind the following points of Table 11.5.

Table 11.5 *Management to prevent and treat hypochondriasis*

1 Initial thorough examination, investigation for physical illness.

2 Careful explanation to the patient of the nature of symptoms (simple reassurance is useless).

3 Exploration of psychological factors and illness behaviour.

4 In discussion, allow the patient to discover a link between symptoms and conflict; do not acquiesce in his view of organic aetiology.

5 Establish limited goals and achieve these without recourse to illness behaviour by patient.

6 Marked progress not possible in all patients, but use of placebo is not justifiable as this will reinforce the patient in his sick role.

Hypochondriasis represents a medical dilemma. Collusion with the patient in his belief concerning organicity, or confrontation to assert psychogenic aetiology are equally unhelpful. Neither will the doctor be allowed to ignore the patient's complaints. Diagnosis is a necessary first stage: physical illness is always considered; the identification and effective treatment of depressive illness occurs in an important minority of cases; and setting up a workable treatment plan for hypochondriacal neurosis is necessary for this. 'The sufferer from hypochondriacal neurosis sees perfunctory or ill-directed reassurance as dismissal, as failure to take it seriously. He does not want to be told that there is nothing wrong; he needs to understand his symptoms as a first step to overcoming them' (Appleby, 1987).

Persistent pain disorder

This is discussed further with liaison psychiatry (Chapter 16). The patient complains of localized, persistent, severe and distressing pain. This cannot be explained fully by any physiological process or disorder. It is associated with emotional difficulties and psychosocial conflict.

Characteristically, pain of psychogenic origin tends to be more diffuse and less well localized than the pain of a physical lesion. It often spreads with a non-anatomical distribution. The pain is complained of as constant, becoming more severe at times, but unremitting. It is often associated with an underlying disturbance of mood which appears to be primary both in time and in causation. Patients have difficulty in describing the quality of psychogenic pain. The pain is very unpleasant, and the patient feels he cannot bear it, but at the same time he can find no adequate words for description. Psychogenic pain tends to progress both in severity and extent over time. This would be unusual for a physically mediated pain.

Other neurotic disorders

Depersonalization-derealization

Depersonalization describes a peculiar change in the awareness of self, in which the individual feels as if he is in some way unreal. *Derealization* denotes a similar change in the awareness of the external world. These two symptoms frequently occur together, and they are often associated with both anxiety and depression. Depersonalization is an experience described also by healthy people, but for patients the experience is intensely unpleasant; not infrequently it is considered to be the most distressing complaint by a neurotic patient. They feel disturbed, altered and incompetent, and this may of itself provoke suicidal ideas. The patient has great difficulty in explaining the subjective nature of the symptom and may feel that it indicates the onset of madness; the perplexed disjointed account of the patient in trying to describe it, in construing metaphors that do not satisfy him, is quite characteristic.

Depersonalization and derealization are surprisingly common symptoms, often overlooked by the interviewing doctor. As the sole complaint, this syndrome is unusual, but as a part of a pan-neurotic picture such symptoms are very common. The individual may describe himself or his surroundings as being changed in their quality so that he or they feel unreal, remote or automatic. His quality of unreality may extend to all his functions, both physical and mental. The outside environment may seem to be colourless and lifeless and appear flat, two-dimensional, artificial or unreal. Such patients may comment that everyone else appears to be living a full and meaningful life whereas they are outside and deficient in some way.

Treatment of these symptoms has proved remarkably difficult, and the treatment of associated anxiety and depression is more rewarding. Explanation to the patient concerning the nature of symptoms, and the fact that they do not indicate the onset of madness or psychotic illness will be of some value.

Dysmorphophobia

In dysmorphophobia, which is not a phobia at all, the primary symptom is the patient's belief that he or she is unattractive because of an external physical defect which is noticeable to other people. In practice, the organ of complaint is not conspicuous to others, who are surprised at the patient's distress. Complaints about the shape of the nose are particularly common; the nose is thought to be very ugly, and the patient importunes for surgery. The symptom is associated with great distress amounting to suicidal ideas on occasions. The dissatisfaction with appearance may be associated with complaints of disturbance in function. The complaint itself is, phenomenologically, an *over-valued idea*. Another common organ of complaint is the shape, and especially the size, of the breasts, which are considered to be too small, or, more rarely, too big. Other external organs are less commonly affected.

The specific symptom of dysmorphophobia is commonly associated with depressive mood, and anxiety symptoms. The patient believes his appearance is unattractive to other people, and this severely affects the capacity for relationship. When it is proved that a patient does not have an underlying psychotic illness, surgical treatment, although not necessarily producing objectively a more satisfactory organ, has resulted in relief of psychological symptoms in a number of cases.

An exaggerated concern with one's self-image and especially with personal appearance is called *narcissism*, after the myth of Narcissus who was punished for his disdain of Echo's admiration by being condemned to fall in love with his own image in a pool of water. The absorption with self-image is usually associated with feelings of insecurity of self, especially a fear that the body is going to disintegrate and shows signs of growing old. The abnormality often reveals an inability to make relationships with others, resulting in the capacity for loving being turned in upon the self. Narcissism has some similarities both to dysmorphophobia and to hypochondriasis: to the former in that there is a concentration upon physical appearance, and to the latter in that there is a fear of progressive loss of physical capacity. This clinical picture may also be one manifestation of an underlying depressive illness.

Further reading

Appleby, L. (1987) 'Hypochondriasis: an acceptable diagnosis?', *British Medical Journal*, 294: 857.
Merskey, H. (1979) *The Analysis of Hysteria*, London: Baillière Tindall.

12

Obsessional states

The word 'obsession' is in everyday use, where it usually implies a high degree of preoccupation with some concern or other. It often conveys an idea of excess: either the person recognizes that the matter has gone beyond reasonable bounds, or someone else takes that view. The technical sense in which the term is used in psychiatry is very similar to the everyday use, but there are certain refinements to its meaning.

The central feature of an *obsession* is the sudden entry into the mind of an unpleasant thought, against conscious resistance. The subject tries to resist but is unable to do so. Such thoughts become repetitive and the subject becomes a victim of recurrent, unwanted, yet intrusive thoughts.

Obsessional thoughts are unwanted not only because they are recurrent and unpleasant but also because they are recognized by the subject as unnecessary or senseless. They often lead to actions which share most of the features of the obsessions, known as *compulsions*. These too are recurrent and resisted, and they make sense only as secondary rituals to counteract or dispel the thoughts. Attempts to ignore or dispel obsessive thoughts usually lead to an intense inner struggle which may absorb virtually all available psychic energy. Marked anxiety, tension and depression frequently arise when obsessive-compulsive activity is resisted, although they may be well concealed.

Although the content of an obsessive thought is felt to be intrusive, it is, nevertheless, always recognized by the subject as coming from within; this distinguishes it from the passivity experienced in schizophrenia, when the patient may feel that thoughts have been inserted into his mind by some external agency. Likewise, an obsessive idea differs from a delusion in that the latter is accepted as true, while the sufferer from an obsession recognizes its absurdity and tries to repudiate it, although this is a painful mental struggle.

The prevalence of obsessional illness is unknown: figures derived from hospital contacts suggest it to be much less common than depression, phobias, anxiety states or schizophrenia; general population epidemiological studies suggest a much higher frequency. Obsessional *symptoms*, however, occurring as part of many other psychiatric disorders, are undoubtedly common. They may be prominent in depressive illness; or may be part of schizophrenia and become interwoven with its other symptoms. Obsessions may also be engendered by organic disorder such as encephalitis or head injury. There is, furthermore, some evidence of an association between birth trauma and the later occurrence of obsessional disorder.

Mildly obsessive thoughts may transiently disturb those who are otherwise normal, especially when tired or under emotional stress. They often take the form of a repetitive or meaningless word, catch-phrase or slogan, or perhaps a snatch of melody which reverberates irritatingly in the mind. Such happenings cannot be considered as pathological so long as they do not interfere with productive mental activity. In contrast, severe obsessions and compulsions must be regarded as amongst the most distressing, and sometimes intractable, of all psychiatric symptoms.

Aetiology

First, it must be said that the cause of obsessional illness is unknown. No hard evidence supports genetic, physiological, psychological or social aetiology. Perhaps the greatest interest in recent years has focused upon the likely pathophysiological role of the 5-hydroxytryptamine (5-HT) neuronal system. However, no simple neurochemical theory will suffice; the dopaminergic system also seems to play some part in the process.

It has, however, often been observed that a substantial minority of patients' relatives suffer from obsessional illnesses or exhibit obsessional traits of varying severity. Clearly, there is opportunity for a child in such a household to learn obsessional ways of behaving; however, separating hereditary from psychologically acquired symptoms is an almost impossible task.

Obsessional illnesses may be characterized by fluctuations in intensity, in which case the possibility of a link with an underlying primary recurrent affective illness should be considered. Many, however, seem to arise slowly and become part of the person's characteristic ways of thinking and behaving – and show little obvious relation to mood.

Obsessional personality

It is a widely held notion that there exists, between the many who experience mild transient obsessions and the few with full-blown obsessional illness, a group of people who exhibit enduring obsessional features sufficient to warrant description as obsessional personality. In place of 'obsessional' the term *'anankastic'* is sometimes used; it is a Greek word with virtually the same meaning.

Some people showing mild yet persistent obsessionality are conscientious, scrupulous, perfectionistic, prone to checking – even when sure that a task is properly completed. Some are tidy in manner, others cannot settle until everything is in its proper place or 'just-so'; a liking for precision may, however, become fussiness or rigid pedantry. Some are beset by unwarranted self-doubt, leading to vacillating indecision. In severe cases, many of these characteristics may be troublesome to the person or to others around him; a need for formality and an inflexible approach may render someone personally inefficient or tiresome to others.

Some sufferers from obsessions live in constant dread that they may have done or have omitted to do something which may have serious consequences for others: for instance, the person who, whilst knowing he has already done so, fears he may have failed to turn off the gas and returns home from a trip out in order to check.

If there is an abiding pattern of obsessional thinking and actions which can be called obsessional personality, what is its relationship to obsessional illness? A substantial proportion – perhaps one-third to one-half – of patients suffering obsessional illness are found to have a background 'personality' of an obsessional kind. We do not, however, know why a large proportion of those who develop obsessional illness as a new event do so in the absence of previous obsessionality, nor why many people with markedly obsessional styles of thinking and behaving never develop full-blown obsessional illness.

Symptoms

Normal children often pass through phases in which they exhibit compulsions to count, touch objects (such as running the fingers over passing railings), or step over cracks in the pavement. The obsessional element in childish games bears a very close relationship to superstitious behaviour and to primitive ceremonial ritual. In the majority of cases, growing-up and exposure to normal social influences leads to the disappearance of such acts. In some, however, obsessional trends become more pronounced and troublesome. In adults, all degrees of severity occur, from an occasional preoccupation with a tune running in the head, a sudden destructive or aggressive impulse usually soon checked, or an unnecessary examination of the gas taps or electric light switches, to more insistent obsessional states which can seriously interfere with comfort and make productive work impossible.

The patient realizes the nature of his obsessions, regards them as foreign to his personality and attempts to subdue them. Thus, he recognizes their futility, but the knowledge provides no help whatsoever.

Obsessional thoughts

Obsessional thoughts often have a quasi-philosophical content, in which the sufferer sets himself quite unanswerable questions concerning the nature of God, the universe, the meaning of life and so on. Not infrequently, high-minded and dignified thoughts may occur in contiguity with the degrading and repugnant. Thus the appearance of a religious idea may be immediately followed by one which is grossly sexual – to the great distress of the patient. States of doubt and indecision (*folie de doute*) may interfere greatly with the patient's activities. Some suffer from seemingly senseless mental rituals such as: inner recitation of words or phrases; absurd mental arithmetic tasks like the adding up of numbers on car registration plates; moving the head or whole body so that various people or objects may line up in an unaccountable way; touching or counting objects in some curious order.

The non-stop repetition of thoughts over long periods is sometimes termed '*rumination*', with the implied meaning of continual 'chewing over' of the ideas. In spite of almost continual preoccupation with a tangle of interwoven thoughts and counter-thoughts, many sufferers of obsessive ruminations are able, over long periods, to keep their inner affliction hidden from even their closest associates. Where obsessional fears or compulsions are prominent, however, secrecy is less easy – although even severe problems may be known to surprisingly few relatives or friends.

Obsessional fears and compulsions

One of the most prevalent obsessional fears is related to cleanliness and contamination. For example, a patient may fear that if his hands are unclean he may transmit infection, thereby causing harm to some other person. This may lead to constant compulsive washing rituals; perhaps wearing gloves and, having removed them, burning them at once. The variety of behaviour patterns is endless but the theme remains the same. Repeated hand-washing, scores of times each day, often leads to contact dermatitis, and recurrent use of powerful fluorinated steroid ointments or creams may lead to thin and atrophic skin. One patient, during a severe episode, repeatedly spent 2 to 3 hours in the toilet, using more and more toilet paper until he could feel clean enough to pull up his trousers and leave. Worsening of situations of this kind may lead to urgent admission to hospital or day unit.

For others there may be a feeling of compulsion to perform certain acts which the patient realizes are foolish, useless or even dangerous. These ideas may emerge suddenly, accompanied by intense anxiety. A mother may be afflicted by the thought that she may give way to a desire to injure or even kill one of her children, or she may fear that she will do so unknowingly whilst sleep-walking. This may lead her to lock up all the kitchen knives before retiring to bed. When such behaviour extends, as it sometimes does, to the avoidance of any contact with the threatening object or, so far as possible, with the environment in general, the patient may become virtually immobilized. These symptoms are occasionally accompanied by visual imagery – adding to the distress.

Although suicide may be an outcome, it seems to occur only in a very small proportion of cases; it is surprising, perhaps, that it does not occur more often. Suicide apart, instances of a patient translating morbid obsessions into action are seldom if ever reported.

Compulsive rituals

Whereas some compulsions are clearly a direct response to obsessional fears, others take the form of quite inexplicable and complex procedures. These rituals have countless themes, varying from a needless compulsion on retiring for the night to check and recheck that all doors are doubly locked, all lights are out and all gas and water taps securely turned off, to almost ceaseless rituals concerned with everyday affairs such as dressing and undressing and other matters concerned with toiletry. These simple tasks, normally taking no more than a minute or two, may all too easily become those of the greatest complexity, so that a patient can take 3 or 4 hours to prepare for bed and get himself up in the morning again. The left shoe must be removed before the right, likewise the left sock; trousers must be removed before shirt and so on. Possible variations are endless. If in the middle of all this the thought occurs that some sequence has not been performed in its proper order, then all must be done all over again, with, of course, no absolute certainty of ever getting it right. One patient, each time she put her car in the garage, spent 20 minutes or more in a tortuous sequence of measures related to closing the car and garage doors. Sometimes, for no explicable reason, rituals of this kind involve significant numbers and counts. For example, an action might be complete when it has been carried out four times, or eight, twelve or so on; three or five times would not be acceptable.

Just as some obsessional patients search constantly for perfection, so do others search for certainty; both elusive qualities. At times, no compromise can satisfy an obsessional patient, which is why he is forced into the futile and repetitive pursuit of making sure of making sure.

Treatment

As described earlier, obsessional patients may have concealed their thoughts and even compulsive acts for many years. Whilst some patients have confidants, a great many do not. Even when relatives or spouses are aware of the nature of the problem, the patient has often shared with them only a little of the complex web of thoughts, fears and actions. Because doctors understand the principles of obsessions and compulsions, and are well acquainted with the many common themes, contact with a doctor who is able to indicate knowledge and understanding of the patient's predicament may be enormously welcome. Many patients ask whether their experiences are unique, or whether they indicate madness. The therapist's ability to ask informed questions and correctly anticipate some symptoms is clear evidence of prior experience of similar problems; demonstration of such a grasp of the patient's plight is often a source of great comfort.

Understanding of this kind may be an important component of therapy, often over long periods. Exploration of past and present difficulties and conflicts, perhaps in the family, is almost always important in psychiatric treatment. Obsessions are not readily relieved by interpretive psychotherapies. Both psychoanalysis and other forms of organized, one-to-one psychotherapy have excluded severely obsessional patients as unsuitable for such treatment.

Obsessional thoughts and compulsive acts may be seen as habits, which once ingrained do not require a further stimulus to be maintained. Not surprisingly, it has been from behavioural psychotherapy that effective interventions have emerged. Although a theoretical case might be made for systematic desensitization (see page 193), that strategy is not effective with obsessional fears. Other techniques have been developed over the last 30 years to help patients relearn normal patterns of behaviour.

It has been found that, paradoxically, many obsessional patients feel more anxious after completing their rituals than if they were prevented from carrying them out. In *response prevention* the therapist seeks to persuade the patient to avoid ritualistic activity by exercising self-control. This may be achieved by such factors as constant surveillance, or by carrying out alternative activity. Response prevention has been successful in compulsive hand-washing by persuading the patient to increase the interval of time between washing his hands and having somebody stay with him while he practises this. For obsessional thoughts, response prevention in fantasy may be carried out; this is more difficult for the patient and less often effective.

Modelling is of some value in the treatment of compulsions when the therapist demonstrates that the required behaviour is harmless. For example, with compulsive hand-washing there is frequently fear of contamination, and any suspicion of dirt will promptly cause the patient to wash his hands. To combat this fear the therapist will, for example, handle the sole of his own shoe and then carry on with normal activities without washing his hands. This technique is often combined with *confrontation* in which the patient is maintained in the stressful situation in which he is tempted to carry out the compulsive behaviour. With exposure, the anxiety, and therefore the stimulus for such behaviour, gradually diminish. Behavioural treatment of obsessional illness is labour-intensive. Many health districts employ non-medical specialist behavioural psychotherapists. These staff usually have psychiatric nursing qualifications and experience but have, in addition, been seconded for a lengthy period of training on a specialist course. They may then work, along with medical staff, treating those patients for whom behavioural interventions are appropriate.

In obsessional neurosis, drugs have been used mostly as an adjunct when there is associated disturbance of mood. Tricyclic antidepressants, especially clomipramine, have been claimed to be effective; they are most likely to be beneficial when depression of mood is also present. Particular benefits are claimed for antidepressant drugs which inhibit 5-HT re-uptake; there is some evidence to support such claims. If in doubt about the coexistence of depression, it is worth using an antidepressant drug as it is sometimes unexpectedly successful in diminishing obsessions. Monoamine oxidase inhibitor drugs have also been reported as useful in obsessional states.

For very severe and intractable cases, psychosurgery by some type of stereotactic subcaudate tractotomy has been undertaken with many reports of benefit. Such operations are rare, even when there has been disability with extreme incapacity for several years. Psychosurgery is only indicated, if at all, for the most severe degrees of intolerable tension.

Many patients crave *reassurance*. However, if given, such reassurance may reinforce the patient's belief that he has something to worry about. Support and encouragement given by the doctor are very important, with emphasis upon the gains made in treatment and the areas of life with which the patient is now able to cope. The doctor's demonstration of an ability to understand and emphathize is invaluable. The patient benefits from trust in the doctor and knowing that at least there is someone who comprehends what he is describing even if he cannot relieve all the symptoms. Of all patients, those who suffer from obsessions may be those who most benefit from a tolerant professional friend who may encourage both avoidance of certain situations which appear to aggravate the obsessional tendency, and the development of tactics for resisting some other obsessions.

Prognosis

The course of obsessional illness may include self-limiting or relatively acute but repeated episodes, remission with subsequent relapse, and chronicity. There is no doubt that behavioural and physical treatments, together with the support derived from a therapist, can accelerate remission and ameliorate suffering.

The prognosis tends to be unfavourable in those with a long-standing history when the onset is insidious rather than acute. Where an obsessional state develops as a symptom in a depressive phase, remission usually takes place as depression yields to treatment. Obsessions in childhood generally have a good prognosis.

Some cases do appear to 'burn themselves out', or possibly the sufferer may achieve some kind of *modus vivendi*. Others, perhaps finding treatment of so little avail, no longer seek psychiatric help. However, even in the worst cases, remarkable and quite unexpected remissions do sometimes occur. This makes it justifiable, and even advisable, to avoid too gloomy a prognosis.

Further reading

Beech, H.R. (1974) *Obsessional States*, London: Methuen.
Cooper, J.E. (1983) 'Obsessional illness and personality', in *Handbook of Psychiatry 4: The Neuroses and Personality Disorders*, G.F.M. Russell and L.A. Hersov (eds), Cambridge: Cambridge University Press.

13

Personality disorder

The concept and classification of personality disorder are both controversial and confusing. Nevertheless, most practising psychiatrists use the category, and an understanding of how personality contributes to disturbance of behaviour and experience is essential for anyone studying the subject. The standpoint taken in this book regards personality disorder *not as illness* (in the medical sense), but as a variation of personality in one or several of its *traits* from what could be considered as a statistical mean.

Terminology

Personality may be considered subjectively (what the patient believes and describes about himself as an individual) and objectively (what the observer notices about the patient's consistent patterns of behaviour). Subjectively, personality is that unique quality of an individual which he knows to be himself and expresses in his feelings, aims and goals. Objectively, the characteristic behaviour of an individual is what makes him different from other people; the way in which his actions can be predicted in any particular circumstances. *Personality* includes prevailing mood, attitudes and opinions, but it is distinct from intelligence, which, like personality, is an abstract concept and not a distinct *thing*. Personality is manifested in social

relationships, and it can only be assessed by observing what people actually do in a social context.

When one describes *normal personality*, one is using 'normal' in the statistical sense of the word; that is, characteristics of the personality are present within a certain range, neither to gross excess nor extreme deficiency. If one were to take the personality characteristic of 'charitableness' then the majority of people would show a normal degree of this quality. However, Hitler and St Francis of Assisi might equally be regarded as abnormal in this character in opposite ways. Abnormal personality is a variation upon an accepted, yet broadly conceived, range of average personality.

Certain aspects of personality are clinically important. These characteristics have been collected into *typological* lists. For example, one was produced many years ago by Schneider, which has influenced the subsequent development of the International Classification of Diseases (ICD-10). This chapter follows the list of types of personality trait and disorder described in ICD-10 (Table 13.1). If these characteristics of personality are present to an abnormal extent and this abnormality of personality causes the person himself or other people to suffer, then we regard this as *personality disorder*. This is, however, not a precise distinction; the social environment is all-important. For instance, a person because of his personality may be a

Table 13.1 *Normal and abnormal personality and personality disorder*

Normal personality	Traits developed within normal limits
Abnormal personality	One or several personality traits accentuated outside normal limits
Personality disorder	One or more traits exaggerated to the extent of causing suffering to individual or others

misfit in one station of life, but when circumstances change, perhaps with the declaration of war, he becomes a great success as a charismatic leader.

Our modern concept of personality disorder has developed from two contradictory ideas. The first is that personality disorder is present when any abnormality of personality causes problems to the patient himself and to others; this is the sense recommended here, and used in the International Classification. In the second, the term 'personality disorder' is used in a pejorative sense; personality disorder implies unacceptable, antisocial behaviour and therefore a person whom we are inclined to dislike and reject. This latter use of the term is enshrined in the word 'psychopath' and is *not* the meaning used in this chapter.

These two quite different meanings for personality disorder can be traced through its history. In Greek medicine, individuals were assumed to have a preponderance of different humours which in their turn resulted in a specific temperament, such as *sanguine, choleric, melancholic* or *phlegmatic*. These have subsequently been developed into the *stable/neurotic* and *extrovert/introvert* dimensions of personality described by Eysenck. In the early nineteenth century, Pinel recognized that there were conditions in which reason remained intact, but the person could yet be 'insane' because his faculties of emotion and will were disturbed. This he called *'manie sans délirie'*. Benjamin Rush (1812) described *moral derangement* as due to either congenital defect or disease, and John Conolly (1830) described 'inequalities, weaknesses and peculiarities of human under-

standing which do not amount to insanity'. The concept of 'psychopathy' has often been ascribed to J.C. Prichard (1835) of Bristol, who defined the condition he called *moral insanity* as 'madness, consisting of a morbid perversion of the natural feelings, affections, inclinations, temper, habits, moral dispositions and natural impulses without any remarkable disorder or defect of the intellect in knowing or reasoning faculties and particularly without any insane illusion or hallucination'.

Although Prichard equated the word 'moral' with 'emotional' rather than intending it to have ethical implication, it was with his cases of antisocial or even criminal behaviour that the term 'moral insanity' and 'moral imbecility' (later changed to 'moral defect') came finally to be associated.

Henderson in 1939 described the *creative, inadequate* and *aggressive* forms of psychopathy, and this contention, that psychopathy was a distinct condition, became enshrined in the 1959 Mental Health Act. Walton (1970) proposed a classification of abnormal personality that was based upon severity. *Mild* disturbance or *character disorder* occurred when the patient complained of symptoms of maladjustment; *moderate personality disorder* was identified clinically; and *severe disorder* or *sociopathy* was usually identified socially. The problem with such categorization is that a person with relatively mild asocial personality disorder may cause suffering to other people, whilst a person with severe anankastic personality disorder (see page 120) may cause suffering only to himself, but to a very great extent. A distinctive contribution to the discussion was made by Barbara Wootton, who described people with psychopathy as 'extremely selfish persons and no one knows what makes them so'. More recently, psychopathy has not been regarded as a separate diagnostic category, but this still poses a diagnostic dilemma with important consequences for forensic practice. It would now be accepted that there are a number of different types of abnormal personality that may result in disorder, and one such type is *dyssocial* or *sociopathic personality*, which conforms closely with the previous description of *psychopathy*.

Reliability of diagnosis

The reliability of the diagnosis of personality disorder – that is, the likelihood of the same diagnosis being given to the same subject on subsequent occasions or by two different clinicians – has been considered to be very low. Different clinicians tend to concentrate upon different aspects of the patient's personality to the exclusion of others, and thereby tend to over-diagnose certain types of personality and ignore others. Several meanings may be attached to the same term used in personality description – for instance, 'hysterical' – and this will cause confusion. There is inadequate definition of the variation present amongst normal traits; for instance, how much *attention-seeking behaviour* is regarded as normal, and at what point it exceeds normal limits. Despite these difficulties, more recent studies, where the precise descriptions of personality types have been used, do show considerable degree of reliability both when the same rater assesses personality after an interval of 12 months and also between raters. For satisfactory reliability to be achieved the terminology of personality disorder must be used precisely.

Differential diagnosis

For the diagnosis of personality disorder, its presence needs to be differentiated from *normality of personality, neurotic disorder, criminality, affective disorder, organic state* and *schizophrenia*. Of course, personality disorder may coincide with affective disorder, organic state or schizophrenia, and it is very frequently found in association with neurosis. *Neurosis* is seen as an inappropriate response to perceived stress, which may be acute or prolonged; it is, therefore, a *reaction*, whilst personality disorder is seen as a long-term effect of the person's constitution and development. Personality disorder is found very much more frequently amongst sufferers from neurosis than in the general population. The distinction from normal personality depends ultimately upon an arbitrary

threshold, and this depends on the definition of normality as discussed earlier.

The distinction from *criminality* is important to bear in mind; that is, all psychopaths are not criminals and all criminals are not psychopathic. To distinguish *affective personality* from disorder it has to be decided whether the abnormality of mood is a temporary state or a lifelong characteristic. The latter points to an affective personality disorder; this is no longer regarded as a separate category in ICD-10.

Various *organic psychosyndromes*, especially *brain damage* following trauma, may result in permanent damage to the personality and its manifestation in social behaviour. This is recognized in ICD-10 in the term 'personality and behavioural disorder due to brain disease, damage or dysfunction'. The contrast between this secondary damage to personality and a primary constitutional disorder of personality may be compared with the situation affecting intellect, where dementia is a secondary effect of illness or injury whilst mental retardation (learning disability) is a primary constitutional impairment of intellect. Sometimes *schizophrenia* may be difficult to distinguish from *schizoid personality disorder*, where a person shows callousness, recklessness, shallow affect and a lack of will or drive. Usually in schizophrenia there will have been a break at some point in the life history; for instance, the adolescent who at some time in development quite dramatically failed to achieve earlier expectations both academically and socially. With *residual* and *deficit states of schizophrenia*, deterioration of the personality occurs secondarily.

Aetiology

What causes personality disorders is obscure. There are some who would see personality disorders as constitutionally and, therefore, genetically determined. To others they are largely if not wholly derived from psychological factors; in particular, those operative during early development such as faulty upbringing, emotional deprivation or undue exposure to parental discord. These views, however, remain theories only, for very little is known about the nature of personality and what factors influence its development.

Hereditary factors

There is some evidence that genetic factors determine the type of personality and therefore to some extent whether personality disorder occurs or not. This information comes from genetic family studies and from comparison of monozygotic with dizygotic twin pairs. It is probable that although the type of personality is substantially determined genetically, whether or not personality disorder develops or abnormal emotional reaction occurs is probably the outcome of environmental influences.

It is very difficult to unravel the relative contribution of heredity and environment in the development of personality disorder, and anyway this is a relatively pointless exercise as usually both factors are present. Even where a child's family environment is clearly unsatisfactory it may still be impossible to disentangle the influence of this from possible genetic influences derived from parents who are themselves disturbed. In psychiatric aetiology, only in the very rarest instances are single factors important; multiple and complex causation is almost an invariable rule. What has to be considered is how and the extent to which each of the factors interacts. Heredity must play some part; it then becomes a question of how adverse environmental factors activate and develop an innate predisposition towards emotional or personality disorder. Similarly, how far a satisfactory genetic predisposition may counter this development must be considered.

Constitutional factors

Personality abnormality may result either from constitutional factors, as a deviation from a 'norm', or as a condition resulting from acquired cerebral disease giving rise to abnormal and sometimes antisocial behaviour. The effects of frontal lobe damage upon personality provide a good example of this. However, whereas the influence of adverse environmental factors clearly has the same effect upon those with normal brains as on those with brain damage, in the latter case the level of tolerance of adverse factors may be lowered.

Encephalitis in childhood may sometimes account for subsequent personality damage. Certain personality anomalies may also be observed in the near relatives of those suffering from manic-depressive and schizophrenic illnesses. In some cases there is reason to believe that such anomalies are attenuated forms of the illness itself.

Developmental factors

Personality disorders may be wholly, or at least predominantly, caused by psychological factors derived from the social environment. It may be learned within families, or alternatively from the deprivation of not being brought up in a family, and what is called 'personality' may simply reflect learned patterns of behaviour in early childhood and through adolescence. Such a behavioural approach would seek to diminish the importance of personality as an independent concept and emphasizes consistent patterns of behaviour, with the implication that a relearning process, if properly conducted under appropriate conditions of reinforcement, would be able to change those patterns. In psychoanalysis, it is considered that conflicts occurring in early childhood have been repressed into unconsciousness only to gain conscious manifestation later as the consistent patterns of behaviour described as 'personality'.

Psychodynamic factors

Fundamentally, psychoanalysis, although never denying the possible role of constitutional factors, construes personality and its disorders as being derived almost wholly from early environmental influences. Psychoanalysis considers that an individual's conscious thoughts and behaviour, which of course contribute largely to his personality, are determined by mental processes which originate in his unconscious. Behaviour and personality are therefore seen as the resultant of a mass of instinctive unconscious tendencies, together with acquired habits and modes of reaction to the environment. According to Freud, these unconscious and instinctive tendencies are of an essentially primitive kind and are governed by the *pleasure principle*. Because this principle is at variance with conscious thoughts and activities, and especially with ideas of morality and environmental pressures towards conformity, it has the effect of putting a person into conflict with himself. How and at what stage of development these pressures are applied is thought to determine personality. Where development does not proceed normally, this, according to psychoanalytic theory, is the result of a fixation in certain stages of psychosexual maturation. From this arises the concepts of *oral* and *anal eroticism* and the *oral, anal* and *genital* types of personality.

More recently, theorists have seen an association between the psychodynamic oral type of personality and asocial personality; that is, there is a need for immediate gratification without taking into account the long-term consequences. Similarly, the anal type has been equated with the obsessional personality. Such persons experience intense personal emotion but are unable to express it in anything more than a formal manner. The tendency of obsessional personalities to have become collectors (postage stamps, money, ritualistic ways of doing things) is also seen as evidence of an anal, retentive type of personality. However, these metaphorical usages of terms about personality should be treated with considerable caution.

Types of personality disorder

The term 'personality disorder' is little more than a convenient and descriptive label. In the ensuing description the terms from the International Classification of Diseases (10th edition) are used. They are not separate diagnostic entities but common aggregations of traits which develop to an abnormal extent resulting in impaired functioning. That they are not diagnostic entities is further apparent in that an almost infinite variety of combinations of one kind of abnormal personality trait with others may be encountered in practice. The types described in ICD-10 are listed in Table 13.2.

Paranoid personality disorder

Such people show, as a personality trait, persistent and conspicuous *self-reference*; they misinterpret the words and actions of other people as having special significance for, and being directed against, themselves. They tend to misconstrue other people and are suspicious of them; they feel that others are antagonistic and derogatory and are preoccupied with conspiratorial explanations for events. The person with a more active type of paranoid personality is often aggressive, quarrelsome, litigious and will go to elaborate lengths to defend his rights and redress real or imagined injustices and insults. He is intensely jealous of what he regards as his own belongings, whether these are people or objects. He may go to fanatical lengths to avenge himself. He often has an inflated opinion of his own self-importance.

The more passive person with this personality is not aggressive in achieving his objectives. He knows with absolute certainty that other people are opposed to him, will make life difficult for, dislike and despise him; but he does not take any action. He accepts as a matter of course that

Table 13.2 *Personality disorders in ICD-10*

Paranoid personality disorder

Schizoid personality disorder

Dyssocial personality disorder

Emotionally unstable personality disorder
  Impulsive type
  Borderline type

Histrionic personality disorder

Anankastic (obsessive-compulsive) personality disorder

Anxious (avoidant) personality disorder

Dependent personality disorder

he will suffer from everyone else's ire and greed. He is suspicious and misconstrues what happens to him.

Schizoid personality disorder

These people show a disinclination to mix with others, appearing aloof and uninterested, and lack the capacity to enjoy life. They are not shy or sensitive concerning other people but simply prefer not to be involved in social occupations, pursuing solitary interests with objects rather than people. Their relatives and neighbours find them to be emotionally cold and detached; they do not respond to praise or criticism. This withdrawal from society may result in a state of callous indifference to others' discomfort and suffering. They show little interest in sexual relationships or other close, confiding situations with others. They are often eccentric in behaviour and do not conform with societies' expectations.

Dyssocial personality disorder

The dyssocial personality (previously psychopathic personality) denoted by Schneider as *affectionless* or *feelingless personality*, is characterized mainly by an emotional blunting or complete indifference towards the rights and feelings of others. For such persons passion, shame and conscience seem to have no meaning. There is some similarity between this condition and the cold, affectionless state of certain schizophrenic patients, and also a similar state which may appear following brain injury. Such people are selfish, egocentric, vain and often cruel; they seek primary instinctual gratification with short-term aims, and social adaptation and hence relationship is unsatisfactory or non-existent. The abnormal sexual behaviour of many psychopaths has been compared with that of small children.

Whiteley has considered the psychopath to be an individual: (1) who persistently behaves in a way which is not in accord with the accepted social norms in the culture or times in which he lives; (2) who appears to be unaware that his behaviour is seriously at fault; and (3) whose abnormality cannot readily be explained as resulting from the 'madness' we commonly recognize, nor from 'badness' alone.

The core defect in dyssocial personality disorder is primarily one of empathy. Such a person does not have the ability to understand other people's feelings, and especially to understand how these people feel about the consequences of his own callous actions which hurt or offend them. He appears not to experience the shame or psychological pain that prevents most of us from carrying out unpleasant actions towards other people most of the time. He is unable to put himself into the position of being at the receiving end of such behaviour. He is unable to tolerate frustration and tends to blame others when things go wrong.

Emotionally unstable personality disorder

(a) Impulsive type

The chief characteristic of these people is a tendency to sudden emotional discharge leading either to sudden impulsive and usually unsuccessful suicidal attempts or to assault on others. Such outbursts may be precipitated by minor frustrations which are quite disproportionate to the reaction which ensues. These are sometimes known as 'short-circuit' reactions. There may be an association with alcoholism, intoxication being a factor which favours explosive outbursts. A previous history of head injury is not infrequent. Such people have difficulty in maintaining long-term goals.

(b) Borderline type

This category should be avoided as it is not a descriptive term about personality but based on theory. There is an unproved implication that such people are on the border between personality disorder and psychosis, showing instability in mood, self-image and social relationships. Impulsive and unpredictable behaviour often occurs and there is usually some disturbance of personal identity. It will be seen that such a description is an amalgam of different personality types; there is no evidence that it precedes schizophrenia. It is apparent from the way different psychiatrists use the term that they are not all describing the same condition.

Histrionic personality disorder

It is important to make a clear distinction between hysterical neurosis with conversion and dissociation symptoms, and histrionic personality disorder. The two may coincide in the same person but need not necessarily do so. People with histrionic personality disorder are egocentric; they show emotional lability, excitability and dependency. Affect tends to be shallow and inconsistent; they make excellent superficial relationships but have considerable difficulty in sustaining long-term exclusive relationships, as in marriage. Attention-seeking, appreciation-needing and affection-craving are prominent. Theatricality, with an air of insincerity, typifies such people's social relationships. There is usually a degree of sexual immaturity with flirtatious display in the initial stages of a relationship, but rejection and coldness typifies the stage when the relationship has become serious. Histrionic personality disorder is said to be commoner in females, and has on occasions been considered to be a female equivalent of the dyssocial personality disorder, commoner in males.

Anankastic (obsessional) personality disorder

'Anankastic' is a better term than 'obsessional personality' as the latter may be confused with obsessive-compulsive neurosis. Although obsessive-compulsive neurosis and anankastic personality do occur together on occasions, the majority of patients with an obsessional neurosis do not have anankastic personality, and the great majority of people with anankastic personality never develop obsessional neurosis. A person with anankastic personality shows prominent sensitive and perfectionist traits. Sensitivity implies heightened feelings of strong emotion with only limited powers for expressing these feelings verbally and a poor capacity for emotional discharge. Anankastic people tend to ruminate continuously about the possible meaning of any experience and, being insecure, are inclined to look upon themselves as the possible cause of all sorts of unfortunate events. Conflicts over sex are frequent, together with a clash between ethical sense and sexual and aggressive drives. They have an over-ready tendency to develop sensitive ideas of reference and to believe that others are inclined to regard them askance. The key experience which releases this reaction is perception of some kind of moral defect; that is, some experience which leads to a feeling of shame or failure.

In order to guard against feelings of failure, the anankast shows scrupulous conscientiousness amounting to perfectionism and rigidity in his work and social relationships. He is excessively sensitive to a whisper of criticism, which immediately awakens his self-doubt, always near the surface of his self-consciousness. The only way he has found to deal with his chronic sense of insecurity is by being always a little more correct and therefore less likely to be criticized than other people.

Anxiety (avoidant) personality disorder

Persistent feelings of tension and apprehension pervade all areas of life, causing the individual to feel self-conscious, insecure and inferior. Such people are very sensitive to criticism, which restricts their capacity for relationships, and they desperately want to be liked and accepted. They are cautious, very aware of risks and tend to live restricted and circumscribed lives in order to achieve security.

Dependent personality disorder

Such individuals appear to succumb to any influence, good or bad, their predominant feature apparently being what, in common parlance, is usually called 'weakness of character'. They show passive compliance, accepting a dominating leadership from another person; for example, parent or spouse. There is a lack of vigour to undertake any activity, especially those that require determination, and they usually establish a life pattern of dependence upon other people and only come to psychiatric attention when these dependent relationships break down; for instance, separation from spouse, redundancy from employment, discharge from the armed services or other loss of a structured environment.

Neurosis and neuroticism

There is clearly an important association between neurosis which is an inappropriate reaction to perceived stress, and neuroticism which is the abnormal state of personality in which neurotic behaviour becomes more likely. This is represented in Figure 13.1. Very severe stress will provoke a neurotic reaction in the majority of people; for example, with prolonged exposure to battle-front conditions. A very marked degree of abnormality of personality amounting to personality disorder will predispose an individual to a neurotic reaction with a relatively minor stress. These factors then have a marked influence upon prognosis.

Personality is lifelong; the traits and characteristics manifested by an individual in adolescence are likely to continue, subject of course to the changes in his environmental and social situation, throughout life. It is highly likely that the pedantic small boy will develop into the cautious and scrupulous middle-aged man and become increasingly perfectionistic, intolerant and rigid in his attitudes as he grows old. Although the basic characteristics of a personality do not change markedly through life, whether these manifest as a personality disorder is quite largely determined by the social context, and as this changes through life there are modifications of the extent to which personality disorder is shown.

There is an increased likelihood for some of those with personality disorder to develop alcoholism, drug abuse and other forms of maladaptive behaviour during adult life; where such dependence is associated with personality disorder the prognosis with appropriate treatment is less optimistic. Those with personality disorder show an increased likelihood for premature death, especially from suicide and accidental death such as road traffic accidents. Those with asocial personality disorder tend, with increasing age, towards less criminal behaviour; perhaps they become less physically aggressive, with diminished physical strength. However, they remain disturbed in relationships within the family and the community.

In assessing the influence of personality and its disorder upon the mental state it is helpful to make the following judgements. Is the person essentially normal in personality, and what are the prominent traits? Are any of these traits of personality developed to an extent that would constitute abnormality? Does the abnormality of personality cause suffering to the individual or to other people, and thus be designated personality disorder? In order to answer these questions the clinician needs to have acquired a good understanding of the range of normal personality and to have learnt the complex skill of assessing personality and its disorder.

Treatment

It is important to stress that in discussing treatment one is considering all forms of personality

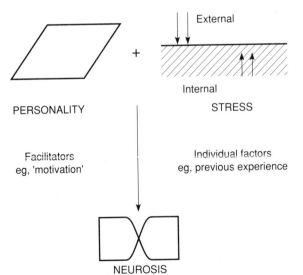

Figure 13.1 Stress, personality and neurosis

disorder and not only asocial personality disorder. Treatment is not aimed at altering the personality itself but at the untoward behaviour or unacceptable symptoms resulting from the personality, and associated with its abnormality.

The most effective forms of treatment will combine various types of psychotherapy. *Individual psychotherapy*, especially of a cognitive type, may be most appropriate for an individual with sensitive or anankastic personality with very marked feelings of low self-esteem and expectations of failure. Between therapy sessions the individual is encouraged to use his obsessionality to examine and record his thoughts of failure and low self-esteem, and to counter these with rational arguments demonstrating that he did in fact to some extent achieve valuable objectives. This record of his thoughts and counter-arguments is discussed at treatment sessions, working from the assumption that persistent low mood follows depressive cognitions rather than vice versa.

Group therapy is helpful in the treatment of some patients with personality disorder, especially when this is accompanied by social anxiety or fear. The composition of the group is a matter of importance, and the theoretical background from which group therapy is carried out will determine the precise nature of sessions and intended goals. The aim for the person with personality disorder is not to change his personality but to help him learn what are the effects of his personality on other people and how to modify his behaviour in a socially appropriate way.

The *therapeutic community*, in which every aspect of daily life and every interaction between patients and staff is used in discussion for treatment, has been employed for those with asocial personality disorder or psychopathy. The aim is to help those in treatment to learn to take responsibility for their own actions using social pressures derived from the group setting. In such a situation an individual has to explain his actions to other people who may resemble him, as they too have some of the same or similar problems. By his behaviour in the group he earns social approval or disapproval from them. The results of this type of treatment are not striking, but they appear somewhat better than other methods that have been used. The social factors operating in a therapeutic community according to Rappaport, are: (1) permissiveness to act in accord with one's feelings without accustomed social inhibitions; (2) communication in sharing of tasks, responsibilities and rewards; (3) democratic decision-making; and (4) confrontation of the subject with what he is doing here and now.

Dynamic psychotherapy such as psychoanalysis is rarely directly useful in the treatment of personality disorders; however, it has formed a theoretical background to many of the more recently introduced types of therapy. *Behavioural modification* has been extensively used, sometimes with *social skills training* (page 194). *Social manipulation* may be beneficial on occasions; in a different environment the person with an abnormal personality may not cause suffering to himself or to others. Most often, an eclectic combination of dynamic, behavioural and social types of therapy will produce the best environment for the treatment of individuals.

The therapeutic potential of institutions needs to be recognized and also the ways in which they may hamper the development of the person with abnormal personality. Hospitals, wards and other closed therapeutic communities, even prison, may be valuable in encouraging a small-group atmosphere to develop which enables disordered people to learn about themselves. The disadvantage may well be that the skills they learn in social interaction are not relevant to the world outside the institution where different values and attitudes will pertain; for instance, it may be quite inappropriate to apply the egalitarian attitudes towards fellow patients and members of staff of a therapeutic community to the much more hierarchical structure operating in a factory. Recently, there has been more emphasis on the development of treatment methods in the community such as enforced community projects for those with a milder degree of asocial personality.

Physical treatments have relatively little place in the management of personality disorders. However, they may be useful for dealing with specific symptoms. Anxiolytics have on occasions been helpful with the anxiety symptoms present with some types of personality disorder; antidepressants have been claimed to have a beneficial effect occasionally in those with dysthymic personality disorder; major tranquillizers have been used to control explosive outbursts, and sometimes small doses have been used prophylactically; drugs such as benperidol and cyproterone acetate have been used to control deviant sexual behaviour. Psychosurgery had a vogue in the past in the control of severe aggressive outbursts but is not used now.

Those with asocial personality disorder do not fit well into a conventional psychiatric hospital setting; on occasions their 'acting out' may interfere with the welfare and treatment of other patients. They may also, if tending to violence, present a security risk. Treatment will normally need to be given under the terms of the Mental Health Act and in specifically dedicated hospitals or units (see Chapter 24).

In general, with the aim of improving the lot of the patient himself and those around him, one need not necessarily be pessimistic about treatment for personality disorders. There are a number of different options for treatment, but it does require adequate provision locally of a range of different types of therapy. It must be accepted that the personality will remain unchanged, but the aim is to achieve the most appropriate conditions for the individual to live at ease with himself without harming other people.

Further reading

Sims, A.C.P. (1983) *Neurosis in Society*, London: Macmillan.
Tyrer, P. (ed.) (1988) *Personality Disorders: Diagnosis, Treatment and Course*, London: Wright.

14

Sexual behaviour and its disturbances

Psychiatrists are often called upon to deal with *sexual dysfunction*. It may present to a psychiatrist either as the main complaint or as a secondary feature of another condition. Sometimes sexual practices against the law result in referral to a forensic psychiatrist. For some of the conditions described in this chapter, the disturbance of behaviour requires behavioural management which may be provided by psychiatrists. The underlying understanding of sexual disturbances needs to be based upon an applied knowledge of physiology, sociology, psychology and social anthropology. Personality disturbance is often associated with sexual pathology, and this also is an area of expertise of the psychiatrist. Not infrequently other psychiatric disorders are also present, and these may make a more urgent demand upon the attention of the psychiatrist than the sexual disturbance which is the presenting complaint.

Sexual dysfunction

It is only the couple themselves who can decide whether they have a sexual problem or not; there are no absolute standards of sexual performance to which people ought to aspire, although there are probably biological limits beyond which they cannot go. Thus, if a couple are contented with their joint sexual practices, however infrequent or bizarre or different these may appear to be to others, providing neither is harmed thereby, then their sexual behaviour cannot be regarded as symptomatic. Indeed, help or treatment may only be required if one or both complain of some perceived sexual dysfunction within their relationship. It is most important, therefore, for all who are involved in helping or counselling others not to set standards of human sexual performance, nor should it be implied that if these standards are not attained, there is something wrong with the relationship or perhaps with one or both members of the pair. For example, all women, almost without exception, are biologically capable of achieving orgasm, but not all do so during the course of their sexual relationship. Of those who do not, some will see it as a problem and seek help, whilst others will not feel it to be an essential part of their lives to achieve orgasm.

A couple's decision about whether or not their sexual performance falls short in some way will be bound up not only with their own subjective feelings, which are difficult to measure and standardize, but also with cultural and educational factors and, most importantly, with each other's expectations. Couples will therefore tend to complain either of a perceptible change in their sexual function or of failing to achieve a desired goal. What for one couple may seem to be a poor sexual performance may, for others, seem completely acceptable.

There are no adequate data on the prevalence of sexual dysfunction in the United Kingdom. In the United States it has been estimated that as many as 50 per cent of couples have some difficulties, even in an established sexual relationship. It is important to distinguish between transient difficulties and more severe and permanent forms of the same problem. Problems of longer standing tend to become secondarily reinforcing, affecting not only the sexual response of each partner, but also the relationship of the couple.

It is usual to distinguish between *primary* forms of sexual difficulty, where the problem has always existed and continues unabated, and *secondary* problems, where sexual functioning is initially normal but later deteriorates for some reason or other. Understanding an individual sexual problem also implies understanding the whole person, his upbringing, his character and personality structure and other aspects of his relationship.

Courtship

As human sexual activity usually starts with courtship, it is here that difficulty often first arises. Some people are so anxious in social situations that they are unable to tolerate any close encounter with a member of the opposite sex. Although they may not present with a sexual problem, their difficulties may prevent a sexual relationship from developing.

The next stage of development in a sexual relationship is the formation of a close link with just one person of the opposite sex. In most instances, a degree of emotional and physical intimacy is necessary before the sexual act itself can take place, although the speed with which this happens is both culturally and educationally determined, and depends also upon the previous sexual experience of the couple involved. Some people, while perfectly at ease socially and capable of the necessary 'chatting-up' skills may still have difficulty with any kind of emotional intimacy such as may lead to the sharing of experiences and having to take responsibility for the feelings of another person. Thus the development of any degree of inter-

dependence may provoke increasing anxiety and lead to a rapid breaking of the relationship. Fears of physical intimacy can also be a barrier to the development of a sexual relationship, particularly in men or women who come from families among whom touching or displaying the body is taboo. The treatment of such problems is usually behavioural, leading to gradual reduction of anxiety.

Difficulties during intercourse

Male dysfunction

In investigating difficulties during intercourse, it is necessary to consider both parties together and to pay due regard to their interaction although, as male and female sexual difficulties show certain distinct differences, it may, in the first instance, be convenient to consider them separately. Those conditions which primarily affect men include *erectile* difficulties, problems with *ejaculation* and *postcoital* difficulties. In *impotence* (or *erectile difficulty*), either no erection occurs or there is difficulty in sustaining full engorgement for long enough to achieve adequate penetration. Those to whom this happens are liable to become discouraged, for, in trying hard to retrieve the situation, they soon discover the well known fact that no man can will himself an erection. Thus fear of failure together with failure itself tends to become self-reinforcing.

Some men who may have little or no difficulty in obtaining or sustaining erection may find that just before, during, or just after penetration they are unable to control ejaculation and therefore may *ejaculate prematurely*. Other, less common, abnormalities of ejaculation include an inability to ejaculate after penetration has occurred; retrograde ejaculation into the bladder, and seepage of semen during sexual arousal without experiencing full orgasm.

In the postcoital phase, at its most pathological the situation may be exemplified by the half-drunken male who, after a period of clumsy love-making or none at all, ejaculates, withdraws, rolls over and starts to snore, leaving his frustrated and disgusted partner sleepless by his side.

Female sexual dysfunction

'Frigidity' is as pejorative a word as 'impotence', particularly as it suggests an overall coldness which may well not be present. A better term is '*generalized sexual dysfunction*', which, as in men, may be primary or secondary, and partial or complete. Although the woman with general sexual dysfunction may derive little, if any, erotic or sexual pleasure from sexual stimulation, she may still obtain a great deal of comfort from the warmth and closeness which the relationship brings with it.

The characteristics of general sexual dysfunction include lack of erotic feeling, interest or pleasure; lack of physical response or denial of feeling in the presence of normal physiological responses; or absence of physiological responses but retention of feeling and even orgasm. A woman's educational and cultural expectations of what her sexual response should be are also of importance, as is the reaction of her partner. All these are factors which will determine whether she sees her disability as a problem or not.

Many women with generalized sexual dysfunction do not reach a level of sexual arousal sufficient to reach orgasm and may thus complain. Many, however, who arouse easily and are sexually responsive, are unable to achieve orgasm however hard or long they try (anorgasmia). This may be the commonest female sexual difficulty. Failure to obtain an orgasm may be primary or secondary and may be situational or with certain partners. Usually this means that the woman is anorgasmic during sexual intercourse itself but can reach a climax either with her own or her partner's stimulation or by the use of a mechanical aid. Many women who suffer from orgasmic dysfunction are otherwise sexually quite normal.

The other main sexual problem in women is that of vaginal spasm (vaginismus), which may or may not be associated with the other difficulties already mentioned. The problem is that during any attempt at penetration of the vagina, there is an intense spasm of the muscles that surround the introitus so that it remains firmly shut. Once spasm has occurred, any attempt at penetration will be painful, so that the experience will reinforce the reflex closure of the introitus at any future attempt at penetration. The tight ring of muscles can sometimes be felt by the patient or her partner and may be misinterpreted as a mechanical barrier. Vaginismus may be associated with non-consummation of a marriage, although almost invariably in prolonged non-consummation due to vaginismus the husband will be found to have his own problems as well.

Some women with vaginismus are still able to allow a degree of penetration. Milder degrees of vaginismus, in which initial introital pain is experienced but lessens as intercourse proceeds, are also common and may reflect the partner's inexperience. The majority of women who describe superficial dyspareunia, or pain on intercourse are actually describing vaginismus. Of course, in all cases of female sexual dysfunction gynaecological causes must be excluded.

Effects of ageing

Normal ageing, both in men and women, is sometimes mistaken for sexual dysfunction. As a man grows older, certain changes take place in his sexual response cycle, usually from his early forties onwards. It takes him longer to achieve an erection than in his youth and perhaps several minutes for a full erection to occur. He tends, however, to be able to retain his erection for longer before ejaculating but may also find he does not ejaculate every time. Following ejaculation, detumescence occurs more rapidly. Likewise, the refractory period lengthens so that it may take some hours before an erection can be re-established after ejaculation. Also, if an older man loses his erection before ejaculation, he may find it harder to regain it. These are normal ageing changes of no pathological significance although they may be easily misinterpreted by middle-aged men.

If women discontinue sexual activity at the climacteric but later try to resume intercourse, they may find that the normal physiological responses tend to be lost and that the vagina has become dry and atrophic. In order to regain normal sexual responses hormone replacement may be needed. However, if a woman continues to have sexual intercourse during the climacteric, these changes do not usually occur.

Taking a sexual history

There are many causes of sexual difficulty, although the majority are psychogenic. It is most important to obtain a careful step-by-step account, remembering that the problem may be presented quite differently when the history is taken from each partner separately.

It is necessary to discover when and how the difficulty began and all possibly associated precipitating events. This should be followed by an account of how the problem has progressed, having regard to the effect of one partner's problem on that of the other. It is not unusual to find that the member of a partnership who presents for treatment is not the one with the primary problem. It is also important to investigate other relationships in order to discover whether the complainant's difficulty is one which has been repeated in every relationship, or whether there is something special about the present relationship which relates to the presenting problem.

Other necessary information includes such matters as the time of onset of puberty, how, when and where the subject gained sexual information, masturbatory habits and details of adult sexual activity. Information about basic sexual orientation is often best gained by enquiring about fantasies during masturbation. Enquiry should also be made about the subject's attitudes to all these matters, and how much they have subsequently been modified in the light of experience. An important part of sexual assessment includes the effect upon the subject of attitudes of his or her parents. It is also necessary to gauge the extent of the patient's sexual knowledge, and that of the partner.

Organic dysfunction

The vast majority of sexual problems are psychogenic, the only sexual problem where organic causes are at all common being impotence. Even then, in only about 5 per cent of men with established impotence is this due to some organic cause. In organic impotence, sexual drive is often unimpaired and the onset is usually gradual, with inability to respond. Organic impotence may fluctuate in intensity before becoming complete.

Impotence may follow impairment of sex drive, as in generalized illness, liver disease and endocrine disorders, exposure to drugs such as opiates, anti-androgens and some steroid preparations, or physical interference with erection. This can occur with the autonomic neuropathy of *diabetes mellitus* affecting the parasympathetic supply to the penis. The same is true of some cases of *alcoholism*, in which autonomic neuropathy may be present although more generalized polyneuropathy may not yet have developed. Impotence associated with alcoholism may also be projected onto the partner, taking the form of *morbid jealousy* (see page 14). Other conditions which affect the parasympathetic supply to the penis include complications of some surgical operations such as abdomino-perineal resection, neurological diseases such as multiple sclerosis, and some drugs such as tricyclic antidepressants. These latter may, however, sometimes have a paradoxical effect by retarding ejaculation where this is premature, thereby improving sexual performance, but this is not a reliable means of treatment. Erection may occasionally be impaired by malfunction elsewhere, such as local penile disease, or by failure of the necessary blood supply to the penis as in the Leriche Syndrome or in sickle-cell anaemia.

An organic cause for sexual difficulty is rare in women. Occasionally generalized endocrine or bodily illness may lower libido and impair sexual response. More frequently, contraceptive measures may have an influence on female sexual response, with the contraceptive pill impairing sexual response in a small number of women by interfering with the metabolism of testosterone.

Depressive illness

Depression is a very common and important cause of impotence, particularly in those who have hitherto had no sexual difficulties but who, as they start to become depressed, may suffer a loss of libido together with other depressive symptoms, such as loss of drive, concentration, appetite and weight. Sometimes when a depressive illness resolves, impotence persists owing to secondary anxiety. It is important, therefore, to emphasize that potency will almost certainly be regained as the patient's condition improves. The treatment in this instance is, of course, the treatment of the underlying depressive state.

Treatment of dysfunction

Behavioural treatments modified from Masters and Johnson's method appear to be the most successful methods to date and are largely directed towards correcting the secondary effects of sexual dysfunction such as anxiety arising in a sexual setting. These methods are effective probably because they can be learnt relatively quickly and do not need long periods of training before being put into practice.

Discussions are held jointly with the partners until clear goals are agreed between them in terms of treatment aims. Because the initial aim is to deal with the secondary effects of the problem, a ban is imposed on intercourse for the time being. The couple then begin a series of exercises designed very gradually to reintroduce physical proximity and touching, and in such a way that they begin to enjoy physical contact again (*sensate focusing*). They are instructed to concentrate on the giving and receiving of pleasure and feedback information to each other about what they are actually feeling, while avoiding setting targets, or goals, for physical encounter beyond those of giving pleasure. Initially, the exchange of touching is entirely non-genital but gradually, as the exercise progresses, genital touching is allowed but in a non-demanding way. When the therapist is satisfied that the couple are relaxed

in each other's company and enjoy giving and receiving pleasure, sensate focus exercises are continued with gradual addition to the repertoire until eventually mounting and penetration occur (during sensate focus, erections almost invariably return). Initially penetration, without full orgasm, remains under the control of the female partner. The technique consists therefore of a gradual reintroduction of penetration and eventual ejaculation with the man concentrating so much on the pleasure that he is receiving that he stops thinking about the goal. The same approach is used for the anorgasmic female.

For premature ejaculation, after the sensate focus the man is instructed to concentrate on his ejaculatory feelings. This may be assisted by the *squeeze technique* in which the penis is compressed to prevent ejaculation occurring. Ejaculatory control gradually develops in this way. For retarded ejaculation, after sensate focus, vaginal containment is suggested, during which additional manual stimulation of the penis is carried out by the partner.

Vaginismus is treated by intensive relaxation techniques aimed at teaching the woman vaginal muscle control. During a therapeutic vaginal examination the therapist also directs the woman to examine herself. There follows graded introduction of vaginal penetration using the partner's finger and a set of dilators. Finally, as part of the sensate focus exercise, the partner's erect penis is used as a dilator by the woman until she has lost her fear of penile penetration. It is at this point that one often discovers the male partner's own difficulties.

The success rate of treatment of problems using this type of behavioural approach is quite high, many clinics averaging an overall 65 to 70 per cent success rate. Certain problems, such as vaginismus, secondary impotence and premature ejaculation, are probably easier to deal with than others. The treatment of primary impotence, anorgasmia and retarded ejaculation is less successful.

Psychotherapy

Psychotherapeutic measures directed at helping

the couple to a better relationship, or helping one or both partners to understand better the roots of their difficulties, may be beneficial, either on their own or as part of a behavioural approach to the sexual problem. It has been shown, however, that the overall success rate of psychotherapeutic methods alone in treating sexual problems is quite low.

Physical treatments

Physical treatments are hardly ever necessary. The use of drugs with supposed aphrodisiac properties, drugs which allegedly delay ejaculation or drugs which relieve sexual anxiety should be avoided.

Masturbation

Masturbation was, in the nineteenth century, believed to produce a variety of signs and symptoms including dyspepsia, epilepsy, blindness, loss of hearing, rickets, acne and, most importantly, insanity! It was even given as a cause of death in American and British mental hospitals. Almost all persons, male and female, masturbate, especially during adolescence, and the realization that this is so has reduced anxiety about this behaviour, so it is usually only those who are markedly unsophisticated who complain about masturbation as a symptom.

Masturbation becomes a symptom only when it replaces the desire for normal sexual relations when these are otherwise available. Some who are sexually disturbed may prefer to indulge in abnormal fantasies accompanied by masturbation rather than to attempt a normal heterosexual relationship. Excessive masturbation, sometimes carried out in public, may occasionally occur as a symptom of schizophrenia. In this event it is the underlying psychosis which calls for treatment.

Masturbation does not have any damaging physical effects. The same applies to spontaneous nocturnal emissions which occasionally cause distress. These are common, particularly in those who are sexually abstinent and who may resist conscious masturbation. Women, as well as men, may be troubled by dreams which are accompanied by orgasm. Although these too may be regarded as normal they are thought to be commoner in those who have emotional difficulties.

Homosexuality

Homosexual behaviour occurs in all races and cultures, and in many is common. Thus about 13 per cent of men will have some kind of homosexual contact leading to orgasm in their lifetime; in women the proportion is probably higher. About 4 to 5 per cent of men and women seem to be exclusively homosexual in that all their sexual relationships are with their own sex. Gradations between complete homosexuality and complete heterosexuality exist. Transient homosexual behaviour in some who are basically heterosexual also occurs, especially in restrictive circumstances such as in prison or on board ship. It can be important to distinguish between transient behaviour where only one sex is present, such as in prison, and that of a more persistent kind. This is particularly true in adolescence, during which many pass through a homosexual phase.

It is important to make the distinction between *ego-syntonic homosexuality*, the individual is relatively content with his or her situation, and *ego-dystonic homosexuality*, where the person is dissatisfied and wishes to alter the situation. The former may not be associated with any psychiatric condition, whilst the latter will be associated with anxiety, depression, self-dislike or other psychological symptoms, and psychiatric help is appropriate, even if this is only aimed at ameliorating symptoms. Human Immunodeficiency Virus (HIV) infection and Acquired Immune Deficiency Syndrome (AIDS) has introduced a completely new dimension to this situation. Homosexuality nowadays is often linked with fear of AIDS which may be shown by those who are of uncertain sexual orientation, those who have experienced definite homosexual arousal, and those in established homosexual practice. Treatment aimed at changing behaviour and orientation should be offered only if specifically requested.

Aetiology and treatment

The cause of established homosexuality is still a matter of debate. It probably arises out of a complex interaction between genetic and constitutional factors with early familial environment. Some consideration may be given to pre-natal hormonal environment, including the presence of androgens at critical periods of uterine development which partly determine the future pattern of sexual behaviour, and later, parental and environmental factors which may lead to reinforcement at or after the time of puberty. There is no evidence, however, that adult endocrine disorders or other physical factors are responsible for adult homosexuality.

Some of those with homosexual orientation may seek help in order to adapt to their sexual role, or less often they may wish to change their sexual orientation. This is more likely to be achieved if some heterosexual urges are also present. Behavioural methods have on occasions proved effective and also psychotherapeutic methods involving working through the experiences of a conflictual or unhappy relationship with one or both parents.

Disorders of sexual preference

There is a wide variety of sexual anomalies, but only a few are considered here. Virtually all these sexual abnormalities are much more common in males. These conditions can be classified according to abnormality of the sexual object or of the sexual act, and they may be homosexually or heterosexually orientated (Table 14.1). Thus *paedophilia* is the condition in which sexual interest of an adult is directed towards a child; the adult is usually male and the child may be of either sex. *Paederasty* is one type of this, in which an adult male has anal intercourse with a male child. Treatment, in so far as it is successful, is either by physically suppressing sexual urges using anti-androgen

Table 14.1   *Sexual preferences*

Object	Abnormality of sexual	Act
Paedophilia		Exhibitionism
Transvestism		Voyeurism
Fetishism		Sadism
Bestiality		Masochism
Necrophilia		Frotteurism

drugs or the butyrophenone, benperidol, or by trying to help the patient along behavioural lines to develop more adult heterosexual skills.

Transvestism

Transvestism is an act in which a person dresses in some or all items of clothing of the opposite sex. Some men, showing this behaviour, masturbate in private and achieve some degree of gratification thereby; others dress themselves up completely and are further excited by parading in public. Transvestism may also occur as part of passive homosexuality. Here, however, putting on women's clothing is not an end in itself but a role-play which is intended to enhance a homosexual relationship ('in drag'). Transvestism amongst females is often a homosexual phenomenon but is on the whole more socially acceptable than transvestism in men. Dressing in the clothes of the opposite sex is usual as a feature of transsexualism (see below).

Fetishism

The phenomenon of fetishism is clearly related to transvestism in that the male subject is sexually aroused by some article of female clothing such as lingerie, stockings, boots or shoes. If such excitement is subservient to the satisfactory performance of heterosexual intercourse, it can hardly be described as deviant, in that it becomes no more perhaps than one of the trimmings.

Bestiality

This is sexual behaviour involving animals. It is most common in unsophisticated young men of low intellectual achievement often living in an isolated, rural situation.

Necrophilia

This is any sort of sexually arousing behaviour involving dead bodies. It is extremely uncommon.

Exhibitionism

Exhibitionism is one of the commonest of all sexual disorders. The male subject exposes his genitals to women, often in a secluded spot, or perhaps in a car parked at the kerbside. The act of indecent exposure may or may not be accompanied by masturbation or ejaculation but is only rarely accompanied by any other overtly sexual act such as indecent assault. Several different aetiological factors underlie exhibitionism, including an immature form of sexual display, a powerful element of compulsion and occasionally, in older patients, depression, in which it is thought that awareness of waning libido may play a part. It is important to recognize those patients who are depressed.

There are some for whom appearance in a court case prevents further occurrence, but others continually repeat the offence. Behavioural methods of treatment aimed at helping the subject to learn to control his impulses may be used.

Voyeurism

Voyeurism is a form of gratification obtained by observing the sexual and related practices of others. While today there are more commercial outlets to satisfy such appetites, the 'Peeping Tom' may still remain a considerable nuisance.

Sado-masochism

Sado-masochism demands the infliction of pain, and the offering of restraint or humiliation either to the sexual partner or reciprocally. Fully fledged sadists are amongst the most dangerous of mentally disturbed patients, as in the case of certain rapists and child stranglers. Masochism can also be a dangerous pursuit, as in the case of adolescents who tie themselves up and carry out hanging and asphyxiation experiments. More minor degrees of pathological sadistic behaviour include clothes-slashing, the making of obscene telephone calls, 'heavy-breathing' and similar pursuits.

Frotteurism

This is the obtaining of sexual gratification from touching or rubbing up against the clothed body of a stranger in a crowd. It is generally more of a nuisance than a danger.

Treatment of disorders of preference

Treatment is difficult and may be unsuccessful. Conventional psychotherapeutic measures are largely ineffective, although in milder cases they may enable a patient to achieve a better level of social adjustment by containing his behaviour at a fantasy level, rather than acting it out. In situations with forensic implications, suppression of sexuality by chemical means, either using benperidol or an anti-androgenic agent such as cyproterone acetate, may be effective.

For fetishists, transvestites and some others who genuinely wish to be treated, behavioural modification appears to offer the best chance of successful management. An operant conditioning approach can be used with careful attention to the positive and negative reinforcements. A programme is arranged, which must be structured for the individual patient, with careful attention to contingencies so that the advantages of loss of this form of sexual behaviour with replacement by a more appropriate outlet outweigh the disadvantages. This is difficult, as the behavioural patterns are firmly established and treatment results are only moderately encouraging.

Transsexualism

An underlying disorder of *gender role* may manifest itself in transsexualism. The individual will probably dress in the clothes of the opposite sex, but this is not fundamentally for sexual gratification but more because the male transsexual regards himself as a 'female person trapped inside a male body', and the female vice versa.

Transsexuals, although physically normal, are convinced inwardly that they are really persons of the opposite sex, believing that by some freak their bodies have developed abnormally and are not in accordance with their 'real' sex. This belief is held with very strong conviction. The phenomenology of the condition is distinct from transvestism and also from homosexuality, although the fantasy life of these patients is predominantly homosexual, as might be expected. Most transsexuals present not by asking for treatment, but for help in adapting to their chosen sexual identity. The aetiology of the condition remains obscure, but consti-

tutional factors, pre-natal hormonal influences, post-natal conditioning and learning factors may be important. No adult endocrine disability has been discovered.

For some transsexuals who have lived at ease in their chosen gender, who are emotionally stable and who bear no responsibilities such as may be entailed by a marital relationship, social change of gender such as changing name by deed poll and registration for employment, endocrinological support and even plastic surgery has been used. However, as such treatment requires the closest cooperation between surgeon, endocrinologist and psychiatrist, it should never be undertaken lightly.

Further reading

Bancroft, J.H.J. (1989) *Human Sexuality and its Problems*, 2nd edn, Edinburgh: Churchill Livingstone.
Bluglass, R. and Bowden, P. (1990) *Principles and Practice of Forensic Psychiatry*, Edinburgh: Churchill Livingstone.
Crowe, M. and Ridley, J. (1990) *Therapy with Couples*, Oxford: Blackwell Scientific Publications.
Hawton, K. (1985) *Sex Therapy: A Practical Guide*, Oxford: Oxford University Press.

15

Eating disorders

What are the eating disorders?

Primary eating disorders, in adolescent and adult psychiatry, are those conditions in which there is a disturbance of eating behaviour associated with psychological or social precipitants or both. *Secondary* eating disorders occur when serious physical illness results in failure to eat adequately because of loss of appetite, difficulty in swallowing or generalized illness. Thus secondary eating disorder may be associated with the cachexia of carcinomatosis, with the dysphagia of a pharyngeal pouch, and with the anhedonia and associated weight loss in depressive illness.

Other eating disorders occur in children. For example, *pica* is persistent eating of substances other than food by very young children, and this may include paint, sand, hair, clothing, string and even insect and animal droppings. There is some association of this condition with learning disability but no association with the eating disorders of adolescent and adult life. Repeated regurgitation of food in early infancy may also occur as a behavioural abnormality and is also on some occasions associated with learning disability. Again, there is no connection with the eating disorders of later onset. *Anorexia nervosa* is, according to ICD-10, 'An illness characterized by deliberate weight loss, induced and/or sustained by the patient herself'. The condition most commonly occurs in adolescent girls and young women. It is an independent syndrome because the clinical features are readily recognizable, there is a high reliability of diagnosis between clinicians, and follow-up studies show that sufferers from the condition maintain the regularly described features.

Bulimia nervosa is 'a syndrome characterized by repeated bouts of over-eating and an excessive preoccupation with the control of body weight, leading the patient to adopt extreme measures so as to mitigate the "fattening effects" of ingested food'. Many of the clinical features are shared with anorexia nervosa: for example, it occurs predominantly in young adult females and it may follow an episode of anorexia nervosa. *Normal weight bulimia* also mostly occurs in young women; however, the age range of affected people is wider and the similarity of symptoms with anorexia nervosa less marked than in the better defined syndrome of bulimia nervosa.

Table 15.1 *Major forms of primary eating disturbance of behaviour (from ICD-10)*

1	Anorexia nervosa
2	Bulimia nervosa
3	Normal weight bulimia
4	Obesity with psychological disturbances
5	Vomiting with psychological disturbances

Obesity is diagnosed when the body weight exceeds the standard weight by 20 per cent. It usually occurs as a combination of constitutional and social factors encouraging over-eating. In most cases psychological factors are not of great importance, but psychiatrists become involved occasionally when excessive eating does appear to be associated with emotional factors or when weight reduction is being hampered by emotional disturbance. Many overweight people have low self-esteem and lack social confidence. As well as treatment for the associated emotional disturbance, psychological methods of treatment have been used for the treatment of obesity. These methods include group therapy, behavioural methods and social support.

Psychogenic vomiting is indicated when there is repeated vomiting without an organic cause. It is commoner in women than men and usually occurs after meals and without nausea. Unlike the vomiting of bulimia nervosa it is not self-induced.

History of anorexia nervosa

A case report by Simone Porta in the early sixteenth century described a girl, aged 10, who stopped eating for forty days, and it was claimed that she lived on air; in 1669 John Reynolds wrote 'A discourse on prodigious abstinence'; and in 1694 Richard Morton, in his book *Phthisiologia, or Treatise of Consumptions*, wrote: 'A nervous atrophy, or consumption is a wasting of the body without any remarkable fever, cough or shortness of breath'. In this condition, which he was distinguishing from tuberculosis, he pointed out that there was loss of appetite, amenorrhoea and extreme wasting without lassitude. In the eighteenth century there were further reports of young women with slow pulse, a switch from self-starvation to over-eating, 'obstinate vomiting', and an eccentric diet such as 'pickled mangoes and tea'. Sir William Gull in 1868 described young women with extreme emaciation who showed a refusal to eat food, and in 1874 he coined the term 'anorexia nervosa'. Meanwhile, in France, Lasègue in 1873 had described eight women

aged between 18 and 32 as suffering from 'anorexie hystérique'.

The classical description of emaciation in women associated with pituitary damage, often postpartum, was made by Simmonds in 1914. This resulted in considerable diagnostic confusion with anorexia nervosa, and it was not until 1936 that Ryle distinguished anorexia nervosa from Simmonds disease. In contrast with anorexia nervosa and its very long history, bulimia nervosa was only described in 1979 by Russell as an 'ominous variant' of anorexia nervosa. The two features of intractable over-eating and self-induced vomiting to prevent weight gain were recognized.

Aetiology

For many years there was debate as to whether anorexia nervosa was primarily an organic disturbance with secondary psychological effects or vice versa. However, there are very few experts who would now look upon anorexia nervosa as other than a fundamentally psychiatric disorder with psychological and social causation. It is perhaps best to have a psycho-socio-biological model of pathogenesis and aetiology, in which the condition, once induced, is seen to be self-sustaining. Biological vulnerability includes some evidence for a genetic contribution to causation. There is marked hypothalamic dysfunction with anorexia nervosa but this is generally regarded as secondary to starvation rather than of primary aetiological significance; however, this hypothalamic change probably contributes to the sustaining of dieting and weight reduction.

Psychological predisposition to anorexia nervosa includes dietary problems in early life, parental preoccupation with food, and feelings in the child of loss of self-identity. Descriptions of their individual psychological state by anorexic patients characteristically stress their need for self-control, the relentless pursuit of thinness, and weight phobia. Anorexic patients frequently show features of anankastic personality (Chapter 13).

Social factors are probably of the greatest significance aetiologically. These include both disturbed relationships within the families of patients and also more general attitudes within society. The families of anorexics, especially the parents, are sometimes over-protective, enforcing rigidity and emotionally constraining, with failure within the family ever to resolve the conflicts that have arisen. The preferred image of an extremely slender young woman propagated by films, television and women's magazines has been considered by many to be important in causation, and to explain partly the increased prevalence of anorexia nervosa in western societies in recent decades. Such ideas and topics of conversation become part of the currency amongst adolescent girls at school and have been reinforced by the opinion of admired adults such as teachers, or the casual criticism of chubbiness by boyfriends. There is an increased risk for the condition in ballet dancers, models, and young women taking part in certain competitive sports, both because of the physical demands of the activity and the element of bodily self-absorption so frequent amongst those involved.

The aetiological factors in bulimia nervosa have not been clearly elicited. However, they appear to be similar to anorexia nervosa. The current cultural preoccupation with thinness is considered important, as is the changing role of women in western society. Feelings of guilt are important in eating disorders, with patients feeling guilty when they have had something to eat and especially after a bulimic binge. Moral characteristics tend to be attached to different food substances so that food is categorized as 'good' or 'bad'.

Clinical features and diagnosis

Anorexia is a misnomer, as loss of appetite is very rare, and more common (at least, early in the condition) is voracious appetite ruthlessly suppressed. Bulimia literally means *ox-* (bous) *hunger* (limos).

Anorexia nervosa

The diagnostic criteria for anorexia nervosa

given by Dally and Gomez (1980) are as follows:

1 Refusal to eat;
2 Loss of at least 10 per cent of previous body weight;
3 Amenorrhoea of at least 3 months' duration;
4 Age of onset between 11 and 35 years;
5 No other illness such as organic disease, affective disorder or schizophrenia is present.

According to ICD-10 the following features are all necessary for the diagnosis:

1 Body weight is maintained at least 15% below that expected or, in pre-pubertal patients, failure to make the expected weight gain during the period of growth;
2 Weight loss is self-induced by avoidance of fattening foods and at least one of: self-induced vomiting, self-induced purging, excessive exercise or use of appetite suppressants or diuretics;
3 Dread of fatness as an intrusive over-valued idea and the self-imposition of a low weight threshold; amenorrhoea in the female and loss of sexual interest and potency in the male; delayed or arrested puberty in pre-pubertal patients.

Typically, the patient is aged between about 12 and 21 years. She is intelligent and attractive and extremely strong-willed. She is physically very active, taking a lot of exercise in order to reduce weight, and she pursues thinness fanatically. She may start dieting on her own or with other girls; however, when they stop, she continues enthusiastically. She may have been slightly over-weight before dieting, and may have a wider face and be slightly plump.

Weight loss is progressive and the patient's emaciation causes concern in her family, at school or college or place of work. However, she denies concern and considers herself still to be too fat. She looks extremely unwell with very thin limbs, cyanosed extremities, hollow eye sockets and cheeks, and lanugo hair, but she maintains her restless activity and may claim that she has never felt better. She often has a great interest in food, calories and nutrition, and she may be expert at cooking for other people. Occupational involvement in catering is common among anorexic patients and this may occur after the onset of the illness rather than before. Patients show enormous self-control in their dieting, but at the same time fear that they will lose control and become obese if they eat normally.

There is a great range of severity of the condition, from the one or two girls in every school classroom of 16-year-olds with some degree of eating disorder to the severe, intractable and sometimes chronic case of anorexia nervosa which may only be terminated by death. Most girls with milder symptoms gradually improve and never come to medical attention. Some take themselves, or are taken by a parent, to see their general practitioner and are managed with dietary advice and regularly weighing. A few patients are referred to a consultant physician and a few, generally more intractable, to a psychiatrist.

The onset of anorexia nervosa is usually gradual, occurring over several months. Physical signs which usually occur in other conditions of starvation include gross cachexia, loss of some hair, and the growth of fine downy lanugo hair on the arms and legs with cold blue extremities. The skin may become dry, cracked and yellow due to carotene deposition; bradycardia and hypotension occur. The secondary sex characteristics are not affected. The patient remains energetic until weight loss is extreme and, apart from the gross cachexia, does not look physically ill.

The usual psychological features of anorexia nervosa are listed in Table 15.2. The characteristic body image disorder is a disturbed assessment of body width in which the patient believes herself to be fat when she is, in fact, desperately thin. She over-estimates her breadth at all levels of her body including her face, but she does not over-estimate her height, or the width of an inanimate object. This over-estimate is greater in anorexic patients who

Table 15.2 *Psychological features of anorexia nervosa*

Body image disorder

Feeding disorder

Gender disturbance

Disturbed relationships

purge and vomit, and it improves as the condition improves. It is not specific to anorexia nervosa, and other girls without this condition have also been shown to have a similar but lesser alteration in body image.

The feeding disorder is characterized by enormous concentration of interest on food, nutrition, recipes, cooking and related topics. The patient's symptom is an *over-valued idea* with preoccupation concerning dieting, the pursuit of thinness and fear of becoming fat. This is associated with an intense interest in food. Many patients have cooking as their major hobby, and can also give a precise estimate of the calorific content of any food and also its other nutritional value; however, sometimes these estimates are wildly inaccurate. One patient whilst starving herself was continuously cooking for her husband until he put on 20 kg in weight. Another patient was fascinated by the eating habits of her medical and nursing staff and used to spy on them in the staff canteen.

Anorexic patients may go to enormous lengths to prevent weight gain. This includes self-induced vomiting, purging and hiding food, persuading other patients to take their food away and disposing of food in all sorts of unlikely places. They may also use elaborate devices to conceal weight loss; for example, by putting weights in their clothes, or by tampering with the weighing machine. They can usually estimate their own weight very precisely. A surprising behavioural disturbance of both anorexic and bulimic patients is the occasional patient who will, in a rather obvious manner, steal food; for instance, a patient who stole meringues from a confectioner's shop, whilst shopping with a member of staff.

Gender disturbance is described in anorexia nervosa. Modern patients do not diet out of fear of pregnancy, but they do frequently show rejection of an adult female role with its usual features of forming a social relationship with a boyfriend, taking on a sexual role, becoming pregnant and mothering.

The family and care group relationships of anorexic sufferers are frequently disturbed. Of course, this could be secondary to the condition and the anxiety engendered in parents and friends, rather than a primary feature of the illness. Typically, the relationship with mother is close, mother being over-protective and extremely concerned about the patient's state. The relationship with father is often difficult; sometimes father is remote, rigid, ambitious, upright and seen as being critical and hostile towards the patient. Obviously, these are stereotypes and there may be many variations on the type of disturbance within the family.

Bulimia nervosa

Characteristic of bulimia is binge eating. Binges may last for about an hour and occur once or twice a day, and often involve more than 3,000 calories consumed in the course of the binge which might include a whole loaf of bread, half a pound of uncooked sausages, enormous quantities of ice-cream, and so on. Characteristically the patient feels extremely guilty before and during the binge, but still feels a strong impulse to eat. Laxative abuse and self-induced vomiting may be associated with a considerable feeling of relief.

In the patient who binges and vomits, erosion and discolouration of the teeth occurs, and there is swelling of the parotid glands due to salivation stimulated by vomiting. Diuretic and laxative abuse may cause gross electrolyte imbalance. A further physical sign described in bulimia nervosa is trauma with callus formation or even ulceration on the dorsum of the hand, usually right hand, used in mechanical stimulation of the gag reflex to produce vomiting. A number of other physical symptoms may be caused by the persistent excessive use of purgative drugs, so that fluid and electrolyte problems are the commonest medical complication in bulimic patients. About 50 per cent of such patients show some electrolyte abnormality: commonly raised serum bicarbonate, lowered serum chloride and potassium, and occasionally serum sodium.

Differential diagnosis

Anorexia nervosa needs to be distinguished from secondary eating disorders and from other causes of severe weight loss. Causes of loss of weight in an adolescent or young adult would include the following: chronic infection such as tuberculosis or brucellosis; gastro-intestinal disorders such as coeliac disease, Crohn's disease, ulcerative colitis and cystic fibrosis; diabetes mellitus; hyperthyroidism; malignancy, especially of the central nervous system and of the ovary; and Simmonds disease. These other causes are generally fairly easy to detect, but in a population where young adults are usually healthy, it is important to consider physical causes and exclude them.

Secondary eating disorders are associated with either physical illness where there is loss of appetite or disturbance in the mechanical process of eating or, alternatively, psychiatric disturbance. Such eating disturbances may be associated with depressive illness in which loss of appetite and weight loss is prominent, obsessional and phobic neurosis, alcohol and drug misuse, and occasionally schizophrenic illness.

Depressive illness is particularly important to identify and treat. Appropriate treatment may result in complete relief of symptoms, including the apparent disorder of eating. It is also very important to realize that severe, treatable, but potentially suicidal depressive illness may coexist with anorexia nervosa.

Bulimia nervosa is generally readily distinguished from organic disturbance of appetite with massive over-eating, and also from organic causes of repeated vomiting. Bulimia nervosa should be distinguished from anorexia nervosa, but frequently it supersedes the latter in the life history of the same patient.

Epidemiology

Anorexia nervosa and bulimia nervosa are most common in developed, affluent societies, where they are diagnosed more frequently than previously. This may reflect a true increase in incidence. In Britain there used to be an association with social class, in that more girls of higher social class were affected. Now the condition occurs regularly in all social classes. In the past the condition was reported more frequently in the South than the North of England, but this may also have been a social class effect. Between the ages of 16 and 18, about one in 100 schoolgirls are severely affected at private schools, but only about one in 300 at schools in the state sector.

Anorexia nervosa has been reported with greater frequency amongst students of nutrition, sport, ballet, fashion and modelling. These occupations appear to carry special risk because of the attention the practitioner, and especially the student, needs to give to body weight and fitness; they may also attract those who are already susceptible. Eating disorders have been only rarely reported from developing countries; for example, from the south Asian subcontinent. However, when schoolgirls in Britain of Asian ethnic origin were compared with the indigenous population, they were found to have symptoms of eating disorder no less frequently.

The onset of anorexia nervosa in females is usually between the ages of 16 and 20, and generally before 30. In males the condition occurs somewhat earlier, at about the age of 12 or 13. Only about one in twenty cases are male. Estimates for frequency of the condition vary from about 0.4 to 4 per 100,000 population per year. The prevalence of bulimia nervosa is not known, but some degree of symptoms may occur in up to 10 per cent of young females in western countries.

Prognosis and course

The clinical severity of anorexia nervosa varies enormously from a mild and relatively transient disturbance in eating behaviour, with weight loss that remits without medical intervention, to a severe, chronic and occasionally lethal illness. Mortality has only been recorded for long-term outcome of severe hospitalized patients and had occurred in 18 per cent at long-term follow-up, either directly resulting from the condition or from suicide. Death may occur from cachexia with intercurrent infection, from gross electrolyte disturbance and from acute gastric dilatation. Severely anorexic patients are, of course,

more prone to other illness; anorexia nervosa has been found with greater than expected frequency amongst diabetic patients; the reasons for this are unknown.

Of the more severe cases who are admitted to hospital it is generally considered that about one-fifth of patients recover fully, another fifth remain severely ill, and the remainder show chronic or intermittent disturbance of eating behaviour. Many patients retain difficulty with eating and show food fads and continuing preoccupation with food and diet.

Disturbance of physiological function may include the following:

1 elevation of plasma levels of free fatty acids and ketones;
2 decreased tryptophan supply to the central nervous system (both these may affect mood);
3 reduced sympathetic noradrenergic activity, and this only normalizes very slowly on recovery;
4 enlargement of cerebral fluid spaces and pseudoatrophy on computerized brain tomography;
5 increased caudate metabolism demonstrated in PET scan of the brain;
6 ovarian cysts, associated with subsequent infertility;
7 carotenaemia.

Management and treatment

The milder cases of both anorexia and bulimia nervosa can generally be managed in general practice; accurate diagnosis is followed by regular appointments to check on current eating behaviour and weight, to give advice concerning diet and lifestyle, and to help in dealing with family and other social problems. Depressive illness may occur with either anorexia or bulimia nervosa and requires appropriate treatment.

Some doctors have an excessively pessimistic view about the treatment of severe anorexia nervosa. This is probably because the most difficult patients are referred to hospital services and the chronic recalcitrant patient makes disproportionate demands on staff time. Essentially, anorexia nervosa is a treatable condition, and the majority of patients who are admitted seriously ill make a substantial improvement even if some do not recover completely.

Those anorexic patients who require treatment in or from hospital will need a different approach to treatment at each of the different stages listed in Table 15.3. It is often extremely difficult to *initiate* anorexic patients into treatment. They may believe that there is nothing wrong; alternatively, they may agree with all the doctor is saying in the outpatient clinic and say that they will start eating as soon as they go home, and do nothing. For those patients who are still living in the family home there is a need at this stage to work with the family; family conflicts may be highlighted by the patient's disorder, and this may hinder establishing a treatment programme. Anorexia nervosa is a potentially lethal condition, and in a few difficult situations the Mental Health Act should be considered with compulsory admission to hospital.

For the *correction of profound emaciation*, the necessary treatment is food in the digestive tract which can be absorbed and digested. Electrolyte imbalance may also be a severe problem, with depletion of sodium, potassium and chloride. Treatment is essentially medical in nature and is aimed at re-feeding. Such a regime will generally need to be instituted if the weight is below 30 kg, and, depending on the height, sometimes if the weight is more than this. The ideal site for such re-feeding is probably as an inpatient on the psychiatric ward of a district general hospital. Psychiatric nursing is generally preferable for the care of severely malnourished anorexic patients, but it is important to have easy referral to an interested consultant physician and to have good biochemical and other medical support services available.

Table 15.3 *Stages in the treatment of anorexia nervosa*

1 Initiation of treatment
2 Medical treatment of profound weight loss
3 Learning to control weight and diet

At a very low body weight complete bedrest is advisable, with total observation by nursing staff and especially supervision of all meals with the nurse present at the bed for at least an hour after meals. The main aim of this regime is to prevent disposal of food. Anorexic patients often take excessive exercise in order to reduce their weight, and bedrest will counteract this.

A high calorie diet is used with nutritional supplements as necessary. However, it is a feature of anorexia nervosa that starvation is predominantly calorific in nature and patients have often maintained vitamins, proteins and other essentials of diet until extreme emaciation. If possible, nutrition should be taken as food, but sometimes the patient will only tolerate a fluid diet and occasionally nasogastric feeding is required. This, however, should be avoided if at all possible, as the aim of treatment is to help the patient learn to control their own nutrition rather than passively to receive it.

If the patient has any degree of depression, treatment with antidepressant drugs is indicated, and some have the additional advantage of increasing weight. Tricyclic antidepressants are generally beneficial. However, constipation is a side effect of tricyclic therapy, and this may exacerbate the constipation of re-feeding. Chlorpromazine or other major tranquillizers in small dose may also be beneficial in lessening agitation and promoting weight gain.

Regular weighing, either daily or twice weekly is required. Attention to the scales is important, as anorexic patients have, on occasions, successfully sabotaged vulnerable weighing machines. Progress should be charted regularly and clearly, but it is generally preferable not to discuss weight, or a target weight, with the patient as the eventual goal is to establish safe and sensible eating habits rather than achieve any particular body weight.

The treatment of severe anorexia nervosa requires a high level of cooperation within a professional and well-trained team each member of which understands the aims of the whole treatment regime and makes an individual contribution. Medical staff will include a psychiatrist, who usually supervises the treatment procedure, and may include a physician to advise on electrolyte balance and the programme of re-feeding. A dietitian makes an important contribution in discussing diet with the patient, giving advice, and ensuring that the diet is palatable and appropriate in calories and other essential ingredients. The heaviest burden of care falls upon nursing staff; treatment requires both forging a therapeutic relationship and close observation. At a later stage in treatment there are important roles for a clinical psychologist to be involved in planning the treatment programme, for an occupational therapist to take an active part both whilst the patient is confined to bed and subsequently during the inpatient stay when she is no longer in bed, and for a social worker to be involved with the family.

The final stage of treatment, and often the most difficult, is helping the patient *learn to control* her *weight* and her *diet*. This requires great skill from nursing staff and excellent cooperation between the different professions involved. Some anorexic patients are expert at manipulating differences in the care plan from different members of staff. Family therapy may be helpful and is in general more effective for patients aged under 19 whose illness is not chronic. Cognitive behavioural therapy may be useful for anorexia nervosa and has been demonstrated to be particularly useful for bulimia nervosa. Nutritional counselling, involving a dietitian, has also proved beneficial, especially for patients who also have food fads.

The role of nursing staff in the management of anorexia nervosa for inpatients and subsequently is particularly important, and it has often proved useful to have one nurse identified as the programme nurse who draws up the programme of care and plans successive phases in treatment, and a therapy nurse, who makes a special relationship with the patient and is involved in individual therapy.

Often in the management of anorexia two doctors are involved: a consultant sets up the treatment programme and insists that the treatment regime is maintained scrupulously; a more junior doctor establishes a therapeutic relationship and, when in conflict with the patient over the established regime, informs her that this has been set up by the consultant. It is, of course, important for the two doctors to work closely together and to understand how the relationship between themselves, and between each of them and the patient, works to the advantage of the patient.

In the management of bulimia nervosa it is important for both patient and doctor to know exactly what is the patient's behaviour; and keeping an accurate diary of bingeing, vomiting, purging and other significant events is helpful. This is recorded as a baseline, noting the time of day at which bingeing and other behaviours occur and also the amount and type of food taken in the binge. The diary is continued through treatment and is a useful permanent record for the patient of progress made. Cognitive therapy has proved especially helpful in the treatment of bulimia nervosa; the condition is often associated with feelings of profound low self-esteem. Treatment for depressive symptoms may also be required. The treatment of bulimia nervosa can generally be managed as an out-patient.

Summary

Eating disorders are a distinct clinical entity, with anorexia nervosa and bulimia nervosa forming clear categories yet with considerable overlap. Psychological factors are probably the most important aetiologically. There are long-term physical consequences of both anorexia and bulimia nervosa; the biochemical abnormalities are probably effects rather than causes of the condition. The psychopathology of both conditions is quite clearly delineated, and the epidemiology of anorexia nervosa has been demonstrated.

Anorexia and bulimia nervosa are treatable conditions, although there is a small but definite mortality associated with anorexia nervosa from the consequences of malnutrition and also from suicide. Treatment requires a multidisciplinary approach with considerable expertise. Ideally, inpatient care should be given by a specialist service. Those with bulimia nervosa may generally be treated as an outpatient, and cognitive therapy has proved especially beneficial.

Further reading

Beumont, P.J.V. (1987) *Handbook of Eating Disorders,* Amsterdam, Elsevier.

Crisp, A.H. (1980) Anorexia Nervosa: Let Me Be, London: Academic Press.

Dally, P. and Gomez, J. (1980) *Obesity and Anorexia Nervosa: A Question of Shape,* London: Faber & Faber.

Fairburn, C. (1981) 'A cognitive behavioural approach to the treatment of bulimia', *Psychological Medicine,* 11: 707–11.

Garfinkel, D.M. and Garfinkel, P.E. *Handbook of Psychotherapy for Anorexia Nervosa and Bulimia,* New York: Guilford Press.

Russell, G.F.M. (1979) 'Bulimia nervosa: an ominous variant of anorexia nervosa', *Psychological Medicine,* 9: 429–48.

16

Liaison psychiatry

Over the last decade in the United Kingdom, there have developed increasing links between psychiatry and the practice of medicine and surgery in the general hospital. One reason has been a growth in the number of psychiatric units sited in district general and teaching hospitals. Along with those developments there has emerged a specialty known as general hospital *liaison* psychiatry, which concentrates not upon patients in the psychiatric wards or clinics but those in medical, surgical, obstetric and other wards or clinics, or in the accident and emergency department.

The liaison psychiatrist will be expected to undertake urgent and routine assessments of general hospital patients on inpatient wards, in accident and emergency and in outpatient clinics. The liaison psychiatrist may be expected to have some expertise with the following groups:

- patients who have harmed themselves;
- patients who have coexisting physical and mental illness;
- patients who have developed organic mental illness;
- patients who have problems adjusting to physical illness;
- patients who have unexplained physical symptoms;
- women who have developed a psychiatric disorder related to childbirth.

Liaison psychiatry is the practice of general psychiatry in the particular setting of the general hospital. It demands expertise with organic mental illness, physical illness and physical symptoms, and the ability to work with general hospital medical and nursing staff, to help them deal with the psychological and emotional aspects of physical disease.

Urgency of referral

With the exception of the sexually transmitted diseases clinic, the only part of the hospital service to offer direct access to patients may be the accident and emergency department. For that reason, patients and their relatives and friends regard it as an appropriate place to seek help in a crisis. Accident and emergency departments therefore receive a steady stream of cases requiring urgent psychiatric assessment. A substantial proportion of such cases are those in which the patient has attempted suicide (see Chapter 17). Some of these patients are assessed by a psychiatrist in accident and emergency, but because the majority are admitted to a medical ward, the psychiatric assessment more often takes place there. The majority of psychiatric referrals from accident and emergency are therefore for reasons *other* than self-harm.

Both in the accident and emergency department and on a general hospital ward, almost any kind of psychiatric syndrome may arise or become evident. The following are examples selected from requests for urgent psychiatric assessment over a few weeks at one teaching hospital:

- a patient whose collapse was thought likely to be due to a panic attack;
- a patient whose increasing disability due to diabetes mellitus had resulted in distress and expression of suicidal intent;
- a patient who had suddenly become severely agitated and behaviourally disturbed following admission for elective surgery (he had developed alcoholic delirium tremens);
- a patient with a fractured femur not yet united, who was insisting that he would remove the traction and walk away from the hospital;
- a patient who had developed delusions of persecution following the treatment of multiple sclerosis with corticosteroids;
- a patient with multiple previous admissions to psychiatric hospital who received regular depot neuroleptic drugs, brought on this occasion to accident and emergency by the police who found him in an excited and incoherent state, wandering by the side of the canal.

Such a list is intended to illustrate the mix of cases seen and the skills which might be needed by a liaison psychiatrist. In the last case, for example, such a patient might very well be assessed at the psychiatric unit, or in a police station, or at his home; it is merely that accident and emergency departments have to deal with every kind of crisis. All of the other examples, however, show strong links between the psychiatric symptoms and physical disease of some kind. Effective management of such referrals usually includes consultation and liaison with other specialists.

Less urgent requests for psychiatric consultations show a similar pattern and a similar need for expertise with physical illness in addition to general psychiatric skills. Here is a selection of referrals of inpatients and outpatients:

- a man with recurrent abdominal pain without clear cause, who was refusing to eat because it exacerbated pain;

- a patient who, following recovery from severe head injury, showed marked change in attitude and behaviour which resulted in great family distress;
- a patient who had recovered from the acute phase of Wernicke's encephalopathy (see page 74), but had developed memory problems;
- a dermatology patient who falsely believed that her skin was infested by tiny insects;
- a patient who several weeks previously had sustained multiple severe injuries in an accident at work had emerged from coma; he had a tracheostomy and was tube-fed; he was unable to talk but could make gestures; his wife and the nurses observed that he was very emotional and wept frequently; it was queried whether depression was impairing his recovery.
- a patient investigated for abdominal pain who wanted help to reduce his excessive alcohol consumption.

Attempted suicide

Assessment of deliberate self-harm forms a significant proportion of the work of a liaison psychiatrist in most hospitals. These patients are seen in accident and emergency as well as on short-stay or medical wards, and with differing need for urgency. The arrangements for assessment and management are described in Chapter 17.

Physically ill patients and organic mental illness

The occurrence together of physical and psychiatric illness is not merely a chance association. Some illnesses have both *physical and psychiatric manifestations* – for example, delirium tremens, thyroid disorder or AIDS. Some *treatments for physical disorders* may precipitate mental disorder – for example, corticosteroids, anticonvulsants or levodopa. These kinds of problems are discussed more fully in Chapter 7.

In addition, however, the distress, disability and threat caused by physical illness may lead to psychiatric disorder – in the form of anxious, depressive or other symptoms. These *adjustment difficulties* are discussed in the next section.

Conversely, *psychiatric illness* or its treatment may lead to actual or apparent physical ill health. There are many ways in which this connection may come about. A common instance is the result of a suicide attempt – whether by poisoning, jumping from a height, or fire. In anorexia nervosa (see Chapter 15) patients may reach a stage where inpatient medical care is required. In dissociative states (see Chapter 11), patients with apparent physical disability may be brought to the attention of physicians or neurologists. Some *psychiatric treatments* can lead to serious physical consequences. For example, neuroleptic drugs may cause a severe neurological disorder known as the neuroleptic malignant syndrome (see Chapter 23), or lithium carbonate may severely exacerbate psoriasis, necessitating urgent treatment.

Whatever the relation between coexisting mental and physical illness, its management often presents a challenge. The use of certain treatments may be contra-indicated: for example, tricyclic antidepressant drugs soon after myo-cardial infarction. The ability of staff on a psychiatric ward to deal with medical conditions and treatments, or the ability of staff on a medical, surgical or obstetric ward to deal with psychiatric problems, is often an issue of concern. These difficulties, which are not always solvable, frequently involve the liaison psychiatrist.

The best option is probably the setting up in the general hospital of a psychiatric ward where the nurses are qualified in both physical and psychiatric nursing and the psychiatric staff are dealing constantly with physically and mentally ill patients. Few such units exist. More often, care is provided by psychiatrists with some expertise in liaison work but without inpatient facilities apart from those of ordinary medical or psychiatric wards – where coexisting physical and mental disorder are dealt with as well as possible.

Although psychiatric symptoms may arise in the setting of any physical illness, there are certain associations to which it is worth drawing attention. Examples are briefly set out in Table 16.1, but are described more fully in postgraduate textbooks of psychiatry (see Lloyd 1991 and the references at the end of Chapter 1). Some of the associations are clear manifestations of organic mental disorders; others involve problems of adjustment to the physical condition.

Table 16.1 *Examples of psychiatric disorder associated with physical illness*

Physical illness	Psychiatric disorders with which associated
Neurological disorders	*Head injury, space occupying lesions, strokes and subarachnoid haemorrhages* are each associated with the development of any of a number of psychiatric syndromes: delirium, irritability and aggression, intellectual deficit, depression, emotionalism, anxiety and other neurotic disorders and, occasionally, delusional and hallucinatory disorder. *Parkinson's disease* is associated with depression, delirium and dementia. *Wilson's disease* may lead to change in attitude and behaviour. *Multiple sclerosis* may be accompanied by mood disorder, delirium, delusional and hallucinatory syndromes, and intellectual deficits. *Epilepsy*, especially *temporal lobe epilepsy*, is associated with many psychiatric syndromes: delirium, hallucinations (especially of taste and smell), mood disorder, delusional syndromes, hysterical non-epileptic seizures; some features are particularly associated with aura, others occur as part of or immediately after seizures, others occur between seizures.
Gastro-intestinal disorders	*Liver failure* may precipitate delirium (hepatic encephalopathy). Ileostomy and colostomy *stomas* may lead to adjustment disorders and depression. *Anorexia and bulimia* are described in Chapter 15.

Table 16.1 *(Continued)*

Physical illness	Psychiatric disorders with which associated
Cardiovascular disorders	*Myocardial infarction* may lead to delirium, adjustment disorder, depression, anxiety disorder, disorder of sexual function. *Peripheral vascular disease* and its disability, particularly following amputation, may lead to adjustment disorder and depression.
Renal disorders	*Chronic renal failure* is a very debilitating condition and may bring about adjustment disorder and depression. Hospital haemodialysis seems to be associated with greater psychiatric morbidity than does home dialysis, continuous ambulatory peritoneal dialysis, or successful transplantation.
Endocrine disorders	*Diabetes mellitus*, particularly insulin-dependent diabetes, may give rise to adjustment disorders and problems with compliance; long-term complications have their own psychological impact. *Hypoglycaemia* may produce symptoms of delirium. *Thyroid disease* has numerous psychiatric consequences. Hypothyroidism is associated with depression, delusional and hallucinatory syndromes and intellectual deficits. Hyperthyroidism is associated with anxiety and other arousal symptoms, less often with delirium or delusional syndromes or mania. *Cushing's Syndrome* is commonly accompanied by depression, less often with mania or delusional symptoms. *Hyperparathyroidism* is a rare condition, but depression is a common accompaniment; occasionally other organic states occur. *Phaeochromocytoma* symptoms include severe anxiety.
Infectious, inflammatory, immunological and connective tissue disorders	*Neurosyphilis* at an advanced stage, causing psychiatric symptoms, is now rare. Depression, dementia and delusional disorders all occur and were once commonplace. *HIV*-related disease is associated with adjustment disorder, depression and, in a small proportion of cases, with delirium, dementia or other organic mental illness. *Systemic lupus erythematosis*, as a result of its chronic and disabling course, may provoke depression. However, the vascular lesions may also cause organic mental illness, leading to delirium and delusional and hallucinatory syndromes. The same may be said of the granulomatous lesions of *sarcoidosis*.
Skin disorders	Some skin diseases such as eczema and psoriasis may be *exacerbated* by psychological stresses. *Disfiguring* skin conditions may lead to adjustment disorders or depression. The skin is a site of self-inflicted or *factitious disease* (dermatitis artefacta), and of complaints of skin disorder when only normal skin can be seen (dermatological *non-disease*). A few patients develop *delusional disorder* concerning infestation of their skin (see Chapter 6).
Malignant disease	Any intracranial malignancy, primary or secondary, may cause any form of organic mental state – delirium, affective disorder, delusional or hallucinatory disorder, dementia. Non-metastatic systemic effects may have similar effects. Adjustment and depressive disorders may also arise as a consequence of the diagnosis, treatment and prognosis of the condition.

Problems in adjusting to physical illness

Physical illness has an impact on the person suffering it, and often on those around. Although each person's reaction is unique, there are some identifiable patterns of response. First, illness may be played down or disregarded as much as possible. This approach has its strengths: it allows the person to carry on with life largely uninterrupted by the physical ailment. On the other hand, when carried too far this stratagem may be harmful. For example, a patient with diabetes may so far ignore the illness that he does not comply with attempts to control blood sugar – by missing insulin injections, or failing to carry out blood or urine tests. The long-term consequence of such action is to risk severe and irreversible organ damage. Similarly, a patient with any kind of heart or vascular disease may not acknowledge the relevance of aspects of lifestyle such as smoking, diet, exercise and work pressure – to the detriment of subsequent health.

An alternative approach to ill health may be to attend closely to the disease. There are great advantages to sensible compliance with treatment; for example, in taking necessary immunosuppressant drugs after a transplant, or anticonvulsants when fits may otherwise recur. Some patients go further and find out a great deal about the condition. They become involved with one of the growing number of disease-related special-interest and self-help groups. In most cases, these organizations provide information about treatment and other practical issues related to disability. The British Diabetic Association, for example, has a large membership which includes, as well as a large proportion of diabetic patients, many doctors, specialist nurses, dietitians and other staff. They have a professionally produced, bimonthly magazine with wide circulation and they arrange many activities. Other groups concentrate not on a disease but on effects of treatment. For example, the Ileostomy Association, by means of a network of those who themselves have a stoma, helps people to become accustomed to a major change in bodily function.

There can, however, be problems for those who attend closely to their illness. It is possible to focus upon it so much that other important aspects of life become over-shadowed. Some patients can become more socially disabled than might be expected from the symptoms and other impairments. Others may seek ever more information and can place their physician or surgeon in an uncomfortable position: clinical judgements are repeatedly questioned and unrealistic demands are made for certainty over prognosis (with or without intervention), side

effects to treatment, and so on. The management of most illness cannot be undertaken without ambiguities over the prognosis and the best course of action. Where the patient finds this impossible to endure, the burden on both the patient and others may be increased; on occasions, decisions about intervention may be made not according to likely benefit and risk, but result from conflict between the patient and staff.

The above descriptions may imply that there are two kinds of physically ill people: those who are too little concerned with their condition, and those who are too much concerned. Not so; the majority of patients, even those suffering severe ill health and disability, fall somewhere between these extremes and deal with their predicament remarkably well. Personal reaction to illness has many components. Some of them were usefully described by Lipowski (1969), and are set out in Table 16.2. All health staff need to have some understanding of reactions and behaviours associated with illness. The psychiatrist in the general hospital will frequently be called upon to assess and help a patient whose adjustment to illness or disability seems to be causing difficulties. It can be helpful to recognize these and other reactions.

While attempting to adjust to illness it is common to develop understandable degrees of anxiety, depression, irritability and anger. From time to time such difficulties become prolonged, and it is therefore worth encouraging resolution of the problems at an early stage. Where these emotions are themselves causing difficulties, they are sometimes termed '*adjustment disorders*' – a rather non-specific term which indicates that a diagnosis of more definite psychiatric illness is not justified by the symptoms.

The problems which result from incomplete adjustment to illness may be manifest through the patient's emotional state or in disturbances of behaviour, such as poor compliance. In either case, the most valuable psychiatric intervention is most often psychotherapeutic. The grief involved in severe disabling or life-threatening illness may require assistance to work through. Many patients are helped by an opportunity to discuss their symptoms, disability, impact of

Table 16.2 *Psychological aspects of physical illness*

• Threat	Often marked at an early stage in illness, and at any other time when either diagnosis or outcome become uncertain or sinister. Features of anxiety may be prominent.
• Loss	May be particularly marked after operative procedures such as amputation, mastectomy, bowel resections with stomas, and others. Loss is not only anatomical – for example, when ill health alters a person's role as an earner. Loss is often associated with depressive symptoms.
• Gain or relief	At first sight it may seem unlikely, but there can be gain from illness. It can allow avoidance of unwanted activity, improve relationships, increase attention paid to the person.
• Challenge	Everyone who works in medicine is soon aware, if they were not already, of the extraordinary way in which some patients rise to the challenge of illness, disability, even impending death.
• Insignificance	Some people seem to be surprisingly untouched by the effects or threats of illness. On some occasions a serious condition is regarded as insignificant because the person is not informed about its nature or likely outcome. In other cases patients may exercise the mental mechanism of denial.

illness and prognosis with a psychiatric physician – in a setting where it is acceptable to express emotions and fears. Interviewing of one or more family members with the patient is often invaluable in both assessment and treatment. Specific psychotherapeutic techniques, such as cognitive therapy, are also widely used.

In some cases, a more severe psychiatric disorder develops – usually an *anxiety disorder* or *depressive illness*. It can be difficult to discriminate between an understandable response and psychiatric disorder. Among all those with significant physical illness, distress is commonplace – with no clear cut-off between those who are abnormal and the rest who are 'all right'. It is important, however, to recognize certain specific and treatable disorders. For example, persistent phobic anxiety may respond well to psychiatric intervention (see Chapters 10 and 21).

Established depressive illness is more serious and may require more urgent intervention. Because it may readily be understood why someone with a disabling condition is unhappy or even wretched, their reversible depressive illness may be overlooked. Why, among all those who are very handicapped by arthritis, does this patient feel so miserable? When the facts are assembled they may reveal that: although she has been very handicapped for many years,

she has only become low-spirited over the last few months; she has only lately begun to tell her husband that he would have a better life without her encumbrance; having been an avid reader she no longer wants her husband to fetch books from the library; she stays on her own as much as possible and she prefers it if even her daughter and young grandson, previously the apple of her eye, do not visit.

In physical illness, depressive symptoms may be present, but they can be more difficult to establish – either because of their 'understandability', as above, or because they are confounded by the features of the physical state. Poor appetite, sleep disturbance, change in libido, loss of energy and other striking depressive symptoms can be useless in the assessment of the physically ill. Nevertheless, careful history-taking and discussion with key informants will usually allow severe depressive illness to be identified from the combination of psychological and physical symptoms. Recognition of depressive and other psychiatric symptoms in physical illness can be impeded by the feeling, either in the patient or the doctor, that there is shame or stigma in such experiences.

Treatment for depression may be particularly challenging. There is often need for adequate drug treatment, sometimes ECT. Both, however, have their contra-indications and these are more often relevant in patients who are physically ill (see Chapter 23).

Unexplained physical symptoms

It is a common observation that there are many patients whose physical symptoms are not adequately explained by demonstrable signs or investigations. In some cases the reason is that the disease is at an early stage, with the clear abnormalities yet to emerge. In other cases the disorder is self-limiting and is improving at the time of consultation. Sometimes, however, the doctor concludes that psychological or emotional factors are the main reason for the clinical picture. Many terms have been used for such circumstances: 'hypochondriasis', 'somatization', 'functional illness', 'functional overlay' and many others. These terms all tend to imply that the 'real' disorder is a psychiatric rather than a physical one. In fact, the physical symptoms are almost always completely authentic and experienced in the way described by the patient.

In some cases a *primary psychiatric condition*, such as depressive illness, accounts for the secondary physical symptoms. One patient, a woman in her late fifties, had twice been admitted to the rheumatological ward over the preceding few months. She complained of severe pain in and around her cervical spine and she had become progressively immobile, spending most of the day at home in bed. She had radiological evidence of vertebral changes in her neck but had responded poorly to analgesia and physiotherapy. She was seen by a liaison psychiatrist after she was readmitted to hospital following a deliberate overdose of analgesics. By that stage she had many depressive symptoms, and antidepressant drug treatment was begun. She made rapid progress in both mood and physical symptoms. About two months later she sent the psychiatrist a postcard from the Spanish Coast to let him know that she had thrown away her cervical collar. Her complete recovery was sustained throughout the follow-up period of one year.

Cases with such dramatic improvement in physical symptoms are not rare. However, it must be said that, even where there is evidence of a psychiatric disorder in addition to the unexplained physical symptoms, improvement in mood is not always accompanied by resolution of physical complaints. In another group of patients, unexplained physical symptoms are found *without* clear evidence of a psychiatric condition. Several questions may then arise. First, do the unexplained physical symptoms constitute a psychiatric illness? Second, is another psychiatric disorder present even though it is not obvious? Third, might a psychiatrist help with the symptoms, regardless of their origin? These issues form the basis of the rest of this section.

Hypochondriacal or somatoform disorders

Although the terminology varies, most psychiatrists agree that unexplained physical symptoms can sometimes be regarded as a psychiatric condition. For many years 'hypochondriasis' was the term most widely used; nowadays 'somatoform' or 'somatization disorder' are often preferred; all are included in ICD-10 terminology. Whatever the name, one or more of the following characteristics will usually be present:

- repeated presentation of physical symptoms, disproportionate to any physical disease detected by examination or investigation;
- persistent seeking of medical investigations and consultations, despite repeated negative findings and assurances by doctors that symptoms are not based on detectable and serious physical pathology;
- an expressed firm belief in the existence of physical disease, despite evidence and assurances to the contrary;
- abnormal behaviour related to the presentation of symptoms, variously described as 'demanding', 'difficult', 'attention-seeking', 'having a large functional element', and so on.

Coexisting or primary psychiatric disorder

A significant minority of patients with persistent or severe unexplained physical symptoms do have another psychiatric disorder – most often depressive illness, with anxiety disorders the next commonest group. As suggested by the case cited above, the psychiatric illness may not be obvious, especially early in its course. Careful enquiry may be necessary to identify symptoms. In such cases treatment of the depression or anxiety, by physical or psychological intervention, may result in marked improvement in physical as well as psychological symptoms.

Treatment of unexplained physical symptoms

With hypochondriacal patients, reassurance has usually failed. However, in practice 'reassurance' may well have meant no more than telling the patient that there is nothing wrong with him. Since this assertion seems to the symptomatic patient manifestly to be false, it is disbelieved. Reassurance should consist of two elements: not only the statement that symptoms are not based on serious physical pathology, but also an accompanying explanation of what pathological or physiological mechanisms *are* responsible for the symptoms. This second element in the reassuring process is sometimes missing, or is not emphasized or repeated sufficiently. Instead, maladaptive beliefs and relations with the medical world develop or worsen. More investigations or consultations are sought by the patient, in the hope of proving that the doctor is mistaken.

Many if not all of these patients develop *dependent yet hostile* relationships with doctors. One patient showed the liaison psychiatrist appointment cards for more than ten specialists she had consulted during the previous two years. Over the first few months of regular psychiatric appointments she spoke of doctors only with praise for their efforts in general and on her behalf in particular. Her less generous sentiments towards the medical profession only became apparent when one day she broke down into tears, talking about the 'countless hours spent waiting for doctors who never came'. When this was explored she had much to say about follow-up clinic appointments when, having hoped to talk with the consultant, she saw instead a great many and ever-changing trainee doctors who were unfamiliar with her case, who seemed often to deal with her brusquely but who always arranged further or repeat investigations.

Physical investigation

There are several problems with extended or repeated physical investigation of patients with unexplained physical symptoms. First, because investigations reveal only what is *not* present, the patient perceives them as invalidating his experience of physical symptoms. Second, when results are abnormal they are often medically trivial, yet result in unnecessary treatments or further 'reassurances' which are not believed; disagreement between doctors about how best to deal with the findings may soon follow. Third, the process of carrying out further tests is not in itself reassuring; it constantly raises the possibility that something *might* be found.

Psychiatric management

The components of treatment are briefly outlined in Table 16.3.

Fatigue syndrome

Recently, increasing attention has been paid to symptoms of disabling fatigue. Various fatigue syndromes have been described, with similar but not identical features and different names, such as myalgic encephalomyelitis (ME) and post-viral fatigue syndrome. There have been attempts to standardize terminology: *chronic fatigue syndrome* and its sub-type *post-infectious fatigue syndrome* are regarded by many as the two important conditions. The principal complaint is of prolonged, severe and disabling fatigue for at least several months, affecting

Table 16.3 *Components of management of unexplained physical symptoms*

Mood disorder	A substantial proportion of patients with persistent unexplained physical symptoms have depressive disorders. These should be identified and treated; antidepressant drug treatment is often of value. Anxiety disorders also require identification and treatment.
Patterns of illness behaviour	For those patients with a pattern of multiple and repeated medical contacts and requests for investigations, time is spent discussing the lack of benefit – indeed, harmful effects – of such action. Attempts are made to agree a strategy of 'no further investigation'.
Attitudes to symptoms	Bodily experiences are often wrongly attributed to physical disease. Akin to the elements of cognitive therapy (Chapter 21), such *misconceptions* about symptoms are carefully identified and, then, challenged by the psychiatrist. *Education* about how these physical experiences may arise is undertaken. Tension headaches, for example, can be used to illustrate that physical symptoms do not always mean physical disease. Most people have heard about phantom limb pains, hypnosis for pain relief, and other examples of the complex way we may perceive bodily experiences. As with cognitive therapies in other settings, it may be helpful to *test out* some of the misattributions and strategies. Muscle tension, patterns of breathing and so on may be brought on to elicit the symptoms, and then methods of control taught to abolish symptoms when they arise.
Possible psychological or social stressors	Many patients resist any attempts by the doctor to attribute physical symptoms to life's events and difficulties. Nevertheless, striking relationships between the onset or nature of symptoms and possible psychosocial provoking factors often do emerge during careful history-taking. Sometimes stresses are only revealed after a long period of contact, and it is counter-productive to attempt to force patients to make associations between stressors and symptoms. In time, patients may begin to recognize for themselves the context in which their symptoms arose.

physical *and* mental functioning but not arising from an established medical or psychiatric condition known to cause fatigue. Some cases clearly follow or accompany infection, but the infection is one not generally associated with chronic fatigue; so the aetiological link is usually uncertain.

The condition is most prevalent between the ages of 20 and 50 years and is found in both sexes, with women more often affected than men. Patients describe worsening of fatigue with mental or physical exertion, and often muscle pain, particularly of a 'burning' quality. Depression and sleep disturbance are common. Fatigue and weakness, when prolonged, may lead to reduced mobility and social handicap. Patients develop restrictions in their occupational, family, social and leisure activities and, in severe cases, in self-care. Many treatments have been tried without conspicuous benefit, both pharmacological and psychotherapeutic (mostly behavioural or cognitive). Many patients whose main complaint is chronic fatigue are reluctant to accept psychiatric referral; psychiatrists are however increasingly involved with other physicians in management. There is interest in treatment programmes which may include diaries to monitor activity and symptoms, graded activity, group sessions, physiotherapy and occupational therapy. Antidepressant drugs have been advocated and widely used even when depression itself is not prominent. Unfortunately the necessary intervention trials of drugs and other procedures have not so far been carried out. Many patients do recover, usually slowly. As in many conditions, some people experience enduring symptoms and increasing disability and social handicap.

Psychiatric disorder related to childbirth

Of all life's events, childbirth has the strongest known association with the subsequent development of mental disorder. This association is often considered as three distinct syndromes, differing in their time-pattern and their clinical features. It is an over-simplification to consider the three as entirely separate, but the distinction is a useful introduction to the topic.

- the maternity blues;
- puerperal psychosis;
- post-partum depression.

The maternity blues

The maternity blues is a mood disturbance which occurs soon after childbirth in perhaps a half or more of women. It is so common that it must be considered as a normal state. The woman's mood tends to be more changeable, more emotional than is usual for her. There may be transient or more prolonged distress: she may, at different times, be tense, anxious, miserable, irritable, sometimes briefly elated, and frequently shows a mixture of these emotions. The change in mood may begin within the first few hours but often takes a day or two to develop. The peak time for mood disturbance is three or four days after delivery. It has been argued that this change is not specific to childbirth but is similar to that seen after other health-related events such as operative surgery. This explanation seems unlikely: for example, in women of childbearing age, distress after gynaecological surgery is most marked immediately after the operation and steadily improves over the next few days.

The maternity blues is a self-limiting state which usually clears within a few days of its onset. If it has any relation with later development of post-partum depression, which has been suggested, the link is by no means a clear one. The condition requires no specific treatment. The most important aspects of management are explanation and understanding, together with practical and emotional support. The woman, her husband, her parents, the midwife, the general practitioner – whoever is involved in her care – needs to be clear that it is self-limiting and should become neither severe nor prolonged. If it does, which is rare, then an alternative diagnosis is indicated (see

below); for this reason it is essential to be sure that the mood returns to its normal range within one or two weeks of delivery.

Puerperal psychosis

Few disorders in psychiatry are as striking in clinical form and epidemiology as puerperal psychosis. The disorder is relatively rare but the rate of admission to psychiatric hospital has repeatedly been found to be about two cases per 1,000 live births. In a large health district such as Leeds (700,000 population), this means about twenty episodes each year. As with most conditions, the true population rate is undoubtedly higher than the hospital admission rate – perhaps three or four times as common. A case vignette is outlined here in order to illustrate some of the features of the condition:

A 31-year-old married, primiparous woman, who had no psychiatric history and had experienced an unremarkable pregnancy, gave birth by normal vaginal delivery to a healthy full-term child in her local hospital on Tuesday morning. She was well through Wednesday, but by Thursday evening her husband expressed to the ward staff concern about her emotional and distressed state. Following a sleepless night, on Friday morning it was agreed that she should remain in hospital for another day or two while she established breast-feeding and to ensure that her mood returned to a more stable state. Instead, she became more weepy and increasingly restless and irritable. By Friday night her mood was constantly abnormal, characterized by misery interspersed with invective directed at her husband and her own parents. She was also over-active, pacing about and rapidly becoming exhausted. Her family were anguished to see her in this state – so unlike her normal self. Of perhaps even greater concern, she had begun to say that her child should not come home with her when she left hospital.

The nursing staff and the obstetrician felt that she was showing signs of definite mental disorder. The liaison psychiatrist confirmed that the patient was in a seriously abnormal state of mood and thinking. Mood was a mixture of depression, perplexity, arousal and irritability. She showed pressure of speech and her thinking was disordered in its form, including many puns and clang associations (see page 43). She had numerous delusions including: that she was a criminal which was why police-car sirens could be heard outside (in fact, the sound was due to ambulances); and that she and the child would be taken to prison where both would become 'jailbirds'. She was disorientated for the day of the week but there was no other clearly evident intellectual deficit; no formal testing was possible due to her other abnormalities of mental state. She had been mildly pyrexial on the second post-partum day but was now in reasonable physical health.

Arrangements were made for her and her baby to be transferred to the special mother-and-baby unit on a psychiatric ward. She agreed because she thought it the only way to avoid her worst delusional fears. At first she continued to develop delusions and became even less coherent in her talk. At one stage her speech was replaced by gesticulation and she believed, despite their protestations to the contrary, that her family and staff knew what she was 'saying' by her gestures.

With active treatment (see below), after three weeks on the psychiatric ward she became well enough to be discharged with her baby. It had been possible for her to continue breast-feeding throughout her hospital stay. Her only symptoms at discharge were those of mild-to-moderate anxiety with occasional episodes of panic. The patient, her family and the health visitor felt that she had sufficient support to manage at home with daily visits from both the health visitor and the community psychiatric nurse. By one month after discharge she seemed entirely back to normal; confirmed by the patient herself and her family. By the time of her child's first birthday she had experienced no further symptoms.

Clinical features

The great majority of puerperal psychotic illnesses arise within the first two post-partum weeks; most within the first week, and many after only a few days. It is rare, however, for there not to be a day or two of normal mood and behaviour before symptoms develop. Primiparous women have higher risk of a first episode than do those who already have children (risk of *further* episodes is discussed below). Every kind of socio-demographic and obstetric factor has been examined for links with risk. There have been many reports of associations, but few if any have been confirmed or sustained. There may be a higher incidence following Caesarean section. However, the most striking feature of most first episodes of puerperal psychosis is its unheralded onset.

The first symptoms are often non-specific features of mild distress – tension, anxiety, poor concentration and attention, and emotionalism; the state may be indistinguishable from the maternity blues (see above). The difference lies in the progression to more sustained symptoms. These are often depressive but may be manic, mixed-affective (such as in the example above), or even like the symptoms typically found in schizophrenia. As the disorder worsens it is usual to encounter almost any pattern of functional mental illness. Depression with guilt and other preoccupations and delusions; mania with grandiose delusions and disturbance of behaviour; and typical schizophrenic passivity phenomena all occur – sometimes simultaneously, sometimes consecutively. Put another way, all four of the following clinical patterns occur: depressive, manic, mixed-affective and schizo-affective. In most cases, the eventual pattern is much more typical of affective illness than of schizophrenia.

Treatment

One consequence of the rapidly developing

psychiatric disorder may be severe disturbance of behaviour. With the baby as well as the mother to consider, it is important that appropriate care is urgently arranged. In general, admission to a psychiatric ward is necessary. The obvious question over such an admission is whether a mother, albeit one who is seriously unwell, should be separated from her new baby. There is no easy answer to this dilemma. In some places no choice is available; if the woman has to be admitted it must be without the child, who is looked after by family, or in a nearby paediatric ward or, more rarely, by temporary foster parents.

Some psychiatric wards have basic facilities for child-care and are prepared to accept the admission of the infant. This is not without problems and risk to the child. A mother who is deluded and behaviourally disturbed may constitute some danger; other severely disturbed patients on the ward may be a greater hazard. These risks are lessened by the establishment of facilities dedicated to the care of mothers and young babies. There needs to be adequate staff, both in number and expertise, to cater for mother and child. Part of the ward is set aside for nursery rooms. Also required are windows between rooms for appropriate levels of supervision, suitable sleeping accommodation and so on. Puerperal psychosis is not a common condition, but the incidence is such that health districts should set up such facilities, preferably in district general hospitals, or should arrange to share a facility with a neighbouring district.

In recent years one or two health districts have pioneered the care of puerperally psychotic women at home, trying to avoid admission even in states of severe disturbance. The disturbance may in any case be less in familiar home surroundings. Often, in the early stages of the condition, 24-hour care and attention will be necessary. In addition to family supervision it is therefore necessary to have on hand a team of staff: a senior psychiatrist, community psychiatric nurses – even, in some cases, one or more experienced and skilled volunteers.

A central principle of care is an attempt to establish or maintain the crucial relationship between mother and child, even where the condition of the mother makes it difficult to do so. Even if the patient's husband or her mother are caring for the baby and bringing the child in to visit daily, or if the child is on a nearby paediatric ward, the separation distresses the patient during all phases of the illness and makes it even harder to take up normal motherhood when she goes home.

The first step in medical treatment will often be the use of sedative neuroleptic drugs. They help both with the behavioural disturbance and with the delusions, hallucinations and motor abnormalities which have caused the disturbance. Chlorpromazine or thioridazine may be used in smaller doses than for an equivalent effect in a non-puerperal patient. Where there are clear depressive symptoms, the usual antidepressant drugs may be effective only slowly, if at all. ECT may be considered at an early stage: if depressive symptoms are prominent; if there is a poor response to neuroleptic drugs; or if there is serious concern about safety because of failure to drink or rest, and so on. Likewise, lithium carbonate may also be considered at an early stage in treatment, particularly where manic symptoms are conspicuous.

The issue of breast-feeding frequently presents a dilemma for patients, relatives and the psychiatrist. Probably a majority of puerperal psychotic patients have intended to breast-feed their child, and will still wish to do so. There are two main problems, assuming that the baby and mother are together. First, breast-feeding always demands great patience in order to sit still for long periods. The mother also has to be available even when tired, fed-up or distressed. To help seriously unwell mothers manage breast-feeding is a considerable challenge to all those involved. Second, the drugs prescribed for the treatment of puerperal psychosis may be excreted in the milk. This is particularly true of *lithium*, which is contra-indicated. Neuroleptics are used in modest doses, but with careful monitoring of the wakefulness of the infant. Antidepressants seem to be safe. Even in severe illness, breast-feeding can often be maintained, but it may be essential to express the milk and feed the child from a bottle on occasions – particularly in the early and most disturbed phase.

Outcome

The great majority of women recover fully from puerperal psychosis. The length of stay in hospital will often be as short as three or four weeks; less often a longer period, perhaps eight or ten weeks, is required. Although the delusions and other psychotic symptoms may go away within a few weeks, there is a tendency for more low-grade depressive features to linger. However, full recovery is the usual outcome. There is a substantial risk of relapse in the weeks following recovery, but this may be diminished by carefully titrated drug treatment over the next few months. As may be expected, considerable support is essential for the woman to become successfully re-established in her own home. Community nurses, general practitioners and others play a vital role in helping the woman and her husband and family.

When, as is sometimes the case, the woman with a puerperal psychosis has had a previous severe mental illness *not related to childbirth*, there are some additional points to make. First, her puerperal episode may have clinical features more like those of the previous episode than of the typical puerperal illness. However, even in someone with a non-puerperal history of schizophrenia, a puerperal episode of illness may often seem to be especially notable for mood symptoms. Second, the prognosis is different. For women with a first-ever episode in the puerperium, the likelihood of psychotic illness unrelated to childbirth is fairly low. This is not so for those with previous non-puerperal illness, where the prognosis remains that of the original disorder.

With further childbirth, the risk of repeat puerperal psychosis is high. Where there have already been two puerperal illnesses, recurrence after another childbirth is very likely. Research efforts are being made to find successful ways of minimizing risk in susceptible women.

Post-partum depression

Maternity blues are very common but generally require no specific intervention; puerperal psychosis is rare but requires active treatment. The third condition, post-partum depression, shares some of the features of the other two – it is fairly common *and* it is important in terms of disability and need for treatment. Estimates of the incidence and prevalence of post-partum depression vary, but several surveys have reported that over 10 per cent of women become depressed to a clinically severe degree in the three months after childbirth; some have found much higher rates.

Clinical features

Generally, post-partum depression does not begin as early as puerperal psychosis. It may start in the first week or so after delivery, but more typically it begins insidiously over the next few months. There is some dispute about whether, compared with non-puerperal women of similar age, the incidence of depressive illness is truly increased in the months following childbirth. There is, however, no doubt that the condition often fails to be diagnosed and is a cause of great, and sometimes prolonged, disability.

The clinical features of post-partum depression are similar to those seen in non-puerperal depressive illness. However, many symptoms such as distress, sleeplessness, extreme fatigue, change in appetite and weight, a succession of worries and preoccupations, and low libido are easily overlooked in the post-partum period because they may be thought to be a natural reaction to childbirth. Other features, such as anhedonia (loss of the pleasure response, see page 37), guilt and ideas of worthlessness, obsessional symptoms, agoraphobia, social withdrawal and so on, may not be noticed and the appropriate diagnosis not made. If the woman were to develop such a constellation of experiences and social disability at any other time of life, a depressive diagnosis might be made more readily.

Treatment of the illness is also similar to that undertaken with non-puerperal depression. Tricyclic antidepressant drugs are usually safe even with breast-feeding and are often effective. Many psychiatrists believe that ECT is indicated at an early stage in treatment because the condition seems to respond particularly well. The special circumstances surrounding a woman with a small child mean that there are many additional aspects to the care. Admission is especially difficult. Even special mother-and-baby units are not always helpful; once the child is more than a few months old, such a unit becomes an inappropriate place. Community nursing, day-care and other non-hospital options are widely used.

The outcome is generally good for post-partum depression that is identified and treated. Although it has a strong tendency to remit even without treatment, the problem with untreated cases is that many months, even years, of depression may ensue in the meantime. Severe, sometimes permanent, damage may be caused to many aspects of family life. Relationships with the partner, the baby and other children in the family may all suffer harm. The important bonding process between mother and child is impaired by prolonged depressed mood. It is therefore very important to identify the disorder and treat it, so that harm is prevented or minimized by every effort to produce early remission. Continuation treatment is also recommended in order to help prevent relapse over the first weeks and months following recovery.

Liaison with general hospital staff

Most of what has been said about liaison psychiatry so far in this chapter has been about specific conditions, symptoms and interventions. However, much of the work of psychiatry in the general hospital is the process of liaison with other staff. A good working relationship with other medical staff depends upon prompt and effective help for patients referred, and clear and helpful communication with the staff. In addition, however, liaison psychiatrists sometimes form definite associations with certain hospital teams. This chapter ends with a brief indication of some of the benefits which can arise from liaison which extends beyond individual patient consultations.

- Patients may be seen in *combined clinics*, in which a psychiatrist and another specialist see the patient together or, more often, hold the joint clinic in nearby rooms. This emphasizes to the patient the role of the psychiatrist as part of the medical management. This can be particularly appropriate in management of certain complaints – for example, unexplained dermatological symptoms – where patients will often be reluctant to visit a psychiatric clinic.
- Where the liaison psychiatrist has an established link with another team, staff other than senior doctors have access to refer cases. An opportunity is thereby created for all members of the team to observe and discuss matters related to adjustment to illness, unexplained symptoms and so on – with potential benefits to patients.
- Some areas of hospital medical practice place particular stresses on the staff; intensive care, oncology and renal units are examples. The regular involvement of the liaison psychiatrist with patients on the unit can provide opportunities for staff to acknowledge some of the difficulties they face when carrying out their work. Regular staff meetings with the psychiatrist present have developed successfully on some units. Where staff are able to accept the emotional difficulties inherent in their work, they may find it easier to acknowledge and identify emotional problems and psychiatric symptoms in their patients.

Further reading

Creed, F.H. and Pfeffer, J.M. (1982) *Medicine and Psychiatry: A Practical Approach*, London: Pitman.

House, A.O. (1989) 'Hypochondriasis and related disorders: assessment and management of patients referred for a psychiatric opinion', *General Hospital Psychiatry*, 11: 156–65.

Lipowski, Z.J. (1969) 'Psychosocial aspects of disease', *Annals of Internal Medicine*, 71: 1197–1206.

Lloyd, G.G. (1991) *Textbook of General Hospital Psychiatry*, Edinburgh: Churchill Livingstone.

Oates, M.R. (ed.) (1989) *Psychological Aspects of Obstetrics and Gynaecology. Clinical Obstetrics and Gynaecology: International Practice and Research*, vol. 3, no. 4, London: Baillière Tindall.

17

Deliberate self-harm and suicide

Non-fatal deliberate self-harm

Suicides have been recorded throughout history, and there is little reason to believe that the present rate is grossly different from that in past generations. The same cannot be said for non-fatal deliberate self-harm, where rates have greatly increased during the last half-century. In the United Kingdom there were few systematic accounts of self-harm until the 1950s; before then it was regarded as a rarity. Some recovered, but it was understood that, particularly when poisons were consumed, acts of deliberate self-harm were intended to be lethal. Self-poisoning as a method of self-harm was uncommon and the use of therapeutic drugs rather than poisons was rare. The recorded number of non-fatal suicide attempts exceeded that of actual suicides for the first time in the late 1940s. Throughout the 1950s and 1960s there continued to be a steady increase in the number of such episodes throughout the United Kingdom and in other western countries. For example, in Sheffield, there was a six-fold increase in self-poisoning between 1955 and 1966, associated with a conspicuous rise among patients aged under 30.

Whereas rates of non-fatal self-harm, particularly self-poisoning, were increasing, successful suicide was decreasing in frequency. The ratio of attempted suicide to completed suicide was therefore growing. While in the first post-war decade it was thought that they occurred equally often, by the 1970s it was suggested that the gap between non-fatal events and suicide had widened to between 10:1 and 30:1.

The law and attempted suicide – changing attitudes

Until 1961 attempted suicide was an offence in England and Wales. Between 1946 and 1955 almost 50,000 attempted suicides were known to the police in England and Wales. Of these, only about one person in eight was brought to trial. However, almost all of these were found guilty; two-thirds were placed on probation and 7 per cent were imprisoned. Custodial sentences continued to be handed down to a minority of cases until 1959, shortly before the law was changed. The law in Scotland was more humane, and attempted suicide was never an offence. Pressure to change the law came from many directions, including a powerful lobby from the medical profession, magistrates, the Church and the press.

During the passage through Parliament of the Suicide Act (1961), the Lord Chancellor announced that arrangements were being made to ensure that persons brought to hospital having attempted suicide were examined by a psychiatrist, who would consider whether treatment or supervision was needed. Accordingly, a short memorandum was sent to Regional

Hospital Boards a few weeks after the passage of the Act. In that document, psychiatric factors were described as being of major importance in most cases of attempted suicide. Hospital authorities were asked 'to do their best to see that all cases of attempted suicide brought to a hospital received psychiatric investigation before discharge'. This recommendation has been the prevailing influence in the hospital care of deliberate self-harm patients since that time, although the Department of Health's recommendations became more flexible in 1984. All hospitals are expected to have a clear policy, but while every patient should receive a 'psycho-social assessment', this need no longer be made by a psychiatrist, but may be carried out by another member of staff with appropriate training and supervision.

Trends in non-fatal deliberate self-harm

During the 1970s, in what was described as an epidemic of self-poisoning, dire predictions were made concerning the future of acute medical facilities. It was estimated in 1977 that there were at least 100,000 admissions in the United Kingdom each year, with almost one in three medical emergencies due to self-poisoning. The prediction was made that if trends continued, all acute medical beds would be required for self-poisoning patients by the year 1984. Fortunately, admissions reached a plateau around 1978 and there was a small reduction in the yearly rate over the next ten years, although rates have increased again slightly in the late 1980s and early 1990s.

Over the last twenty years the pressure due to the numbers of cases has led in many parts of the country to a change in assessment policy. A number of physicians have felt that it was unreasonable to refer to a psychiatric team every case admitted under their care. There has been decreasing availability of acute medical beds, and research has suggested that non-psychiatric doctors, nurses and social workers, when given satisfactory and specific training, are well able to assess these patients. It may be, therefore, that some of the reduction in admissions results from general practitioners referring

fewer patients to hospital, or accident and emergency departments admitting a smaller proportion to medical wards.

Whatever the current pattern, there is still a very large number of such patients attending doctors each year. It remains one of the commonest reasons for emergency consultation at hospital – the most frequent medical reason for admission of females, and the second commonest reason for admission of men (behind coronary heart disease). All hospitals should have in place a policy about the assessment and admission of such patients.

Deliberate self-harm: clinical epidemiology

At present, about 90 per cent of episodes of deliberate self-harm are due to poisoning. Self-inflicted injury – for example, skin laceration – is responsible for less than 10 per cent of cases. Throughout the rest of this section on non-fatal deliberate self-harm, information largely refers to self-poisoning, although in many cases it also applies to self-injury. The pattern of substances ingested has varied over the years. In recent times there has been an increase in the use of non-opiate analgesics, such as aspirin and other non-steroidal anti-inflammatory drugs, but most noticeably *paracetamol*. These drugs now constitute the single largest category, and well over half of all patients take such a drug. Minor tranquillizers are the next commonest group. Antidepressant drugs account for a substantial proportion of cases (see Figure 17.1). Almost a quarter of patients take miscellaneous drugs such as oral contraceptives, antibiotics and many others. About one-third of self-poisoning patients consume more than one drug. There is a relation between age and drugs taken; analgesics are particularly popular among younger patients.

Alcohol consumption is commonplace around the time of self-poisoning. When seen at hospital, about half of the men and one-third of the women have taken alcohol in the preceding few hours. Deliberate self-poisoning is much more common amongst young people than amongst the elderly (see Figure 17.2). In the 1960s and 1970s self-poisoning was much more

Drug type

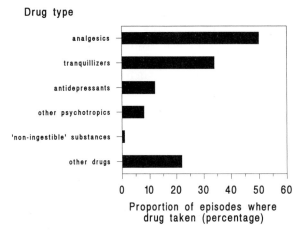

Figure 17.1 Drugs taken in deliberate self-poisoning episodes

proportion of episodes (%)

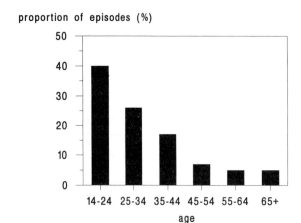

Figure 17.2 Age and self-poisoning

common in females than males – often reported in a ratio of 2:1 or more. Since then there has been a gradual equalizing of the sex ratio. For example, of all the self-harm patients referred to psychiatrists in Leeds General Infirmary for the year 1991, exactly half were male. Most reports, however, still suggest a slight excess of females. In general, the female to male ratio lies between 1.5:1 and 1:1.

Rates of self-poisoning are inversely proportional to socio-economic status; those of lowest social class have the highest rates.

Clinical aspects of self-harm

Reasons for self-harm

Episodes of self-harm often arise soon after stressful events. Conflicts, rows and splits within close relationships are much the commonest precipitating events. Others include problems at work, school or college, and involvement as the victim of accidents, violence and crime.

Occasionally, such events seem to have been the sole reason for the self-harm. Much more often, however, long-standing difficulties are also present. Common and important problems include:

- unemployment;
- work dissatisfaction;
- marital disharmony;
- conflict with parents or children;
- debt;
- housing problems;
- legal problems;
- social isolation;
- physical health problems;
- bereavement.

A minority of episodes are a consequence of psychiatric illness; in such cases depressive illness is much the commonest condition, but self-harm quite frequently occurs in schizophrenia.

Outcome

Many patients repeat self-poisoning. Research studies show that between 12 and 25 per cent do so during the year following an episode. Repetition is most likely over the first few weeks or months. It is more likely amongst those who already have a history of previous episodes, and in those who have had some kind of psychiatric care, whether recently or in the more distant past. Patients with alcohol or drug problems, those who are unemployed, and those in whom there is evidence of antisocial or criminal behaviour are also more likely to repeat.

Fortunately, a much smaller proportion of self-harm patients proceed to successful suicide.

Over the year following a self-harm episode the suicide rate is about 1 per cent. Recent figures suggest that this proportion rises to about 3 per cent over eight years of follow-up (Hawton and Catalan 1987). Although comparatively small, this risk is far higher than that of the general population and, because deliberate self-harm is so common, accounts for many cases. Subsequent suicide is more likely amongst those with a history of previous episodes, past psychiatric contact and past admission to a psychiatric ward. It is also more likely in men, those who are older, those in poor physical health, those who are unemployed and those who live alone.

Assessment of deliberate self-harm patients

When the physical aspects of deliberate self-harm have been dealt with, each patient requires a *psychosocial assessment*. There are two essential prerequisites for an adequate interview. First, the patient should not be physically unfit – for example, drowsy, delirious or vomiting. Second, the person carrying out the assessment – whether a psychiatrist, another doctor or other professional – needs to be properly equipped for the task. That means that the setting must allow for private conversation, and the assessor must be specifically trained as well as have appropriate supervision and time.

The objectives of assessment are:

- to understand what happened before and during the event;
- to evaluate the suicidal intent of the episode;
- to estimate the degree of further risk;
- to identify treatable psychiatric illness;
- to identify continuing social, emotional and interpersonal problems.

These aspects of the case overlap. In practice it is important to take a history which has the elements of the usual psychiatric history and mental state examination (see Chapter 3). In addition, particular attention is paid to the circumstances of the self-harm when appraising the *suicidal intent* of the episode:

- Was the subject alone and likely to so remain for some time?

- Were precautions taken against being discovered?
- Did the subject seek any help during or after the attempt?
- Was the attempt planned and prepared for before it took place?
- Did the subject make any final arrangements (wills, financial accounts and so on) or leave any messages for others?

In addition, it is important to gain a clear idea of the patient's own view of intent. Did he hope to die? Did he think it likely? The Beck Suicide Intent Scale (Beck *et al.* 1974) can be useful in clinical practice (it is reproduced in Hawton and Catalan 1987). Of course, the assessment is not complete until the patient's *current* wish about living or dying has been established.

It is always important to gain as much information as possible from an informant, relative or friend, but especially when a patient is very drowsy or in coma.

Management

When the assessment is completed it will be clear that some patients require no additional help. More often, however, continuing problems, further risk, mental illness or a combination of these will have been identified. The next step depends on the features identified.

- A minority, especially those with clear psychiatric illness such as depression or schizophrenia, will require *psychiatric inpatient care*. Psychiatric admission may also be required where high intent and continuing risk are prominent – even when psychiatric illness is not evident. In some cases admission may be a valuable way of clarifying the degree of illness and risk. Very occasionally patients will need admission on a compulsory basis (see Chapter 24). Quite often, a psychiatric day hospital may provide a suitable setting for further assessment and treatment.
- Psychiatric *outpatient follow-up* is useful on occasions, but because appointments made are often several weeks hence, and with a doctor different from the person who carried

Table 17.1   *Examples of helping agencies*

Agencies	Characteristics
Self-help organizations	offer help to people with specific problems (e.g., CRUSE for those who are widowed); families in which there are medical problems (e.g., the Huntington's Disease Association for Huntington's chorea sufferers and their families); facilities to help carers (e.g., Alzheimer's Disease Society).
Crisis centres	provide a rapid response to crisis, offering intensive short-term counselling; may be funded by Social Services or other public funds.
Counselling centres	offer counselling, usually brief, but sometimes longer-term; may be targeted at specific groups (such as women) or at particular types of problem (such as distress associated with past sexual abuse).
Citizens' Advice Bureaux	offer many services, including welfare rights information, legal advice and help with tackling debt.
Community Mental Health Teams	In some areas mental health teams will rapidly assess and offer help from an appropriate team member, such as a social worker, psychologist, community nurse or psychiatrist.

out the initial assessment, these appointments have a high rate of default and can be of limited value unless special care is taken over the arrangements.

- Often of more practical benefit is the offer of *immediate help for the problems* identified. The person who carries out the assessment may either arrange for help to be provided by others or undertake the work personally. There is a substantial role for a wide range of other agencies, such as those set out in Table 17.1: each of these offers special kinds of help. The effective assessor is aware of the facilities available in his or her own geographical area, and how to contact them so as to arrange a rapid response.

Suicide

Epidemiology

The epidemiology of completed suicide differs from that of non-fatal deliberate self-harm in several important ways. First, suicide is much less common. The overall annual rate per 100,000 UK population (averaged for five-year periods) rose from about 13 after World War II to 15 in the late 1950s, dropped to a low point of 10 in the early 1970s and has been rising

slightly since. Over this same post-war period, males have been continually over-represented by a ratio of up to 2:1. Suicide rates are higher in older age-bands, with a peak in those aged 65–80 years. In recent years, the rates amongst women have fallen slightly, while rates amongst younger men have risen. Altogether, suicide accounts for about 10 per cent of all deaths in England and Wales.

Methods used for suicide show striking sex differences. In the 1980s for England and Wales the three commonest methods amongst *men*, in descending frequency, were: hanging (and other methods of asphyxiation), carbon monoxide poisoning, and poisoning by ingestion (mostly therapeutic drugs). Amongst *women*, poisoning by ingestion was much the commonest method, followed by hanging and asphyxiation. In both sexes all other methods were relatively rare.

In social terms, suicide is commonest among those in the lowest socio-economic group (V) and also more frequent than expected in the highest socio-economic group (I). It has been observed for a long time that the rate is high among the medical profession. Durkheim, the French sociologist, proposed in 1897 that suicide was related to social cohesion in society; his views remain well respected. Modern studies tend to affirm such connections; broadly speaking – less social cohesion, more suicides.

Psychiatric disorder and suicide

Studies of completed suicides have repeatedly found that in a high proportion of cases, the person has been affected by psychiatric disorder. In perhaps a half of suicides there has been previous psychiatric contact; many have been psychiatric inpatients in the past. Many have a psychiatric illness at the time of the suicide. Three conditions are particularly important. First and most prevalent is *depressive illness*. Second, *schizophrenia* is also well represented. However, although suicide occurs in a substantial minority of patients, because schizophrenia is much less prevalent than depressive illness, it leads to fewer suicides. Third, *alcohol dependence* has a strong association with suicide. Not only psychiatric disorder, but also *physical illness* has a higher than expected prevalence amongst suicides.

In the case of patients with any of these three conditions, it is important to keep the possibility of future suicide under consideration. The doctor must be able to discuss the matter when the occasion demands it. This issue was discussed in some detail in relation to depressive illness (see page 46). Remarks made there are equally relevant when talking with patients with schizophrenia, alcohol dependence or any other disorder.

Suicide is at all ages a significant cause of death. It has an important relation to both psychiatric illness and to non-fatal episodes of self-harm. Rising European rates of suicide and non-fatal self-harm are among the thirty-eight targets for the World Health Organization's 'Health for All 2000' initiative. Suicide reduction is also a target in the United Kingdom Government's 1992 'Health of the Nation' programme. There can be little doubt that, whilst it is difficult to plan how to reduce rates of non-fatal self-harm, suicide rates can be minimized by appropriate identification and treatment of depression and other psychiatric conditions. It is also likely that improved intervention with non-fatal, deliberate self-harm patients will reduce repetition and suicide.

Further reading

Beck, A.T., Schuyler, D. and Herman, J. (1974) 'Development of suicidal intent scales', in *The Prediction of Suicide*, A.T. Beck, H.L.P. Resnick and D.J. Lettierite (eds), Maryland; Charles Press.

Hawton, K. and Catalan, J. (1987) *Attempted Suicide: A Practical Guide to its Nature and Management*, 2nd edn, Oxford: Oxford University Press.

Hawton, K. and Fagg, J. (1992) 'Trends in deliberate self-poisoning and self-injury in Oxford 1976–90', *British Medical Journal*, 304: 1409–11.

House, A., Owens, D. and Storer, D. (1992) 'Psychosocial intervention following attempted suicide: is there a case for better services?' *International Review of Psychiatry* 4: 15–22.

Morgan, H.G. (1982) 'Deliberate self-harm', in *Recent Advances in Clinical Psychiatry*, vol. 3, K. Granville-Grossman (ed.), Edinburgh: Churchill Livingstone.

18

Psychiatry of old age

Throughout this century, in most countries, demographic changes have led to a great increase in both the actual number of old people and their proportion of the population. There are at least two reasons why these demographic trends have resulted in the development of special psychiatric services for old people. First, compared with younger age-groups, old people have different and often extra problems – for example, physical health problems and social difficulties. Second, in old age there are mental disorders which have greater prevalence and sometimes different features. This chapter will examine these aspects of the psychiatry of old age.

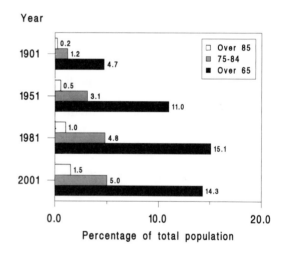

Figure 18.1 Proportion of old people in the population

Demographic trends

At the beginning of this century people aged 65 or over accounted for about 5 per cent of the UK population; the proportion now is three times greater. Figure 18.1 illustrates this trend; projections for the near future suggest no further increase. However, the proportion of the population who are 85 years and over is still increasing: at the beginning of the new century the proportion will be 50 per cent higher than it was at the start of the 1980s.

Physical problems in old age

All the physical disorders whose prevalence increases with advancing age – heart disease, respiratory disease, malignancy, arthritis and so on – have psychological and social repercussions. Some health problems – especially failing hearing and eyesight, and increased immobility due to locomotor or other debilitating problems

– are particularly associated with increasing *isolation*.

Infirmity results from disease but also from treatment; many drugs taken by old people for therapeutic reasons have unwanted and disabling effects. The list of such drugs is almost endless but includes treatments related to physical illness (for example, digoxin or antihypertensives), psychiatric illness (for example, antidepressants or anticholinergic agents), and no illness at all (for example, benzodiazepines for insomnia).

Social difficulties in old age

Some people do not respond well to *retirement*. Work not only passes the time and provides income, it also brings a person into daily contact with other people. Where there are few family roles and little in the way of hobbies or other outside interests, retirement can lead to a sense of futility and lack of purpose. The enforced change in daily pattern brought about by retirement requires adaptation not only by the retired person but by other members of the household; friction – temporary or sometimes permanent – between wife and husband is not uncommon. For some, *loss of earnings* can be considerable. Even amongst some of those who have contributory pensions, the rise in the cost of living can soon erode a fixed income or one which is subject only to meagre increments. Real *poverty* can and does occur – for some, for the first time in their lives. Living standards, *nutrition*, ability to travel and meet family or friends may all decline.

Social isolation readily develops in old age. For some, with family already living at a distance, it may come about gradually as friends move away or die. For others it may happen more suddenly with the arrival of *widowhood*. Some people retire to another part of the country, often one with a better climate or a rural or coastal setting. This action sometimes results in loss of availability of friends or family, difficulties in striking up new and constructive relationships, and often poor mobility due to geographic isolation.

Of those aged 65 years and over, a little over one-third live with a spouse in a two-person household, whilst a little under one-third live alone. Seven out of ten, therefore, live in households with no one else under that age. However, those in any form of residential accommodation – hospital or residential home for the elderly – are numbered at well under 10 per cent of the total. Infirmity affects a substantial proportion of over-65s: one in three cannot carry out a household task which requires climbing steps; one in seven are unable to do their own shopping; one in ten cannot leave home and walk down the road alone (General Household Survey, 1980). The proportions with such difficulties are, of course, greater in older age-bands.

The mental disorders of old age

In old age, almost all the mental disorders of adult life may occur. In most cases, the disorders have already been considered in earlier chapters. Emphasized here are those which are common, or different in form, or easily overlooked.

First, as pointed out above, old people are particularly likely to suffer *physical disease*. It is an important axiom that mental disorders are closely associated with such ill health. For example, physical disease may *cause* delirium or dementia, *precipitate* depressive illness or *result from* alcohol dependence. The mental disorders directly arising from organic disease are considered first.

Delirium

Delirium (synonyms: acute confusional state, acute organic reaction, acute brain syndrome) may occur at any age (see Chapter 7) but is particularly prevalent amongst old people. It is most likely when a degree of dementia is already present.

Clinical features

In medical training it is a familiar aphorism that it is the *history* rather than the examination or special tests which holds the key to diagnosis; nowhere is this principle more true than in the assessment of a confused patient. Of course, the history will often need to be taken from a relative rather than from the patient. Of all the features of the case, it is the short duration of confusion which most suggests a primary diagnosis of delirium. Because many causes of delirium are reversible, and because there may be a tendency to regard confusion or memory difficulty as signifying the presence of dementia, this point requires emphasis when dealing with old people.

In the elderly the clinical findings are similar to those in younger adults (see Table 18.1). The presence of some of the clinical features outlined in Table 18.1, together with a history of brief duration, may be enough to establish the presence of delirium even when no cause is apparent. However, there will often be clear indications why delirium has developed. There are many causes, and Table 18.2 sets out some of the common or important ones in old age (Table 18.2 is an abbreviated version of Table 7.5).

Management

Identification and treatment of the underlying physical disorder is clearly fundamental. This process will often require inpatient care, preferably on a ward where there is medical as well as psychiatric expertise and ready availability of laboratory, neurophysiological and radiological investigation. Elderly patients with delirium require nursing care in the same manner as described for other patients (see Chapter 7). The course depends a good deal upon the primary condition; delirium may clear as the patient improves from the physical disorder. On the other hand, the underlying physical disease is sometimes serious and may lead to further deterioration or, in some cases, to death. A proportion of patients develop a chronic state; in such cases it often emerges that there was an undetected element of dementia prior to the onset of delirium.

Dementia

Dementia (synonym: chronic brain syndrome) is a clinical syndrome, resulting from disease of the brain, in which there is impairment of many of the identifiable components of higher cortical function. It may occur at any time in adult life, but it has a much higher incidence in old people,

Table 18.1 *Clinical features of delirium*

Consciousness and attention	From mild inability to focus or sustain attention through to severe drowsiness or coma; often fluctuating in severity
Perception	Distortions, illusions or hallucinations; in any sensory modality, but most noticeably visual
Thinking	Impairment of comprehension and grasp of abstract concepts
Belief	Transient delusions often occur
Memory	New learning and recall of recent memory are impaired. Remote memory may be relatively unaffected
Orientation	Disorientation, especially in time but also in place and person
Motor activity	Restless over-activity, apathetic under-activity and fluctuation from one to the other; perseveration of action; apraxia; visuo-spatial deficits
Language	Dysarthria, aphasia, perseveration of speech, comprehension deficits
Sleep pattern	Disruption of any kind, but especially nocturnal wakefulness followed by daytime drowsiness
Emotion	Distress – whether anxiety, fear, depression, irritability, hostility or perplexity; euphoria is less common

Table 18.2 *Some common or important physical causes of delirium in the elderly*

Traumatic	head injury
	sub-dural haematoma
Neoplastic	primary cerebral tumour
	cerebral secondaries
	systemic non-metastatic effects
Vascular	stroke and transient ischaemic attacks
	sub-arachnoid haemorrhage
	myocardial infarction
Metabolic	uraemia
	hepatic encephalopathy
	hypoglycaemia
	anoxia
	dehydration and electrolyte disturbance
	thiamine (B1), vitamin B12 or folate deficiency
Infective	chest infection
	urinary infection
	intra-cranial infection (meningitis/encephalitis)
	viraemia and septicaemia
Epileptic	aura preceding seizure
	complex partial seizure
	post-ictal state
Endocrine	hypothyroidism and hyperthyroidism
Drug toxicity and withdrawal	anticholinergic drugs (including tricyclic antidepressants)
	all tranquillizers, especially benzodiazepines and barbiturates
	steroids
	L-dopa
	anticonvulsants
	antihypertensives
	digoxin
	diuretics
	Substance use: for example, alcohol
	Poisoning: many substances, including carbon monoxide

where prevalence is directly associated with age (Table 18.3). It is usually chronic and progressive.

The most common cause of dementia in old people is *Alzheimer's disease* (synonym: senile dementia of the Alzheimer type), accounting for around half of all cases. *Vascular dementia* (synonyms: arteriosclerotic dementia, multi-infarct dementia) and *mixed cases* of Alzheimer's and vascular dementia account for most of the rest. In the elderly, other causes of dementia outlined in Chapter 7 form only a small proportion of all instances.

Table 18.3 *Age-specific rates of dementia*

Age	Prevalence of dementia (%)
65–69	2
70–74	3
75–79	6
80+	22

Source: Practical Psychiatry of Old Age (Wattis and Church 1986)

Clinical features

Dementia results in many neuropsychiatric abnormalities (Table 18.4). In some patients there will be global impairment of all these

Table 18.4 *Clinical features of dementia*

Orientation	Disorientation in time, place and person.
Attention/concentration	Poor ability to attend to a task or manipulate information.
Thinking	Impairment of comprehension, grasp of abstract concepts and judgement.
Memory	New learning and recall of recent memory are impaired. Remote memory is also affected, but may be relatively spared during the early phase of the illness.
Language	*Aphasia*: characterized in the early stage by mild expressive problems such as word-finding or naming difficulty; later, in more severe cases may include receptive difficulty. *Writing* and *reading* may also be affected. *Perseveration* may occur.
Visuo-spatial function	Spatial disorientation; deficits in distinguishing left and right.
Motor activity	Either restless over-activity or apathetic under-activity may occur (rapid fluctuation from one to the other is usually associated with coexisting delirium). *Apraxia* may occur, such that simple tasks like dressing or eating become impossible.
Consciousness	Not usually affected unless there is coexisting delirium.
Sleep pattern	Nocturnal wakefulness is common.
Perception	*Recognition* of places and persons may be impaired. Distortions, illusions and hallucinations are not usually present unless there is coexisting delirium.
Belief	False beliefs, if present, are usually directly attributable to failures of grasp and recognition.
Emotion	Emotions may be relatively normal or increasingly labile; some patients become very distressed.

elements but, especially in early cases, the deficits may be patchy. Unlike delirium, it is not usual for consciousness to be diminished or fluctuating.

Except in advanced cases, many of the features of dementia outlined in Table 18.4 may be apparent only on careful enquiry or testing. Forgetfulness, noticed either by the patient or by others, is often the first prominent sign of the illness. What has seemed to be merely absent-mindedness worsens. Memory deficits become more striking and later disabling or dangerous. For example, a person may first become unreliable at remembering appointments or arrangements, then repetitive in questions or anecdotes, and only later a safety risk with cookers and fires.

Occasionally, dementia may come to light through loss of self-control leading to uncharacteristic acts such as violence or inappropriate sexual actions. Shop-lifting by an elderly person with no previous record may reveal the presence of dementia.

Advanced dementia is usually associated with physical changes. Weight loss can be considerable and may be accompanied by acceleration of loss and depigmentation of hair, and development of wrinkled, inelastic skin. Movement is often weak and poorly coordinated. Extrapyramidal abnormalities such as rigidity and tremor of limbs and head, and dyskinesias (especially bucco-lingual-masticatory dyskinesias) are common. Epileptic seizures occur in a substantial minority of patients with chronic dementia. Amongst the most unfortunate features of advanced states are incontinence of urine and of faeces.

Specific types of dementia

Alzheimer's disease is characterized by an

insidious onset, often indistinguishable at first from normal ageing, and by a slowly progressive course. Localizing neurological signs are not usually evident until the disease is at an advanced stage. The pathological process is of unknown cause. There is substantial loss of neurones throughout the brain, especially in limbic, temporo-parietal and frontal areas. Neuro-imaging has demonstrated in live patients what has been apparent for many years post-mortem, that there is clear shrinkage of brain substance with widening of sulci and enlarging of ventricles. Histopathological examination reveals neuro-fibrillary tangles and plaques of amyloid. There is also deficiency of cholinergic neuro-transmitters.

Vascular dementia typically has abrupt onset, is accompanied by neurological deficits at an early stage, and shows step-wise rather than steady progression. The intellectual deficits are often more patchy than with Alzheimer's disease, and emotional lability may be a striking feature. Some patients show fluctuations in conscious level, particularly at night. In a typical case the patient may have established hypertension and may previously have suffered transient ischaemic attacks or completed strokes. The dementia results from multiple infarcts and is but one manifestation of more widespread vascular disease. The diagnosis may sometimes be confirmed when neuro-imaging reveals evidence of these infarcts.

Distinguishing these dementias is difficult in practice for two reasons: there is overlap of clinical features, and coexistence of the two disorders is common. The clinical features of the less common dementias are described in Chapter 7.

Management

Apart from measures to reduce risk of further vascular episodes, for most cases of dementia there is no pharmacological intervention of established benefit – neither to treat the disorder nor to prevent additional impairment. The two principles of management are *identification and treatment of reversible disorders* and *practical social measures* to avert unnecessary deterioration.

Reversible conditions such as delirium or depression may coexist with dementia. If so, their successful treatment will reduce disability, despite continued presence of dementia. However, both delirium and depression can also produce a clinical state of confusion which may be *mistaken* for dementia. It is therefore imperative that the doctor considers these alternative diagnoses before deciding in favour of dementia. Depression imitating dementia is described in the next section. Almost any coexisting physical ailment may compromise function in dementia, but hypothyroidism, vitamin B12 deficiency, anaemia and constipation are all relatively common and important; they should be identified and treated.

There are many practical steps which may help prevent unnecessary worsening. For example, it is important to ensure that *hearing* and *eyesight* are functioning at maximal level. Disorientation in dementia is worsened by a *change of environment*; for example, by removal from home to hospital or residential care. Provision of services to the home of the patient with dementia is often preferable to care elsewhere. Nevertheless, inpatient or day-hospital care may be required for assessment or other reasons. Social Services day centres may provide regular hours of respite for a spouse, daughter, son or other carer. Longer periods of respite care, for one or more weeks, are sometimes provided by residential homes or hospitals. Whatever the setting, familiar people and familiar possessions help orientation. Conversely, much damage to function can result from an institutional environment without personal effects.

Wandering can lead to danger and an intolerable burden on the vigilance of carers. Together with restless agitation, and occasionally aggression, it may be an indication for sedative drug prescription. However, all sedative drugs have the propensity to reduce function further and, on occasions, worsen confusion and agitation. Other methods for reducing unwanted behaviours should therefore be tried before resort to medication.

Depression

The standard symptoms of depression in younger adults are also commonplace in old people. However, it can be more difficult in the elderly to decide when these experiences add up to depressive illness. For example, it is not unusual for an old person who is widowed to gain little enjoyment from day-to-day activities, to be rather pessimistic about the future, to worry about safety, health and finance, to sleep and eat poorly, and so on. As with younger patients, care in eliciting the circumstances of the case will usually determine whether depressive illness is present. Depressive illness is common in old age; it is the most prevalent psychiatric disorder treated among patients aged 65–75.

Clinical features

In general, the clinical features of depression in old age are similar to those in younger age-groups. Somatic physical complaints are probably more frequent in older patients. Suicide is also more common (see Chapter 17). Compared with younger depressed patients, in old age a higher proportion of patients develop *psychotic symptoms*: particularly delusions, agitation and psycho-motor retardation.

Delusions of poverty and illness are particularly prominent themes in severely depressed elderly patients. One elderly man, whose wife had died of a carcinoma of the oesophagus one year previously, when he became depressed developed the conviction that he could not swallow solids or liquids, despite radiological evidence to the contrary. This delusion, which led to serious difficulties in managing his fluid balance, disappeared when the depressive illness was treated.

Although some depressed elderly patients become retarded, mute or stuporose – as may younger patients – it is their propensity to develop a state of restless *agitation* which is especially notable. The agitation affects thinking as well as activity. In a typical case, the patient may constantly worry about minor matters, to the exclusion of normal activities. Such a state is often accompanied by motor restlessness. One elderly man with recurrent depression on each occasion developed pacing, muttering and hand-wringing, together with worries about his pension which became delusional in intensity (this patient's delusions were described in more detail on page 39).

An important aspect of depression in old age is how it may mimic dementia. Particularly where there is retardation – with inhibition of mental functioning such that concentration, memory and other intellectual faculties are impaired – the depressive illness can easily be mistaken for dementia. Even careful history-taking can be misleading because the depression may have an insidious onset, and sadness and other aspects of mood may be masked by the intellectual and motor abnormalities. This condition, sometimes termed *'depressive pseudodementia'*, may resolve completely when the underlying depression is successfully treated.

Management

The treatment of depression in old age is similar to that in younger patients. The important point to stress is that whilst older patients are more likely to develop side effects of antidepressant drugs, they are nevertheless likely to respond to effective treatment. Careful titration of dose of suitable drugs is required.

ECT is beneficial in some cases. Compared with drug treatment there may be fewer side effects, it is more effective in treating psychotic symptoms and it acts more rapidly. There are therefore occasions when it may be the treatment of choice, especially when stupor or severe agitation are endangering life. Compared with younger depressed patients there is probably a higher risk of suicide – another pressing indication for active treatment.

Mania occurs in old age but it is not common. It may arise as a first-ever event or in patients who have suffered bipolar affective disorder for many years. Its clinical features and the principles of its treatment are similar to those in younger patients; drug doses are much lower.

Persecutory states

For many years there has been argument about the nature of a persecutory disorder which develops in a small but significant proportion of old people. This disorder, known by some (including Kraepelin) as *late paraphrenia*, has features in common with schizophrenia, persistent delusional disorders and organic delusional disorders. It is not surprising that some regard it as a separate syndrome, others as merely the way in which schizophrenia presents for the first time in later life, and others as an essentially organic disorder. The issue remains unclear; the condition will be described here and called 'paraphrenia', but no attempt will be made to define its disease status. In ICD-10, it is not accorded a separate category but is included with persistent delusional disorders.

The typical patient with paraphrenia develops the disorder for the first time in old age. The patient's general character is unchanged and mood is not conspicuously abnormal. The complaint lies in persecutory beliefs, often in the form of a system of delusions. There may also be hallucinations, including clear-consciousness voices commenting on the person's actions, and there may be passivity experiences (see Chapter 6). One patient came to believe that tiny people were following her around; she could not see them but could hear them conversing, saying abusive things about her. She called the tiny people 'silent robbers' and thought that they flew around on miniature tape-recorders. In all other ways this lady was normal; she had a lively and friendly demeanour and intact intellectual function. A common theme in cases of paraphrenia is of interference from neighbours, involving processes such as surveillance devices, and rays which shine through the walls and affect the patient's body in some way.

These syndromes are more prevalent among those who are socially isolated, including those who have had a tendency to isolation or poor relationships throughout adult life. There have been many reports suggesting a greater frequency in those who have impaired hearing. Persecutory delusions can also occur in affective and organic psychoses; a substantial proportion of persecutory states in old age are due to one or other of these.

Where the disorder does not seem secondary to mood or organic disorder, the treatment is usually with neuroleptic drugs – seeking to avoid sedation and to minimize extra-pyramidal symptoms. Some patients gain remission, many experience improvement, but there is a sizeable minority for whom the symptoms continue with some force.

Other disorders

Many of the conditions encountered in psychiatric practice are manifest early in life; some persist over many years. It follows that among a population of old people are some who have behind them many years of psychiatric problems. It is relatively unusual for certain conditions, such as anxiety, phobias or obsessions (and almost unknown for others, such as anorexia or bulimia) to *develop* in old age. Where they do, they often turn out to be symptomatic of another disorder – particularly depressive illness, which *does* often begin in old age.

One difficulty warrants a special mention because it is so readily overlooked in the elderly: harmful use of and dependence on *alcohol*. In all age-groups alcohol problems are very often concealed, perhaps especially so in the elderly. It may be falls or other accidents, subdural haematomas, or alcoholic dementia which draw attention to the problem.

Further reading

Office of Population Censuses and Surveys. *General Household Survey, 1980*, London: HMSO.
Wattis, J. and Church, M. (1986) *Practical Psychiatry of Old Age*, London: Croom Helm.

19

Child and adolescent psychiatry

Although the similarities are obvious, so also are the differences between the practice of adult and child psychiatry. The relationship between the two is rather like that between paediatrics and medicine; some of the conditions treated are similar but many are quite different, and the approach to the patient is necessarily conducted in a different way. However, the essential academic bases are held in common. This chapter is only a minimal introduction, and the reader is strongly advised to read a textbook of child psychiatry for further information as it is impossible to convey either the interest or the complexity of the subject in a brief account. Some of the diagnostic terms used in child psychiatry are shown in Table 19.1.

We hope that the reader is already convinced that the social situation is always important in psychiatry, and this is especially true for child psychiatry. Social influences and their psychological consequences are especially important in the cause and course of childhood disorders. Of particular significance are discordant relationships within the family including hostility, violence, quarrelling and tensions, and also over-involvement of the parents with the child. Lack of parental control is also seen as a significant factor. The stresses and disturbances that occur at school may also be causative.

Essential for the understanding and evaluation of child patients, whether in paediatrics or child psychiatry, is a good working knowledge of normal development. It is not possible to separate completely the three elements of physical, intellectual and emotional development which respectively will account for such important aspects as motor skills, the development of language and the capacity for social interaction. Each of these elements affects development at each stage; for the child patient comparison is made with what would be expected. It is useful to have a plan for purposes of comparison, although the range of normal variation is huge. The developmental stages that are commonly recognized are listed in Table 19.2.

When commenting on a child's condition it is always important to note age for comparison with the normal developmental stage, but these stages occur at different ages in different children. As the child develops, grows and alters, his interactions and relationships with others, as also the parents' attitudes and those of siblings, change. Other influences are, also, continually coming to bear upon the family, partly associated with the children and partly from outside. Temperamental, constitutional, intellectual and physical features of the child are partly inherited and partly determined by early experience. These affect both the child's psychological functioning and also his later development as an adult. The child is influenced by the family in attitudes and beliefs, and also contributes these to the family.

To a large extent child health services work quite separately from those serving adults.

Table 19.1   *Classification of child psychiatric disorders in ICD-10*

DISORDERS OF PSYCHOLOGICAL DEVELOPMENT

Specific developmental disorders of speech and language
   Specific speech articulation disorder
   Expressive language disorder
   Receptive language disorder
   Acquired aphasia with epilepsy

Specific developmental disorders of scholastic skills
   Specific reading disorder
   Specific spelling disorder
   Specific disorder of arithmetical skills

Specific developmental disorder of motor function

Pervasive developmental disorders
   Childhood autism
   Rett's Syndrome
   Over-active disorder associated with mental retardation and stereotyped movements
   Asperger's Syndrome

BEHAVIOURAL AND EMOTIONAL DISORDERS WITH ONSET USUALLY OCCURRING IN CHILDHOOD OR ADOLESCENCE

Hyperkinetic disorders
   Disturbance of activity and attention
   Hyperkinetic conduct disorder

Conduct disorders
   Conduct disorder confined to the family context
   Unsocialized conduct disorder
   Socialized conduct disorder
   Oppositional defiant disorder

Mixed disorders of conduct and emotions
   Depressive conduct disorder

Emotional disorders with onset specific to childhood
   Separation anxiety disorder of childhood
   Phobic disorder of childhood
   Social anxiety disorder of childhood
   Sibling rivalry disorder

Disorders of social functioning with onset specific to childhood or adolescence
   Elective mutism
   Reactive attachment disorder of childhood
   Disinhibited attachment disorder of childhood

Tic disorders
   Transient tic disorder
   Chronic motor or vocal tic disorder
   Combined vocal and multiple motor tics (Tourette's Syndrome)

Other behavioural and emotional disorders with onset usually occurring during childhood or adolescence
   Enuresis
   Encopresis
   Feeding disorder of infancy or childhood
   Pica
   Stereotyped movement disorder
   Stuttering (stammering)
   Cluttering

Table 19.2 *Normal developmental stages*

Babies (up to 6 months)
6–12 months
12–24 months
2–5 years
Middle childhood (latency)
Adolescence

Links between hospital- and community-based services are particularly important. The hospital-based child and family psychiatric unit works closely with both the paediatric department and the child development centre where developmental delay is assessed and remedial action undertaken if necessary. For all child health services cooperation within multidisciplinary teams is essential; the team in a child psychiatry unit normally includes child psychiatrists, psychiatric nurses, occupational therapists, clinical psychologists and play therapists. Social work input is also required. The child psychiatrist links closely with community-based services including the general practitioner and practice staff, the Social Services Department, especially social workers and youth workers, the school psychological service and teachers and others in schools. The contact with teachers, educational welfare officers and school medical officers is an important and distinctive feature of the work of a child psychiatrist.

In any year between 5 and 15 per cent of children will suffer from psychiatric disorders that impair their capacity for normal living; for the inner city the rate is twice that of rural populations, yet only a very small proportion are ever seen by child psychiatrists. Most child psychiatric disorders differ quantitatively rather than qualitatively from normal, and so in assessing its presence and extent, the appropriateness of the behaviour is assessed in terms of developmental stages, social setting, presence of life events as precipitants, severity, and duration. Does the behaviour cause suffering to the child or others, or is it socially restricting? In child psychiatry it is always important to determine whether it is the child who is complaining or, as is more frequent, parents or teachers.

Whereas it is helpful in general psychiatry to have further comment upon and corroboration of the history from a relative or close friend, it is *essential* in child psychiatry to interview the parents or other care-givers. Particular emphasis is given to the role of other members of the family, family relationships and the developmental milestones. Of course, progress at school, the child's attitude to school, and relationships with teachers and other children are also of considerable relevance. Contact is made with and information is often sought from schools as part of the evaluation. The interview technique is necessarily different at various ages. For instance, an assessment largely based on play is required for the pre-school child, and much of the physical examination may be carried out by observation of the child playing rather than with formal testing. Making a relationship with an adolescent is a skilled activity and requires experience. Part of the evaluation to be made at the time of history-taking and examination is an assessment of the family.

Multiaxial classification, as described in Chapter 4, is particularly appropriate for child psychiatry formulation. This is exemplified as follows:

Axis 1 Clinical psychiatric syndrome; e.g. *conduct disorder*;
Axis 2 Specific developmental delay; e.g. *specific reading retardation*;
Axis 3 Intellectual level; e.g. severe *learning disability*;
Axis 4 Medical condition; e.g. *cerebral palsy*;
Axis 5 Abnormal psychosocial situation; e.g. *inconsistent parental control*.

Clinical syndromes

There are very few conditions in child psychiatry that present with precise symptoms representing known histopathology. Most diagnosis is by syndrome; that is, a frequently found pattern of symptoms and behaviour. Psychiatric symptoms may complicate organic disease or mimic physical symptoms, and psychological symptoms are frequent consequences of serious physical illness.

Specific delays in development

Whereas learning disability represents a global deficiency in intellectual level (Chapter 20), there may also be specific delays in development, of which the two most commonly occurring are *specific reading retardation* and *specific speech and language delay*. Reading retardation is commoner in the deprived, inner-city child than in rural areas, and in boys than in girls. It may be associated with conduct disorder and with perceptual and motor problems. There is not infrequently a family history. Specific speech delay is also commoner in boys and may manifest either in the production or the comprehension of speech, or both; the child is able to play normally, demonstrating satisfactory motor development. It is generally recognized by the age of 5.

Conduct disorder is defined as persistent and excessive, aggressive or destructive behaviour; this may be fighting, stealing, disobedience, lying, truancy, theft or assault. Conduct disorder occurs predominantly in males, and is associated with lower social class, larger family size, marital disharmony and evidence of child abuse. At pre-pubertal age such disorder is generally *unsocialized*, with the boy acting on his own, whilst after puberty it is more often *socialized*, taking place in a group with peer rules and values. Certain schools become associated with high rates of delinquency and conduct disorder and many affected children have learning difficulties.

Socially isolated boys tend to watch more television on their own and may be provoked by television and video violence into aggressive and antisocial behaviour. Conduct disorder with aggression through childhood leads in some to adolescent delinquency and even in a few to adult sociopathy with criminal behaviour. Management may include parental counselling, family therapy and behavioural methods at home, working with teachers and behavioural or group treatments at school. In a minority of cases, the involvement of Social Services with foster parents or even residential care is required.

Hyperkinetic syndrome

The hyperkinetic syndrome is characterized by persistent and gross over-activity occurring despite the inappropriateness of the situation. This starts before the age of 3 and is much commoner in boys than girls. It is often associated with learning disability. The child has a short attention span, is readily distracted and shows disinhibition. There are often fluctuations in mood, aggressiveness and impulsive behaviour. Understandably there are often difficulties between the child and other members of the family. Generalized delay in development is frequent, and epilepsy and other neurological disorders may be present. There are no treatments of proven specific efficacy; however, counselling for the parents and behavioural management for the child may ameliorate the consequent social difficulties. Amphetamine has been used, but is not always effective and has serious disadvantages.

Emotional disorders

Emotional disorders are common in child psychiatric practice. It is common to encounter a mixture of symptoms, which may include anxiety, misery, shyness, sleep and eating problems, and tantrums. The child may be tearful, socially withdrawn and demonstrably unhappy, with difficulties in relationships both within the family and at school. More clearly differentiated anxiety state, phobic disorder, hysteria or obsessive/compulsive disorder may also occur in childhood, with symptoms approximating to those that occur in adult neurotic disorders. However, the content of these disorders is appropriate to the age of the child (for example, fear of ghosts in an 8-year-old), and family disturbance may have a marked role in perpetuating symptoms.

Depressive illness

Although misery and unhappiness is commonly complained of by children, there is controversy about the frequency of diagnosis of established depressive illness in childhood. The clinical picture is different from that presenting in adult life. Provoking circumstances are usually associated with the family, and its dynamics and problems. Depressive disorder with a recognizable clinical picture becomes more readily diagnosable, and therefore more frequent, with increasing age from childhood into adolescence. Deliberate self-harm and suicide also become more frequent in adolescence.

Treatment of emotional disorders

The treatment of emotional disorders in childhood is likely to involve several different approaches. These include behavioural management for anxiety and phobic states; other forms of psychotherapy, usually involving play, to explore causes and facilitate coping; and family therapy to explore the family interactions and assist the parents and child in dealing with the condition. Pharmaco-therapy is not often used, but occasionally antidepressants may be of considerable benefit when depression is marked, and anxiolytics may be of benefit in the short term. Working with the other professionals involved in helping the child is always important, and this will include the general practitioner, teachers, social workers and sometimes the paediatrician. The child psychiatrist may perform an advisory role to other professionals involved in actually helping and treating the child rather than carrying out treatment directly.

School refusal and truancy

School refusal may be subdivided into two groups, which may overlap: school refusers and truants. *School refusers* usually have a satisfactory school record, and are more likely to come from a stable family background, with over-protective and often anxious parents. They may express fears of going to school and therefore either stay at home or return home after a short time at school. They may show other anxiety and depressive symptoms and phobic avoidance of other stressful situations.

In contrast, *truants* are more likely to have a poor school record with frequent change of school. The family may be disturbed, with absence of one or other parent and inconsistent parental control. The child is often hostile, rejecting school and tending to spend the day away from home with other truants, often involved in socialized but disordered behaviour; there is a strong association with subsequent delinquency. Although these patterns are different, some children will show features of both. Of aetiological significance for school refusal are personal factors, including the temperament and previous experience of the child; family factors, including the emotional state and psychiatric illnesses of parents; and school factors, including change of school, the behaviour of teachers and bullying in the playground.

Management of school refusal will involve exploration of causative factors and then as rapid a return to normal school attendance as is possible. The child himself, and the parents, will require support in achieving this. Chronic school refusal may lead to poor social adjustment and neurotic disorder in adult life.

Enuresis and encopresis

Nocturnal enuresis is persistent bed-wetting at night after the age of 5, most frequently without any period of established continence. It is a common condition and affects boys more than girls. It is more frequent in children of large families of lower socio-economic class and with a family history of bed-wetting. Children of lower intellectual level are over-represented, and those brought up in an institution are especially prone. Other developmental delays are commonly associated and there may be evidence of stressful events predisposing. There is usually no evidence of structural abnormality nor urinary infection; neither is there other psychiatric disorder.

Most children with a bed-wetting problem are never referred for treatment and the condition eventually remits. Such children have often been dealt with at home by fluid restriction in the evening and lifting for micturition during the early part of the night. *Behavioural* treatments used with some success include star charts, relying on social rewards, and pad and bell, waking the child immediately after voiding. *Pharmacological* treatment is used by only a minority of child psychiatrists; imipramine has proved effective for its anticholinergic action, but a major disadvantage is that patients tend to relapse.

Diurnal enuresis is a much less common problem, and is more likely to be associated with physical abnormalities. Many day-time enuretics also wet the bed at night.

Encopresis is faecal soiling after the age of 4. It is also commoner in boys than girls. There are several different behavioural patterns, including the situation where the child has never gained bowel control; cases where adequate bowel control is known to exist but the child deposits normal faeces in inappropriate places; soiling due to excessively fluid faeces, usually associated with gastro-intestinal disease; and toilet phobia when the child has become fearful of the toilet and therefore shows phobic avoidance. Possible physical factors should be investigated, and constipation in early life predisposes to the condition. Psychological factors are also found on occasions, especially rigid parental attitudes towards bowel-training. Treatment depends upon a careful assessment of the type of behaviour pattern and causative factors, and then a judicious combination of behavioural and medical methods of treatment with reassurance and reinforcement of approved behaviour. The condition understandably creates negative views of the child both in the family and at school, and this also requires therapeutic work.

Tics

Tics are quick, involuntary, apparently purposeless and frequently repeated movements. They are not caused by neurological disorder.

However, they need to be differentiated from the involuntary movements of organic disease and the more complex stereotypies and mannerisms that may occur in learning disability and autism. The face is most commonly involved, but other parts of the body including arms and legs may also show tics, which most commonly affect one muscle group. Tics may start at any age during childhood. They are commoner in boys than girls. There is some evidence for a genetic component. They often start at times of family stress. Most tics disappear during adolescence but a few become persistent.

Gilles de la Tourette Syndrome is a combination of vocal tics with tics in other parts of the body. Vocal tics include both staccato, ejaculated, meaningless sounds and monosyllabic swear words which are uttered explosively and inappropriately; this latter is sometimes called *'coprolalia'*.

Treatment for this is initially with reassurance and family counselling. Other techniques, including family therapy, anxiety management, behavioural modification and, sometimes, haloperidol, have been used with effect.

Childhood autism

Autism is a rare condition usually starting between the ages of 2 and 3 in which gross abnormalities in social relationships develop. Sometimes progress is normal until this age and only then ominous deterioration is observed. There is abnormality in communication, with a lack of language or stereotyped use of speech, and also stereotyped patterns of behaviour, with ritualized mannerisms and resistance to any change in the environment. It is most probably an organic condition in which there is disturbance to the central language-processing system. It is commoner in boys than girls; although there is often learning disability, this is not invariable and the two conditions are distinct.

Management aims to maximize the potential for the individual leading a normal life and acquiring language, and includes behavioural management, family therapy to help parents and others involved with the child, and sometimes drug treatment with haloperidol to reduce stereotyped behaviour. Residential treatment with special schooling may be necessary. About a half of autistic children make no substantial improvement and require long-term care.

Other *childhood psychotic disorders* occur but are extremely rare; some of these, especially in older children, are like schizophrenia. All these children require specialist treatment, including child psychiatric assessment.

Pre-school problems

Pre-school problems are very varied in nature, and have a number of different causes which may depend upon the development and personality of the child, early interaction with the parent and family, and social difficulties. The child may be difficult to control, aggressive and attention-seeking and show sleep problems. There may be separation anxiety, delay in acquiring language, and poorly developed play and social skills. Severe pre-school problems may lead on to emotional disorder in mid-childhood. Treatment includes looking for particular causes in the development of the child or in the family, and the use of a combination of family therapy and behavioural strategies.

Sexual abuse

Sexual abuse is the involvement of a child in sexual activity. The child does not understand what is happening and cannot give consent. The perpetrators are more often men and usually known to the victim; many were victims of abuse themselves. The victim may be of any age, male or female, and is often from a family that is both socially isolated and disorganized; sometimes the family members do not seem to have distinctive roles.

Identification of physical and behavioural signs of abuse requires a high degree of skill, and the consequence of mistaken diagnosis in either direction is serious for the child, the family and the person accused. Management requires adequate assessment of the situation,

and ideally will involve intensive work with the family whilst maintaining its stability. In practice, this is difficult to achieve; the whole process depends upon excellent cooperation and mutual trust between the many different professional services involved, and the family.

Adolescence

At an older age the conditions presenting to adolescent psychiatry merge with those seen in the rest of general adult psychiatry. For this reason, *anorexia nervosa, deliberate self-harm* and *psychoses* are not described further at this point, but reference should be made to the relevant chapters.

Child psychiatric treatment

Most treatment in child psychiatry is carried out on an outpatient basis, either in a hospital unit or in the community, but inpatient units are also necessary, especially for the more seriously disturbed child and for those whose difficulties are provoked at home. There is a need for the multidisciplinary team to cooperate with one another and for the child psychiatrist to be able to use a number of different methods of treatment and theoretical models.

Although *drugs* are not widely prescribed in child psychiatry, it is important for the doctor to be skilled in knowing when prescribing will shorten treatment and improve functioning of the patient, and hence the family. Often a combination of medication and other, psychosocial, treatment will be beneficial; making this therapeutic decision and prescribing is a distinctive contribution of the child psychiatrist to the multidisciplinary team.

Behaviour therapy is useful in the reinforcement of desired behaviour, the treatment of avoidance such as school refusal, and management for undesirable behaviour. *Cognitive therapy* has been used with older children and adolescents with the intention of changing attitudes towards self and belief systems. *Individual therapy* carried out with the child usually involves play, with comments and interpretations made whilst the child is absorbed by his imaginative play and toys. *Group therapy* may involve children, adolescents, parents and families. *Family therapy* attempts to see how the individual's problem has been maintained by family dysfunction, and how the family can work together to function more appropriately and hence help the individual member who has an identified problem.

A large part of the work of the child psychiatrist is in *consultation* with schools, residential care staff, social workers and others involved with children. Child psychiatrists may also find an involvement with the law and probation officers in the many forensic cases that involve children.

Further reading

Barker, P.A. (1988) *Basic Child Psychiatry*, 5th edn, Oxford: Blackwell Scientific Publications.

Rutter, M. and Hersov, L.A. (1985) *Child and Adolescent Psychiatry: Modern Approaches*, 2nd edn, Oxford: Blackwell Scientific Publications.

Stone, F.H. and Koupernik, C. (1978) *Child Psychiatry for Students*, 2nd edn, Edinburgh: Churchill Livingstone.

20

Learning disability

Within the population there is a wide range of ability to learn and to adapt. People who have severe difficulties in these areas form the subject of this chapter. They tend to have problems with intellectual functioning, communication and social skills, and activities of daily living. Severe difficulties of this kind have usually been present from early life, often evident as developmental delay. Some of those affected also have severe, and sometimes multiple, physical impairments.

Attitudes are changing towards the care of those who have marked difficulties with learning. Over the last few years there have been two important trends. First, we have begun to alter the terms used to refer to those who have problems of this kind. Second, there has been a move towards greater integration with the rest of the population. Why have these processes occurred together?

Terminology

Many terms have been applied to those with significant learning difficulties. The tenth revision of the International Classification of Diseases (ICD-10) refers to 'mental retardation'. The present UK Mental Health Acts refer to 'mental impairment', which was called 'mental subnormality' in the previous Act until 1983. 'Mental handicap' continues to be widely used.

These terms are less derogatory than those used in the 1913 Mental Deficiency Act: the feeble-minded, idiots and imbeciles. However, many of those affected and their families resist all of these labels, probably because they lead to descriptions of *people* as 'mentally handicapped', 'mentally retarded' and so on.

Generally speaking, when we give a name to a medical disorder we define the features of the condition, and not the people who suffer from it. Thus we define diabetes rather than what people who might be called 'diabetics' are like. This distinction may not seem especially important in the case of diabetes; for epilepsy, on the other hand, categorization of people as 'epileptics' clearly has some undesirable effects. For those with learning difficulties, the terms described in the previous paragraph have not only picked them out from other people but have helped to shape the policies to deal with them. Doctors, psychologists, educationists and other professionals have all played their part in this process of categorization and 'management' . As we move towards the end of an era in which it was usual for people with learning difficulties to be dealt with separately from the rest of the population, terminology and labels continue to exercise considerable influence on policy.

As an alternative to any of the terms described above, only 'learning disability' will be used in the rest of this chapter – for two reasons. First, it contains few if any assumptions about expected level of function. A term like 'mental handicap', on the other hand, implies limits to a person's development. It has been argued that it leads us to collect those with mental handicap together, to put them in specially designated settings, and then to expect little of them. Second, in the United Kingdom 'learning disability' is the term used increasingly by the many professional disciplines working in this area, despite an alternative term in ICD-10.

Separate facilities for care

Until recently it was usual for many of those with learning disability to be removed, sometimes permanently, from wider society and to be accommodated in large hospitals, often located away from the main urban areas. Others, if they lived at home with their own family or foster parents, were educated at special schools. Beyond school age, any work undertaken would usually be carried out in specially designated sheltered units (such as Adult Training Centres) rather than with an employer on the open market. Even basic health care has been subject to special arrangements. For example, management of epilepsy is usually undertaken by the general practitioner and a physician or neurologist; for those with learning disability it is not uncommon for it to be dealt with instead by a consultant in mental handicap, whose training is largely psychiatric. Much of this separate approach to care and facilities continues, but substantial moves towards greater integration have taken place and are described later in this chapter.

Definition of learning disability

When defining learning disability it might be thought that intelligence is the gold standard. Unfortunately 'intelligence' cannot be defined in a precise way and is made up of at least the following components: cognition, language, motor skills and social abilities. Attempts to sum intelligence numerically, such as with Intelligence Quotient (IQ), are sometimes of little practical use. This was illustrated some years ago by a survey of admissions to a mental handicap hospital. In the past, and in ICD-10 an IQ score of 70 has been widely regarded as indicative of learning disability. Of the people admitted to the hospital surveyed, more than half had IQs above 70, whilst a quarter recorded scores above 80, and 7 per cent fell between 90 and 100. It seems likely that some patients were wrongly placed in the hospital. However, the finding also suggests that others may have had only mild intellectual impairment, but it was other difficulties that led to hospital-based care. In practice, disturbances of social behaviour have often been key reasons for hospital admission.

Causes of learning disabilities

Is categorization of patients according to the cause of their disability more useful than IQ? Certainly, there are genetically and environmentally caused medical disorders which may have profound effects on physical and mental development. Such conditions include, for example: Down's Syndrome (a chromosomal abnormality), tuberose sclerosis (a single-gene error), cytomegalovirus (due to infection), and fetal alcohol syndrome (resulting from pre-natal environment). A good account of these and many other disorders will be found in chapters 10 to 12 of Craft *et al.* (1985). In practice, however, clear-cut diagnoses of causes such as these account for less than a quarter of those with learning disability. For the great majority of those affected we cannot determine the cause, nor give a name to the underlying condition.

Most of those who have *severe* or *moderately severe* learning disability are, however, affected by chromosomal abnormalities, severe and rare genetic conditions, or clinically manifest brain damage. They often show evidence of physical signs of central nervous system (CNS) disorder, biochemical abnormalities, or sensory impairment (for example, visual or hearing impediments). However, this group have a prevalence of only about 3 or 4 per 1,000 population. About ten times more prevalent (around 3 per cent of the population) are those with milder learning disability. Very few of this group have evident CNS, biochemical or sensory abnormalities. Instead, their striking characteristic is that almost all come from the lower socio-economic groups in the population. Evidence suggests that social circumstances play a major part in determining those with this degree of learning disability. Some believe that the social environment during childhood is the main determinant. Others take the view that social factors are exerted through biological events, such as a higher prevalence of CNS damage in the perinatal period in lower socio-economic groups, or through the genetic consequences of assortative mating. These issues remain unresolved.

There are several reasons why it is important to establish any definite cause of learning disability. First, where the condition involves chromosomal or single gene abnormalities, there may be need for genetic studies and counselling of parents. Second, it is important for parents, carers or staff to be alert to the possible occurrence of other features of a condition; being aware, for example, that over-eating and obesity are common accompaniments of Prader-Willi Syndrome, or that young adults with Down's Syndrome seem prone to development of Alzheimer's dementia. Third, learning disability may sometimes be prevented or arrested by specific measures; for example, by appropriate diet in phenylketonuria or replacement treatment in hypothyroidism of infancy. Fourth, parents have a strong tendency to apportion *blame* and may, therefore, benefit from careful counselling about cause. Often, blame is self-directed in the form of guilt. Many parents erroneously blame themselves for things they did or did not do – whether before conception, during pregnancy, at delivery, or in infancy or childhood. Increasingly, blame is being focused on the perinatal period, and there has been recent increase in litigation directed at obstetric practices.

Relatives and carers may want to know about cause in order to establish a prognosis. Identification of a chromosomal or genetic disorder may help to explain or predict various impairments. Conversely, knowing that a person suffers from a specific condition holds two dangers. First, not all available information about such disorders is accurate. For example, parents may read or be told that children with Turner's Syndrome are especially prone to intellectual impairment, although it is not so. Second, it is well established that the attitudes of significant people such as parents, carers, teachers and doctors can exert a powerful influence on the performance of children and adults; if limitations are deemed likely because someone has a specified condition, then there is a risk that correspondingly low expectations may lead to functioning below full capability.

Psychiatric illness and learning disability

Just as a person with learning disability may sustain an orthopaedic condition such as a broken leg, he may also become depressed, anxious, deluded, hallucinated and so on. Psychiatric assessment, however, with language and behaviour as its main components, is especially difficult in people who have learning disability. Furthermore, susceptibility to psychiatric disorder is substantially increased among those with learning disability because of such diverse factors as brain abnormality or damage, altered rearing practices in childhood (whether parental or institutional) and social rejection. Although there is undoubtedly a significantly raised prevalence of mental illness among those with learning disability, few specific links have been demonstrated with particular psychiatric disorders. The only important established connection is between Down's Syndrome and development of early Alzheimer's dementia. Although many other links have been proposed, none has proved robust when placed under scrutiny.

There is a growing move to provide psychiatric services for patients with learning disability within the ordinary psychiatric services. As the large mental handicap hospitals close, it may become regular practice for the standard day- and inpatient psychiatric facilities to cater for those with learning disability who also have a mental illness. There is disagreement whether this trend is to the patients' benefit. Such a move is certainly in line with the general drive towards use of ordinary services as far as possible in the community – for health, social services and education. However, there is a real risk that the present special provision will not be replaced by more integrated facilities but will be dismantled without adequate alternatives. Statutory services (health, social services and education) must not be allowed to use the move towards greater integration as an excuse for cutting costs, leaving the most vulnerable and needy to survive as best they can within ordinary facilities which are already over-stretched.

Although psychiatric services for those with learning disability may become increasingly mainstream, it must be emphasized that extra knowledge and skills are required, beyond those acquired during training in general adult or child psychiatry. For example, a person with learning disability who becomes depressed to a point which would benefit from treatment may well not express verbally the low state of mood. Clues may emerge instead from behaviour; for example, in aggressive disturbance or by becoming more withdrawn or less independent. In order properly to diagnose the condition, these clinical features need to be put together with other, more usual depressive symptoms such as change in weight, sleep loss, retardation, guilt feelings and occasionally even delusions or hallucinations.

Treatment

Physical treatment of psychiatric illness in a person with learning disability is broadly similar to that for other patients. There are, however, particular difficulties with psychological treatments. Nevertheless, psychiatrists who work in learning disability are increasingly undertaking psychotherapeutic interventions. Although special skills are required, none of the psychiatric treatment techniques described in Chapter 21 is contra-indicated with patients with learning disability. *Behavioural therapy* has long been used in this setting. *Cognitive techniques*, as for all patients, need to be adapted to the person's capacity through a process of negotiation between therapist and patient. *Counselling* and *interpretative psychotherapies* usually focus on emotionally charged issues; those with learning disability are certainly not immune to distress, nor are they incapable of benefiting from being guided through it by support and interpretation. For those with learning disability, psychological therapies are increasing in demand, and there are often long waiting lists to see a psychiatrist or clinical psychologist. In common with counselling and psychotherapy in other settings, sexual issues and sexual abuse in particular are frequently occurring themes. It is encouraging that when therapy has been successful in reducing distress, it is not unusual for carers or staff to report improvement in function – both behavioural and intellectual.

Services and facilities

As an ideal to aim at, it has been said that a person with learning disability is someone who, because of a developmental abnormality, needs special facilities to lead an ordinary life. In practice, as with physical disability, even with every facility the disability still exists. However, large-scale institutional care and separate provision in education and work do not promote this ideal. The rest of this section outlines the range of services currently available aimed at minimizing the social handicap of people with learning disability. There follows description of special provision and discussion of how those with learning disability may use ordinary services:

- long-stay hospitals;
- social education centres;
- residential provision;
- community teams and specialist staff;
- education.

Long-stay hospitals

It has been government policy since a 1971 White Paper, accelerated by a further government statement in 1985, that long-stay mental handicap hospitals should be replaced by community-based services. There have been substantial moves in this direction, although over 30,000 people remain in NHS hospitals despite community care initiatives. In the long term, it is intended that people with a learning disability should only be in an NHS facility when they have medical or nursing needs which cannot practically be met elsewhere. Ultimately, it is hoped that only when learning disability is accompanied by severe psychiatric illness or multiple physical disability will someone fall into this category.

Social education centres

These establishments were previously called adult training centres (and still are in some areas). They date from the early 1970s and were initially intended to resemble industrial work-places. More than 30,000 places exist at these day centres. People with learning disability attend, often Monday to Friday, from their living accommodation in family homes, group homes or hostels. There has been a shift from a training and occupational ethos towards programmes comprising skills for daily living, social activity, work and leisure, and education.

Although these centres have played a key part in the community care for people with learning disability, they are subject to a number of inherent problems. First, they provide their facilities apart from the rest of the population. Most people would expect to develop social, daily-living, educational, work and leisure skills in a range of settings rather than in any one 'centre'. Second, many of the buildings are 'institutional', even industrial, in design, and are therefore poorly suited to the broad aims of social education. Third, they concentrate people with learning disability in one place, which is necessarily far from the homes and true community of many of those attending. More about their work and philosophy can be found in the book by Craft *et al.* (1985).

Residential provision

In general, until recently there were only two widely available types of residence for people with a learning disability: the family home or a large institution. Smaller *hostels* and smaller *hospital units*, more locally based, have been a feature of the last twenty-five years. In the last five to ten years the trend has been towards further reduction in size of *staffed homes*, with perhaps no more than three or four residents. Another recent development has been an increase in the *fostering* of children with learning disability and the development of schemes for *family placement* of adults. More innovative have been schemes for *group homes* in which several (three to six) adults with learning disability share a house in an ordinary residential street, often with only a modest amount of external support. Two developments represent even greater integration with the general population: first, support for *co-residence* of adults with and without learning disability in ordinary houses or flats; and second, visiting support for those in *independent housing*.

Multi-disciplinary and community teams

It should be clear from the above description of residential provision that 'community care' requires a great deal of coordination between the various disciplines. Community nurses and social workers are the most numerous members of the community team. Others may be regular members of the team or may be asked to contribute as required: they include psychologists, psychiatrists, speech therapists, physiothera-pists and occupational therapists. The general practitioner also has an important role. Each discipline has its special skills but, in addition, each staff member will have a range of general skills. Thus one staff member (the 'key-worker') is able to coordinate a person's care, providing personally much of the professional help required. Other team members will provide their specialist help when asked to do so by the key-worker.

A *consultant psychiatrist* is likely to undertake a range of tasks. They will frequently stay in the same post for longer than most other team members, often at the head of a multidiscipli-nary team. The psychiatrist is therefore at the centre of planning care, and will be arranging and carrying out treatment – especially for those with mental illness and those with severe behaviour problems. Increasingly, psychiatrists are developing psychotherapeutic interventions for people with learning disabilities.

A *community nurse* may have many roles, even with just one individual's care. They might: advise the person or a carer about physical disability, intercurrent illness or menstruation; arrange visits to hospital; carry out a behaviour modification programme or social skills training; act as a counsellor with an individual or a family; or liaise with a school or college about special educational or other needs.

A *social worker* may have a very similar role – probably with less emphasis on health matters and more on practical help like day-care, family holidays and other aspects of local authority and voluntary provision. Social workers may also have a substantial role in direct counselling with individuals and families. It should be emphasized that much social work in relation to a person with learning disability is similar to other social work: it is about relationships, family, finance, housing and so on.

Education

Of all areas of provision for learning disability, it is perhaps in education that some of the most radical changes have been made in recent years. It now seems astonishing that people with severe learning disability were considered 'ineducable' in the 1944 Education Act, and that this position was not reversed until as recently as 1971, when in another Education Act children with severe learning disability gained the right to school education with the setting up of schools for the educationally sub-normal (ESN).

The education of adults and children was considered by an influential governmental Committee of Enquiry chaired by Mary Warnock in 1978. The report suggested a new term to be used for various categories of physical and learning disability: 'special needs education'. Second, it was proposed that those with special needs should receive their education in a less segregated way. The 1981

Education Act followed these precepts and considered learning difficulties as only one aspect of special needs education, dropping the term 'educationally sub-normal'. It also made it a statutory requirement for a school leaver's needs to be assessed – which has helped to promote continuing educational provision for young adults with learning disability. This was emphasized further when, in 1989, another Education Act insisted that local authorities pay particular attention to *adult students* with special needs due to learning disability.

People with learning disability now have statutory rights to education until the age of 19. Colleges of further education in many towns and cities now provide access to their colleges for adult students with special needs. These students take part in courses with non-disabled students. There are also specially designed courses for those with special needs, but even so the wider facilities of the college are open to them, as they are to all other students. Although provision remains patchy, adult colleges of further education are relatively unusual in providing a setting where the general population meet and mix with those with learning disability.

The segregation of the large long-stay hospitals was diminished by provision of hostels and day centres. The integration of adults with learning disability with the wider population has taken a further step forward with their inclusion into local colleges. Many colleges of further education enrol large numbers of students with learning disabilities (up to several hundred in some colleges) who attend the college each week.

Current philosophy and future developments

Two principles are guiding present developments and policy towards those with learning disability: first, integration with ordinary people in ordinary facilities; second, the provision of support to help people do what others can do unsupported. The objectives will vary according to the level of disability; for some they may be practical tasks such as dressing or eating unaided, for others they will be more academic. At present someone with several different needs may be separately assessed by different professionals, each assessing eligibility for a particular kind of support. More recent community care legislation has emphasized *needs-led* assessment under which there should be only one assessment of the person's needs, in a coordinated way – drawing together all the professionals involved. Another term – 'care management' – is also developing as a logical progression from needs-led assessment. A single *care manager*, who might be a social worker or a community nurse or any professional involved, will be responsible for identifying the necessary components of care and arranging for them to be carried out.

One other important change is beginning. Rather as with health service reforms, the government is separating 'purchasing' and 'providing' roles within Social Services Departments. Care managers, coordinating the support and facilities for an individual with learning disability, will belong to the purchasing side of the Social Services Department. It is envisaged that funds will, therefore, be directed by the care manager towards the facilities that an individual really needs rather than to maintaining provisions just because they exist at present.

It is impossible to foresee what these reforms will lead to. It is clear, however, that services for learning disability are at a time of great change.

Further reading

Craft, M., Bicknell, J. and Hollins, S. (eds) (1985) *Mental Handicap: A Multi-disciplinary Approach*, London: Baillière Tindall.

Sutcliffe, J. (1990) *Adults with Learning Difficulties: Education for Choice and Empowerment*, Leicester and Buckingham: National Institute of Adult Continuing Education (NIACE) and Open University Press.

21

Treatment (1): Psychological

In the next three chapters psychological, social and physical aspects of treatment are considered. This distinction is arbitrary, as many patients will require all three. A person requiring anti-depressant drug treatment will also need an appropriate psychological approach to help reduce loss of self-esteem, and social methods of treatment for the disturbance in relationship which may occur. Psychotropic drugs may produce better results used with psychotherapy, and social circumstances are always relevant, whatever the condition and however it is treated.

Psychological treatment is fundamental to the discipline of psychiatry. It is the application in treatment of that other distinctive psychiatric skill – phenomenology. The psychiatrist's concern with evaluating the patient's subjective state leads on naturally to methods of treatment. With psychological methods of treatment, the patient's own psyche is both the recipient of therapeutic endeavour and also an agent in carrying this out. The patient is not merely passive but contributes to change, and so it is important to achieve insight as to how this change may be made, and also confidence that it is possible. He is helped to see that small successes in daily living are possible and that these can be built upon to make progress in more refractory areas. Patterns of behaviour comprise constituent parts, and, when these are modified, behaviour can be changed.

Deciding what are appropriate goals of treatment is not always straightforward. In psychiatry there are rarely physical measures against which to gauge efficacy. Subjective improvement described by the patient is not always reliable and is difficult to quantify. The aims of treatment are to relieve specific symptoms, to produce an overall improvement in the patient's condition, and to optimize the capacity for independent action despite residual disability.

Most important in any type of psychological treatment are the personal qualities of the therapist. His skill and training should determine how complex are the cases which he takes on for treatment. Whilst some people are intrinsically helpful in personal relationships, they are, without further training, unlikely to be able to judge the limitations for improvement in a particular patient and are ignorant of the potential damage they may do. Knowledge of psychiatry is important for the therapist in order for him to avoid using psychological methods alone when this is not indicated.

Those involved in psychological treatment will inevitably become role models for their patients, who will tend to imitate their behaviour and fantasize about their private lives. As this cannot altogether be avoided, *modelling* must be recognized and used as an aspect of treatment; clearly, this has important implications for the recruitment of staff. In the selection or self-selection of psychotherapists, those who become involved with patients in order to solve their own problems should be excluded; they are likely to become over-involved, and more destructive than helpful.

General principles of psychological management

Considerable research evidence now shows psychological management to be effective in many treatment situations, but the ingredients of treatment that are effective are more controversial. There is considerable skill in listening to the patient's account without interrupting and without expressing boredom or disgust which might prevent the patient from continuing. The therapist needs to know when to talk and how much (more often, how little) to say. The art is to steer the patient's own account, using the patient's own material, rather than dominating the encounter. Inevitably, the doctor will need to give some direction as to what is the likely goal of treatment. He cannot be completely *non-directive*. At the same time it is important for patient and doctor to agree on what each of them can and should do; a treatment *contract* is established which may even be worth putting in writing.

Considerable attention should be paid to helping patients develop *coping skills*, for often during the course of a psychiatric illness *demoralization* occurs, in which the patient may feel he cannot handle problems which others expect him to solve. This increases lack of self-esteem and feelings of alienation from others. Treatment concentrates upon goals which are within the patient's capacity to achieve whilst supported by his therapist, so that he learns that more of his behaviour than he previously believed is actually under his own *control*.

A patient needs to understand how his problem relates to other aspects of his behaviour or personality, to gain *insight*. He also needs to realize how other people respond to him and how this affects his relationships. Arising from this, he may be able to take on new attitudes and change his behaviour, although often behavioural change may have to precede change of attitude.

Patients should be helped to gain insight and relief from symptoms, while the therapist avoids either *collusion* or *confrontation*. A patient showing *illness behaviour*, with physical symptoms resulting from a psychological cause, usually wishes to believe that the cause of his condition is physical. Collusion is prevented by the therapist resisting this belief in such a way that the patient does not feel rejected. Although there are times when confrontation is helpful, it is best avoided whilst the therapeutic relationship is being established. A vital part of psychological treatment is the need for patients to *internalize* – that is, to make the effects of treatment their own by repeated practice between sessions of what they have learned. A large part, for example, of the value of behaviour therapy accrues from this process.

Coping and achieving independence is the most effective way to deal with demoralization. As the patient learns to cope, even with quite minor situations, this is pointed out to him and he is shown how he can capitalize upon small gains.

An important part of treatment is to help the patient to realize that he is able to exert, at least within limits, *self-control*, and thereby to take personal responsibility. To achieve this, situations that he previously thought were outside his control are shown to be, in fact, within his control.

Learning *social skills* is a prerequisite for establishing better relationships with other people and hence developing friendships.

The patient's *feelings of guilt* need to be taken seriously and discussed. They should not be dismissed as 'merely neurotic' or 'symptomatic', but accepted as 'real' guilt which the patient needs to deal with within his own frame of reference.

Psychotherapy

Psychotherapy in its widest sense is the basis of all psychiatric treatment and certainly, in one form or another, the oldest. It has been defined as "essentially a conversation which involves listening to and talking with those in trouble with the aim of helping them understand and resolve their predicament … a personal relationship with a professional person in which those in distress can share and explore the underlying nature of their troubles, and possibly change some of the determinants of these through experiencing unrecognized forces in themselves" (Brown and Pedder, 1989).

Psychological factors also play a profound part in the treatment of many physical disorders, whether deliberately or unconsciously applied. For instance, the manner in which a drug is prescribed and administered in part determines its efficacy. The more non-specific the remedy, the more likely is this to be true. Healing, when based upon religious or magical rituals, also appears to depend upon psychotherapeutic processes. Three features are common to different types of psychotherapy in treatment: relationship, insight and incorporation.

The *relationship* between the subject and the doctor, social worker, priest, healer or professional psychotherapist is obviously important for effective work to be done.

For *insight* to be achieved, a patient arrives at a fresh understanding of how he got into his present difficulties, how he himself played a part in the evolution of his problems, how his personality tends to determine his consistent behaviour, and how other people react to him. He may not make all these discoveries at once; enlightenment may only dawn very slowly and even then he may not be able to put it into words. However, in order to be beneficial, insight must be more than intellectual; the patient must understand how his emotions and will are also involved. *Knowing* must be accompanied by *feeling*. Indeed, of the two, the latter is much the more important. This is why some forms of treatment such as 'moral treatment', explanation, persuasion, reassurance and re-education have met with only very limited success.

Incorporation is essential. It is not enough that the patient relates well to his therapist and begins to understand how his symptoms developed. He also needs to learn how to develop more appropriate behaviour, both during and after therapeutic sessions, so that this becomes an intrinsic part of himself. Whether the

theoretical basis of the treatment is psychodynamic, cognitive or behavioural (see below), such incorporation is essential.

Simple psychotherapy

All of medicine depends upon the relationship and communication between doctor and patient. The level of psychotherapy carried out most frequently in general practice, and in the communications of medical and surgical specialties, may be termed '*simple psychotherapy*'. This is useful for patients with emotional problems of short duration with or without coexisting physical symptoms, and also for patients who need help in coming to terms with the consequences of long-term illness. Primary care physicians and practitioners in all medical specialties can be of service to their patients and also prevent wastage of scarce health service resources by learning about and practising the general principles of psychological management. In this way many patients with minor emotional disorders may be effectively treated in primary care; also the psychological component of physical disorders will be recognized and dealt with adequately.

There are two meanings to the word 'counselling'. It refers to the specific method developed by Carl Rogers in which the therapist takes a passive role, 'reflecting back' the emotional significance of his conversation. It is also used in a more general sense to refer to brief courses of treatment with limited goals undertaken by people of good sense and intelligence but without specific training in psychotherapy; for example, marital counselling, bereavement counselling, and so on. Such counselling is greatly in demand and the psychiatrist has a role in helping to train and support the counsellors.

Supportive therapy: short- or long-term

The most frequent form of therapy used by psychiatrists is *supportive psychotherapy*. The aim is to help the individual through a temporary crisis caused by the distress of physical or mental illness, or by social or psychological problems. Long-term supportive treatment is also sometimes of value for individuals with personality disorder to cope more effectively and live more congenially. The underlying personality cannot be radically changed, but the individual can be shown how his personality affects his behaviour and consequent relationships, and how to adapt to this.

The capacity for listening to the patient, encouraging him to talk about his emotions and maximizing his coping skills is essential. It is also necessary to help the patient to accept the inevitable and to achieve as good a quality of life as possible, both psychological and physical, despite disability.

Explanation and *advice* may be helpful but require skill and experience in knowing how and when and how much to speak. Similarly, *reassurance* may be useful on occasions, and *suggestion* also has a use. When the authoritative role of 'doctor' is employed it must be done carefully and with due consideration to the patient's current mental state. The relationship between patient and doctor is, of course, all-important, and the doctor must merit the confidence the patient puts in him. In this way it is possible to support individual patients – for example, with refractory depressive illness – over many years and help them to maintain social competence.

There is a danger with supportive therapy that it will be supporting or *reinforcing* the patient in a sick role, thus tending to make symptoms persist. In order for supportive therapy not to reinforce unhealthy behaviour and attitudes, the therapist should constantly be looking for opportunities for the patient to effect change for the better. It is often appropriate for a consultant psychiatrist to arrange for supportive therapy to be provided by other mental health professionals or by a self-help group.

Crisis intervention

A particular form of supportive therapy assists the individual going through a crisis to function appropriately during the critical period and avoid long-term psychological disability as a consequence. A number of techniques have been developed, and it has been particularly used in the aftermath for victims of severe trauma (*post-traumatic stress disorder*). The precise method depends upon the nature of the trauma, its duration, whether it was individual or took place in a group, natural or man-made, whether the individual was intimately or only peripherally involved in the disaster, and whether his underlying personality structure was vulnerable or healthy. The basic coping skills of the individual are used to encourage problem-solving behaviour. The crisis may involve loss, or threat of a loss, change of role, problems in relationships and difficulties in making decisions.

Crisis intervention concentrates on making sense of the disaster through the victim's own understanding. The principles are as follows. Early intervention can reduce current distress and disturbance and reduce long-term morbidity; it needs to be presented in a manner that is acceptable to the particular cultural group affected; comprehensible information is vital to help people 'make sense' of their experiences; involvement with other people lessens both isolation and stigma, and reinforces feelings of 'normality'; and helpers need to set specific, limited and attainable goals.

In the initial stages treatment will involve dealing with excessive anxiety or depression. There may also need to be extensive social arrangements made for the welfare of the individual. Otherwise treatment involves the principles of supportive psychotherapy in listening, maximizing the individual's own potential for coping, and helping him to find solutions and cope effectively with disability.

Brief psychotherapy

This type of treatment aims for substantial change in a relatively short time, perhaps a maximum of 6 months or twenty-five sessions. The most suitable patients are those who are well motivated and have predominant problems with relationships.

A full psychiatric history is taken first, and there is discussion of the problems identified by the patient and the aims of treatment. The proposed length of treatment is agreed upon early. There is then an attempt to help the patient find solutions to difficulties, and as in other forms of therapy it is important for the therapist to listen to what the patient is saying.

During treatment specific problems are looked at in more detail. The role of the therapist is to facilitate the patient's exploration of his own emotions and begin to find answers concerning the development of symptoms. The patient is encouraged to talk about emotionally painful subjects, to look for recurrent patterns of behaviour, and to see what are the antecedents of current problems. Alternative modes of behaving and thinking are explored.

During treatment non-verbal cues are observed carefully as they may be clues to areas that the patient cannot express in words. The relationship between patient and therapist is also explored (see below).

As the end of treatment approaches, the aim should be as far as possible to free the patient from emotional dependence upon the therapist and also to achieve resolution of the problems. The therapist may by then be spacing the appointments at longer intervals. It is important for patient and therapist to discuss what has been achieved in treatment and for both to realize that the limited goals recorded at the beginning of treatment have in fact been achieved.

Psychoanalysis

Psychoanalytic psychotherapy is very time-consuming, involving several sessions per week over several years; the *analyst* also requires many years of training. The treatment is designed to explore, interpret and, in due course, modify unconscious mental processes which are considered to have given rise to symptoms. It makes use of *free association*; that is, the patient talking whilst freely allowing ideas to come without particular direction. It also involves *interpretation of dreams* and of *fantasy material* produced by the patient. The avoidance the patient shows in not talking about certain areas of life which appear to be important is considered to be *unconscious resistance*, and this is interpreted also. At times the patient is unable to express his feelings in words but may do so in action, often outside the therapeutic sessions; this is described as *acting out*. This may also be interpreted during treatment.

The nature of the relationship between patient and therapist is important. The theory is that the patient transfers to the therapist feelings and attitudes that were originally experienced in relation to other significant people with whom he had a close relationship in early life, especially parents. This relationship is described as *transference*. When the initial relationship with the parent was good it is called *positive* transference; when the relationship was previously poor, it is *negative* transference. It is also accepted that the therapist, in his attitudes towards the patient, reflects his previous experience of relationship towards other figures earlier in his own life. This is called *counter-transference*, and again can be positive or negative.

The ultimate aim of psychoanalysis is not only to give the patient an insight into his problems and to free him from his emotional entanglement with these, but also to release him from any dependence he may develop towards the analyst or may already have had towards other authoritative or over-protecting persons, so that he is able to conduct his life without any sense of inferiority.

Because of its time-consuming nature, psychoanalysis is not generally available within the National Health Service. It is, however, a useful training technique for the analyst and from it are derived many more recent forms of psychotherapy.

Value of psychotherapy

Does psychotherapy work, and, if so, what part of it is the effective ingredient? There is great difficulty in designing measures to demonstrate efficacy which can be agreed upon by different psychotherapists. It is also extremely difficult, and perhaps unethical, to set up controlled studies which both maintain the untreated control group for assessment at follow-up whilst at the same time not offering them some form of treatment that could be considered psychotherapeutic. In practice, a number of trials have now been carried out using different types of psychotherapy for different groups of patients. The findings of such studies have usually shown distinct advantage over no treatment at all, but it has not been possible to demonstrate major differences in outcome between different types of treatment. We are therefore left with the indications for psychotherapy being largely based upon clinical experience. It has also been shown that psychotherapy, like all other effective methods of treatment, is capable of making some patients worse. This is particularly likely where treatment is conducted by a powerful, dominant therapist upon vulnerable, isolated, self-deprecating patients.

Group psychotherapy

Man is a social species who lives in families, usually works with other people, and often finds recreation in companionable ways. Because disturbed relationships are often the most severe of psychological symptoms, treatment of more than one individual may be helpful. Also, because individual therapy is very expensive of both time and money, treatment in groups has the advantage of being more economical. Treatment may be with couples, with small groups, with large groups or in self-help groups.

The optimal size of group in therapy is about eight people. Sessions of treatment may last for an hour and a half and take place once or twice a week. Various insights can be learned and more appropriate patterns of behaviour may be better rehearsed in a group setting. A group member learning how others react to one another may be helped to understand how *natural* groups, such as his own family, interact. In seeing other patients resolve their difficulties, he begins to learn how improvement can occur and how his own involvement is necessary. He is able in the safe situation of the group, with a skilled therapist conducting it, to experiment with ways of communicating with other people.

There are some patients who are unable to benefit from group therapy. However, many do extremely well, often better than in individual therapy, perhaps because the transference relationships and the dependency problems of individual therapy are diluted amongst all the members of the group. For some patients an initial short period of individual treatment precedes group therapy, whilst others may start in a group immediately following initial diagnostic assessment. Groups may be *open*, receiving new members and discharging those improved as appropriate, or *closed*, in which all the members start, continue and finish in treatment together. The composition of the group requires considerable care; mixed-sex groups of roughly equal proportions are often considered best.

Group therapy is particularly suitable for those with difficulties in relationships; this may be associated with neurotic, emotional and/or personality disorder. Definite depressive illness requires other types of treatment and group therapy could be harmful. Similarly, with severe degrees of anxiety state the anxiety must be controlled before the patient can take advantage of group treatment. Obsessional and phobic neuroses similarly require specific treatment and only benefit from group treatment if there is also disturbance in relationship (however, there usually is). Some schizophrenic patients receiving pharmacological treatment for their condition may benefit from group treatment in addition. It is important to realize that, like other potent forms of treatment, groups can be harmful as well as beneficial if used for the wrong patient or conducted with an inappropriate style of leadership.

Sometimes therapeutic groups are too verbal and intellectual to suit some patients referred by family doctors. A combination of group therapy technique with role-playing or *psychodrama* is sometimes beneficial. Here the members of the group take a situation of conflict for one of them and role play the drama by representing the characters involved and trying to explore their probable states of mind. Insight may be more readily achieved in this setting than in an orthodox group.

Large group psychotherapy may take place in a *therapeutic community* or as part of the programme of a psychiatric ward. The large group, perhaps fifteen to thirty people, comprises all the members of the community including its staff. Matters of concern within the community are aired in the group, where it is intended that conflicts should be resolved. Members learn about relationships whilst being supported by other members of the group and also by staff. An important role for the staff in such a situation is to protect the more vulnerable members of the group from the enthusiasm and hostility of the more voluble. The guiding principle of the therapeutic community is that every activity or event occurring within that group of people should be able to be used in treatment; for example, a member's refusal to carry out domestic chores might be interpreted when the group is together.

In *self-help groups* the organization and leadership is by patients or ex-patients themselves. Mutual support and encouragement is given, and the intention is to maintain the members of the group in a satisfactory state of coping. *Alcoholics Anonymous* is such a group, and it has established its own ethos and method of working over the years. Although some sufferers may feel excluded from such a group and therefore gain little benefit, there are many others who feel that it gives them vital support and a social milieu of other people who understand them.

Family therapy

Family therapy is based on the observation that the patient who presents for treatment is not necessarily the only disturbed member of the family from which he comes, nor even the most disturbed. Indeed, when a family constellation is thoroughly explored, it may be perceived that the patient has, in effect, become a scapegoat, and the emotional stability of another family member, or perhaps of the entire family, is only preserved at his expense. For effective treatment of the individual patient with symptoms, it may be necessary to involve the whole family group both to try and deal with disturbance in other members of the family and also to enlist these other members in helping the individual with symptoms. Symptoms, especially in children, often develop within the family, and the family can make a useful contribution in their resolution.

After considering carefully what happens when the whole family is seen together, the difficulties experienced by the symptomatic members and their antecedents within the family may become apparent. It then becomes possible to apply better methods of dealing with problems within the whole family. This technique has been of particular use in child psychiatry, where not only the affected child and both parents but also other siblings and even grandparents may be involved to good effect. The technique of handling a family group is difficult and demands much tact and skill. Careful training is therefore required, and co-therapists are also usually involved.

Marital therapy

As with family therapy, dealing with marital partners together may be effective in helping with problems. Treatment is given because marital conflict is considered to be the cause of emotional disorder in one of the partners, or because the marriage appears to be in danger of breaking up and both partners wish to save it. Treatment is directed at the interaction between the partners. While one or other is likely to be referred initially as 'the patient', it is important to interview the other to corroborate the story, ascertain the conflicts within the marriage, find out how the spouse evaluates the patient, assess the personality resources of the spouse, and, following this, decide upon a treatment plan taking both partners into account. In some cases the best plan may be for the therapist to see husband and wife together; in others, it may be preferable to involve a second therapist, perhaps a therapist of each sex, so that neither partner feels that he or she is under attack from an alliance of their spouse and therapist.

If one or both partners intend to separate, joint interviews are unlikely to be beneficial, although there may be a need for supportive psychotherapy for the partner who does not wish the marriage to end. Such therapy may be invaluable in helping a patient through this acute crisis.

Hypnosis and relaxation

Hypnosis is a state of induced relaxation associated with heightened suggestibility. There is voluntary suspension of initiative, restriction of attention to a narrow field and reduction in self-consciousness and critical appraisal. The technique for inducing hypnosis has had a long history and has waxed and waned in popularity. The word was first used in 1843 by James Braid, a Manchester surgeon, and he demystified the technique and introduced it into British medical practice.

Hypnosis has been used both as a method of treatment and a research tool. Its application in psychiatric practice is limited. It can be used for inducing light trance as a form of relaxation. It has also been used to produce deeper trance to enhance suggestion in order to relieve symptoms, especially certain hysterical states such as paralyses, aphonias and amnesias following psychological trauma. However, it is unwise to apply hypnosis for the mere removal of symptoms without a thorough prior exploration leading to some knowledge of their cause. Failing this, at best the effect may be temporary only, with a return of symptoms in the same or other form; at worst, the patient, deprived of his defences and unable to cope with his basic problem, may become severely depressed, even suicidal. Most authorities regard hypnosis as useless in obsessional states and in those with psychotic disorders who, in any event, are difficult if not impossible to hypnotize.

Hypnosis is, perhaps, most useful in certain psychosomatic states, such as some dermatological disorders in which it may be effective in controlling itching, and in gastrointestinal and other disorders where relief of emotional tension may be of benefit. A patient with acute retention of urine was able to micturate following hypnosis during which she had been encouraged to fantasize herself in a calm, tranquil setting where she could urinate! Hypnosis can also be used in chronic painful conditions, even when these are due to some demonstrably organic cause; for instance, when there is a need for repeated burns dressings or dental procedures. It may also be used to induce relaxation before and during labour; adequate training can be given in the antenatal clinic where group hypnosis has been applied to save staff time.

In suitable subjects the induction of hypnosis does not present undue difficulty providing both patient and doctor have confidence in the procedure. For details of the technique, special manuals on the subject should be consulted. Lesser forms of relaxation, not amounting to deep hypnosis, have been developed for *anxiety control training*.

Anxiety management

Recurrent anxiety can often be effectively brought under control using cognitive-behavioural methods developed from autogenic training, as described by Schultz (Schultz and Luthe, 1969). The essential elements are listed in Table 21.1. A practical account of this method will be found in Sims and Snaith (1989).

The process of treatment is explained to the potential patient and also how anxiety has occurred as part of his problem. The motivation for change is assessed. A system of exercises involving light hypnosis and progressive relaxation of different parts of the body is learnt during treatment sessions. Once the patient has learnt reliably how to relax and thus relieve anxiety, he is then exposed, in fantasy, to further anxiety which he then brings under control. A process of cognitive restructuring of attitudes follows, with the patient carrying out an internal dialogue with himself. Finally the

Table 21.1 *Elements of anxiety management*

1 Explanation and motivation for change
2 Relaxation or meditation
3 Exposure to anxiety
4 Restructuring of attitudes
5 Self-control

technique helps the sufferer to achieve self-control of his anxiety.

Abreaction

This is a technique for encouraging under close supervision the unrestrained expression of massive emotion. It has chiefly been used in military psychiatry for relieving acute symptoms a few hours after severe emotional trauma such as battle stress. Abreaction can be brought about with powerful suggestion causing the victim to relive the traumatic events and experience the violent emotions associated with this. It may be facilitated by hypnosis or a sedative drug intravenously. During World War II it was an effective way of treating acute psychiatric symptoms in order to return soldiers to their duties rapidly.

Behavioural and cognitive therapy

Behaviour therapy is an application of experimental psychology to change symptoms and *behaviour*. *Cognitive therapy* aims to change maladaptive ways of *thinking* and thus produce improvement from psychiatric disorder. Both methods of treatment have been developed in the second half of this century. Behavioural treatment aims at changing the patient's behaviour, but there also needs to be change in attitudes; in cognitive therapy the primary change in cognition must be followed by a secondary change in the patient's behaviour. Although these two methods are here described separately, they are often used together as cognitive-behavioural therapy.

Behaviour therapy

There are a number of different behavioural treatments available, but for them to be implemented, a *behavioural analysis* of the patient's symptoms is required. This involves a detailed record of the patient's symptoms, their antecedents and consequences and the ways in which the patient tries to deal with them. The principles underlying modern behaviour therapy techniques are largely based on *learning theory*. Treatment is aimed at the removal of symptoms rather than dealing with underlying conflict, the symptom being regarded as a *conditioned response* which may be removed by appropriate relearning. Behavioural modification has a great advantage over psychoanalytic forms of treatment in being less demanding of time.

Below are some of the many behaviour therapy techniques in current use.

Desensitization (reciprocal inhibition)

The basis of desensitization in imagination is that anxiety aroused by a specific situation can be suppressed by the simultaneous evocation of other, physiologically antagonistic responses. In essence, the procedure involves training in progressive relaxation to a point where imagining the anxiety-producing stimulus ceases to arouse anxiety. This is achieved by constructing a hierarchy which grades, from the least to the most disturbing, those circumstances which cause the patient to become increasingly anxious. Either using imagery or in a real-life situation, the patient starts at the bottom and, as he becomes able during each session to overcome his anxiety at each step of the hierarchy, he progresses gradually up the scale. The treatment appears to be particularly successful in mono-phobic states, but less so where phobic anxiety is more diffuse, as in agoraphobia.

Operant conditioning

This term was introduced by Skinner. It involves the systematic manipulation of environmental events to produce desired objectives by the skilled use of *reinforcement*. The subject's behaviour is altered by the use of *contingencies*; for example, praise of a desirable action on the part of the subject is likely to result in the repetition of that act. This use of reinforcement is often described as *behavioural modification*. The principle is that if behaviour persists it is being reinforced by certain of its consequences, and therefore by altering the consequences the behaviour also may be changed. The principles of operant conditioning have been successfully applied to the rehabilitation of the chronically mentally ill, in the training of mentally handicapped adults, and also for behaviour disorders in children, where parents have been trained to act as therapists.

Exposure

In exposure techniques for the treatment of phobic disorders the patient is prevented from leaving the situation which provokes anxiety until the anxiety begins to diminish. When exposure to situations provoking severe anxiety is sudden, it is known as *flooding*, and the patient remains in the phobic situation with full force until anxiety subsides. Exposure techniques are useful for agoraphobia and more effective than desensitization. However, their efficacy is made even greater by combining with cognitive methods of treatment. With exposure techniques the patient will be taken by the therapist into the specifically anxiety-provoking situation – for instance, a supermarket – and they both remain there until the patient's anxiety subsides. There are other techniques available also for dealing with patients' high levels of anxiety.

Response prevention

This has been used with success in patients with obsessive-compulsive symptoms; for example, a ritual hand-washer is strongly discouraged from washing his hands for increasingly long intervals after carrying out activity which he regards as contaminating. Although the level of anxiety initially rises after 'prevention', it gradually subsides with persistence. This treatment is sometimes combined with *modelling*, in which, in the above example, the therapist will handle what the patient regards as a contaminated object before encouraging the patient to do the same himself.

Social skills training

This uses behavioural modification to improve functioning of socially unskilled patients. The patient is taught a more appropriate way of acting after the behaviour has been carefully analyzed in a social situation. It is best carried out in a group with reinforcement, usually in the form of approval from other group members, being given for successful behaviour in improving relationships or with specific social tasks (see page 202).

In *assertiveness training* the subject is encouraged to give direct but socially acceptable expression of thoughts and feelings. This is particularly useful for people who are socially awkward or inhibited. It involves enactment in a treatment situation of the required behaviour so that by rehearsing it the subject is able to carry it out in a real-life situation.

Biofeedback

In this technique subjects are taught to control physiological responses mediated by either the voluntary or the autonomic nervous system. Specially designed electronic apparatus is used to give the subject information about specific bodily reactions, such as blood pressure, over which they would otherwise have little or no control. The physiological monitor records and provides information which is then transduced into a form that the individual can easily apprehend, such as a tone of varying pitch or a visual display. The individual then tries to alter the displayed measurement by regulating the relevant function; for example, relaxing, after being taught how to do so, in order to control blood pressure.

This procedure demonstrates a general principle of behaviour therapy – it depends upon enabling patients to learn to control their own behaviour and feelings. Thus *self-control* techniques are fundamental and two stages are recognized: *self-monitoring* and *self-reinforcement*. In self-monitoring the individual records the problem behaviour and the circumstances in which it occurs. Self-reinforcement involves the subject rewarding himself when desired behaviour occurs or when the unacceptable behaviour or feelings have been controlled successfully.

Cognitive therapy

Patients with depression and other emotional disorders show recurring patterns of thought, often associated with low self-esteem and social embarrassment. Cognitive therapy works on the hypothesis that if these recurring thoughts could be controlled, the conditions themselves might be alleviated. Thus the therapist attempts to change disordered ways of thinking; for instance, the unreasonably self-deprecatory and pessimistic ideas of a depressed patient. By changing these cognitions, the hope is that other aspects of the disorder will then also be ameliorated.

The false assumptions are identified by careful interviewing in which patients are asked for the reasons they would give for their actions and the expectations they have from events. A daily record of such *attitudes* and their provoking circumstances is made. These false assumptions are then challenged and, it is hoped, prevented. The therapist may in treatment sessions help the patient to see the logical errors in their attitudes and the patient is then encouraged to record in their diary between treatment sessions more realistic ways of thinking.

Cognitive-behaviour therapy has been developed by Beck and others, and is especially used for depressive disorders. The aim of treatment is to modify the depressive thoughts and attitudes that are always associated with the emotional disturbance. The patient records between treatment sessions the negative, depressive thoughts that occur, the events that led up to these thoughts, and the mood that accompanied them. During treatment sessions these thoughts are examined, and how they logically arise from their antecedents is questioned. The patient examines these ideas himself between sessions and is encouraged to set up alternative hypotheses concerning these thoughts about himself. At the same time he is encouraged to find ways of spending his time that promote feelings of achievement.

Cognitive techniques have been developed and evaluated for the treatment of phobic disorders, generalized anxiety disorders, for panic attacks, eating disorders and even for hypochondriasis. In practice, many psychiatrists will use a combination of cognitive, behavioural and also psychodynamic methods of treatment.

Further reading

Balint, M. (1957) *The Doctor, his Patient and the Illness*, London: Pitman Medical.

Bloch, S. (1986) *An Introduction to the Psychotherapies*, 2nd edn, Oxford: Oxford University Press.

Brown, D. and Pedder, J. (1989) *Introduction to Psychotherapy: An Outline of Psychodynamic Principles and Practice*, London: Routledge.

Gelder, M., Gath, D. and Mayou, R. (1989) *Oxford Textbook of Psychiatry*, 2nd edn, Oxford: Oxford University Press.

Hawton, K., Salkovskis, P.M., Kirk, J. and Clark, D.M. (eds) (1989) *Cognitive Behaviour Therapy for Psychiatric Problems: A Practical Guide*, Oxford: Oxford University Press.

Hodgkinson, P.E. and Stewart, M. (1991) *Coping with Catastrophe*, London: Routledge.

Holmes, J. (1991) *Textbook of Psychotherapy in Psychiatric Practice*, Edinburgh: Churchill Livingstone.

Schultz, J.H. and Luther, W. (1969) *Autogenic Therapy: Autogenic Method*, New York: Grune and Stratton.

Sims, A. and Snaith, P. (1989) *Anxiety in Clinical Practice*, Chichester: Wiley.

Stern, R. and Drummond, L. (1991) *The Practice of Behavioural and Cognitive Psychotherapy*, Cambridge: Cambridge University Press.

22

Treatment (2): Social

Perhaps the most distinctively British contribution to psychiatric practice has been in the development of *social psychiatry*; that is, concern for the context and environment in which the mentally ill person lives, and the use of the social milieu as part of treatment. A discussion of social methods of treatment in psychiatry is necessarily related to the particular society and culture in which it occurs; this chapter deals with circumstances in the United Kingdom.

The only hospital for the mentally ill before the eighteenth century was Bethlem Hospital in London, founded in 1247. The Vagrancy Act (1744) distinguished between 'lunatics' and 'paupers' for legal purposes, and from about that time onwards they were dealt with separately. A ward for the mentally ill was established at Guy's Hospital in 1728, and specialist hospitals began to be provided from the latter part of that century. Four generations of the Tuke family served the mentally ill at The Retreat (Hospital) in York, which was founded in 1792 and emphasized humane care rather than harsh custodianship. The so-called *moral* methods of treating insanity, developed in the nineteenth century, included careful attention to environmental factors and the establishment of a *therapeutic milieu*.

In mental hospitals more liberal and humane management has developed, and over the last forty years there has been a much greater emphasis played by Social Services. This has been facilitated by significant legislation and

government reports including the National Health Service Act (1946); the Mental Health Act (1959), extensively revised to form a new Act in 1983; the Local Authority Social Services Act (1970); the government White Paper, 'Better services for the mentally ill' (1975); and the National Health Service and Community Care Act (1991). Mental illness is not specifically defined in the Mental Health Act but is broadly comprehensive and considered to include those conditions which might reasonably be discussed in a psychiatric textbook.

A typical example of inpatient numbers in a large mental hospital was described in Chapter 1. Most of the county lunatic asylums were established in the first half of the nineteenth century. High Royds Hospital, Menston, West Yorkshire was built in 1888 as an overflow to the original West Riding Asylum in Wakefield. The numbers of patients in hospital increased progressively during the nineteenth century. They reduced a little during both World Wars but finally reached a peak in the mid-1950s. From that time there has been a progressive decrease in numbers which has accelerated over recent years, with the intention eventually to close most of the mental hospitals and replace them with smaller units in district general hospitals.

It should be noted that the distinctions drawn between *medical* and *social* aspects of psychiatry are more apparent in theory than in practice; there is much overlap. Similarly, a psychiatrist will not confine practice to either biological or psychosocial methods, but in most instances will combine both.

Statutory health and social services

Since the setting up of the National Health Service in 1947, statutory services for mental illness have been in three parts: general practitioner, local authority and hospital-based consultant services.

General practitioner services

Every citizen is entitled to a general practitioner, and the vast majority of the population are registered with a general practice. About 50 per cent of doctors who qualify enter general practice, and there are about 25,000 practitioners providing a wide range of services to, on average, about 2,000 patients each. Most practitioners now work in a group practice rather than on their own.

The majority of patients suffering from major psychotic disorders, such as schizophrenia, manic-depressive psychosis, or from dementing illnesses, will be referred by the general practitioner to a consultant psychiatrist. There will then very often be a period of inpatient care in a hospital under the care of the consultant, and following discharge from hospital care is usually shared by the general practitioner and consultant. However, overwhelmingly the commonest mental disorders occurring in the community are the neurotic disorders, involving anxiety and lesser degrees of depression; the majority of such patients are seen in general practice but are not often referred to specialist psychiatric services.

Figure 22.1 shows the 'pathway to psychiatric care'. As the severity of illness increases, the intensity of care becomes greater, but to a decreasing number of people. Goldberg and Huxley estimated that of 1,000 adults in the general population, 250 if assessed in random samples will show some degree of psychiatric morbidity during any year; 230 of these 250 will present themselves with psychiatric morbidity to their general practitioner during the year; 140 of these will be recognized by the general practitioner as suffering from *conspicuous psychiatric morbidity*; 17 of these will be referred to psychiatric services; but only 6 will be admitted as psychiatric inpatients. These authors have likened the situation to a 'filter' acting between each pair of levels preventing a number of the patients involved from progressing to the next level.

Social Services

Social Services are, ideally, complementary to health-service provision. They fall into three broad sectors: local authority Social Services Departments, probation and after-care services, and voluntary agencies. Each of these has some association with the mentally ill. Local authority Social Services Departments provide residential services for the elderly and homes for those with physical and learning disability. They also provide field-work services, including child-care social work which gives counselling to parents and children, oversight of children at risk (especially from non-accidental injury) and implementation of the social work component of the Mental Health Act (see Chapter 24). Local authority support services include running day centres for the elderly, the mentally ill and those with learning disability. Amongst hospital services provided by social workers employed by the local authority are counselling for patients' relatives, environmental assistance and work with other professional staff towards the discharge of patients, providing practical help and liaising with other agencies to facilitate continuity of care. Social workers often have a specific role in carrying out the social component of a care programme for a mentally ill person discharged from hospital.

Probation and after-care services are responsible to the Home Office and are involved with a variety of mostly court-based activities. A proportion of their clients are mentally ill offenders (see Chapter 24).

Voluntary agencies have been particularly useful in providing services for specific interest

	The community		Primary medical care			Specialist psychiatric services	
	Level 1	**Level 2**		**Level 3**		**Level 4**		**Level 5**
	Morbidity in random community samples	Total psychiatric morbidity, primary care		Conspicuous psychiatric morbidity		Total psychiatric patients		Psychiatric inpatients only
One-year period prevalence, median estimates	250	230		140		17		6 (per 1000 at risk per year)
		First filter		*Second filter*		*Third filter*		*Fourth filter*
Characteristics of the four filters		Illness behaviour		Detection of disorder		Referral to psychiatrists		Admission to psychiatric beds
Key individual		The patient		Primary care physician		Primary care physician		Psychiatrist
Factors operating on key individual		Severity and type of symptoms; Psychosocial stress; Learned patterns of illness behaviour		Interview techniques; Personality factors; Training and attitudes		Confidence in own ability to manage; Availability and quality of psychiatric services; Attitudes towards psychiatrists		Availability of beds; Availability of adequate community psychiatric services
Other factors		Attitudes of relatives; Availability of medical services; Ability to pay for treatment		Presenting symptom pattern; Socio-demographic characteristics of patient		Symptom pattern of patient; Attitudes of patient and family		Symptom pattern of patient, risk to self or others; Attitudes of patient and family; Delay in social worker arriving

Figure 22.1 The pathway to psychiatric care: 5 levels and 4 filters
Source: Goldberg and Huxley, 1980

groups; for example, the National Schizophrenia Fellowship and the Manic-Depression Fellowship, which inform and help patients and their relatives involved with those conditions. There are also many self-help groups, such as Alcoholics Anonymous. The National Association for Mental Health (MIND) has run hostels for discharged patients and also carried out other socially supportive activities.

Consultant-based mental health services

National Health Service mental health services are partly provided in the hospital and partly in the community. The government White Paper 'Better services for the mentally ill' (1975) recommended that inpatient psychiatric beds would most appropriately be sited in district general hospitals. There has been a substantial move towards this, and there are now many psychiatric units in such hospitals. With appropriate beds sited in a geographically convenient place with satisfactory wards and facilities, and an adequate number of consultants, other medical staff and members of other professional disciplines, it is possible to provide a good service with fewer psychiatric beds than were necessary in the past.

Outpatient clinics should also be available, perhaps at a district general hospital or in a community health centre, general practice premises or other place easily accessible to patients. Day hospital treatment facilities are also required. These are particularly useful for the rehabilitation of patients with long-term mental illnesses, and also for the treatment of those with severe neurotic disorders for whom admission to hospital may be counterproductive. These two groups of patients may require separate facilities.

Increasingly, psychiatrists are working for at least part of their time in the community, and this involves a close working relationship with general practice. Working practices vary – a consultant psychiatrist may hold an outpatient clinic in a general practitioner health centre, and this is most satisfactory when there is considerable communication between the psychiatrist and general practitioner. Sometimes, the psychiatrist is involved with the general practitioner and practice staff in a case conference discussing particular psychiatric problems within the practice. Some psychiatrists lead mental health teams whose practice is to assess almost all new referrals by visiting patients in their own homes.

Rehabilitation services increasingly extend outside hospital into the community. There may, for example, be provision of a ward in the hospital as a preparation for living outside. After patients have been through this part of the programme, they may then progress to living in a mental health hostel or group home in the locality from which they originally came. Group homes foster independence but may also provide intermittent support from staff and other residents which may enable each individual to make a smooth transition from long-term inpatient care to a fulfilling life in the community. For this to be effective, professional supervision of the group home is required, and the patients must be carefully selected so that they can live amicably together.

Principles of psychiatric care

It has to be decided what setting would be best for the treatment of each individual patient; for instance, whether admission to hospital is necessary or desirable. If the patient is acutely disturbed, is suicidal or a risk to others, there may be no alternative to admission. If such a patient will not accept informal admission, even when this is offered tactfully, compulsory admission under the Mental Health Act may be required (see Chapter 24). Around 90 per cent of admissions are informal. Much depends on the patient's degree of insight. For instance, some depressed patients regard themselves as wicked and protest that they are unworthy of care or attention, and for this reason they may refuse admission. Manic patients may believe there is nothing wrong with them and so resist medical intervention. Patients with persecutory delusions may believe that the hospital authorities intend to harm them. Those with organic states, confusion, delirium or loss of awareness may be unable to make their intentions known, and compulsory admission may be necessary. Their underlying physical illness may require hospital care. Reasons for *informal* admission include unsatisfactory home circumstances or family difficulties preventing satisfactory treatment at home. Some patients may require admission for complex physical investigations to be carried out in order to determine whether there is underlying organic pathology.

Where admission is indicated there should be consideration as to what type of ward or unit would best suit the patient's condition. Most patients can be cared for adequately on an acute psychiatric ward, probably best sited in a district general hospital. The great majority of patients can be looked after on such an open unit although there are a few patients, usually potentially or actually violent, who may require more secure conditions. The best form of security is an adequate number of well-trained, confident staff, as locked doors and the trappings of restraint tend to promote further violence.

Many patients can be treated by day-care without admission; such treatment is particularly suitable for those whose relatives can adequately care for them at other times. Emotionally disturbed patients, unable to work on account of their symptoms, are also often best treated in this way. In fact, admission may be harmful as it may lead to undue dependence, which may impede treatment and prolong the condition.

There are also many patients who do not need admission to hospital at any time and can be quite adequately treated as outpatients, particularly those requiring individual or group psychotherapy. There are some in whom admission to hospital is contra-indicated, including certain patients who, although needing treatment, are able to continue at work. In particular, those with obsessional symptoms, on being forced to stop work, are inclined to fill their time with compulsive rituals.

During the course of a patient's treatment in hospital consideration must be given to preparing for discharge. A *care plan* should be agreed with other members of staff during inpatient treatment and then carried out, ensuring that on discharge the patient has acceptable and adequate accommodation and the necessary level of support from relatives or carers. On discharge, the after-care plan should be agreed with the Social Services Department if further treatment involves a social worker. Community care is only meaningful if care is actually provided after discharge; this implies provision of facilities in the community and cooperation between health and social services to make sure that the patient can take advantage of them. Care plans should be written in the case notes indicating which member of staff will carry out which activity.

It is also important to make sure that missed outpatient appointments or treatment sessions are not ignored. A period of attendance at a day hospital before being referred to the outpatient clinic may be useful, or alternatively going to a Social Services day centre may be more appropriate. There has been a substantial change from predominantly long-term inpatient care, with more than 150,000 patients resident in British mental hospitals in 1955, reducing to fewer than 60,000 in 1990. The number of admissions over this time has increased, but the mean duration of inpatient stay has been enormously reduced.

Deciding when to discharge a patient can often be as difficult as when to admit. There is a temptation to discharge patients with depression prematurely, as often, following appropriate treatment, they feel so much improved that they press for discharge. However, if this is allowed prematurely, relapse may ensue, and under these circumstances the risk of suicide may be high. The depressed patient may wish to leave hospital for understandable reasons, but not be able to be involved in social life at home, and in particular not be ready to return to work. Discharge may need to be delayed until lasting improvement is assured so that previous activity can be gradually resumed. Where weight has been lost, weight gain is a good guide to secure recovery.

Care should be taken to ensure that patients with schizophrenia are not kept in hospital longer than necessary owing to their tendency to become institutionalized. However, the manner of their discharge and after-care should also be carefully planned. Supervision, especially where long-acting drug therapy is deemed to be desirable, must be arranged either at a specifically organized clinic or under the supervision of a general practitioner and a community-based psychiatric nurse. A *service register* is particularly useful for ensuring that contact is retained and relapse thus prevented amongst outpatients. The type of continuing treatment is recorded so that if a patient fails to attend, the appropriate person, usually a psychiatric nurse, is immediately informed and will seek out the patient at home. Such a system, kept scrupulously up to date, can prevent deterioration of a patient's mental state passing unnoticed with possibly disastrous consequences.

Return to his own family is not necessarily always in the best interest of a patient with schizophrenia. Where his family members show *high expressed emotion* towards him, with either excessive solicitousness and anxiety, or, alternatively, harsh scrutiny of his everyday activities, relapse becomes more likely. In this case, a period in a hostel or a group home with others who understand and can tolerate his eccentricities may be of benefit. There has been some experience recently in training relatives of schizophrenic patients so that their high expressed emotion becomes reduced when the relapse rate also appears to diminish.

Those with less severe depression and neurotic disorders may also present a problem for discharge, in that, perhaps having become unduly dependent on the hospital, they are liable to develop fresh symptoms whenever the possibility of discharge looms. One way of overcoming this difficulty may be by carefully defining the limit of stay soon after admission. Even though the patient may protest strongly that he has continuing symptoms at the time of discharge, he may be found on follow-up to have improved much more than might have been anticipated. The message should be conveyed in such a way that discharge is not perceived as rejection but the next logical step in caring treatment.

The therapeutic milieu

Over the last few decades, there has been greater emphasis upon patients using their own internal resources to ameliorate their psychiatric condition. This has found expression in *group therapy*, where individuals have been able to learn and practise more in a group than on their own; in *family therapy*, where the resources of the whole family to help their emotionally disturbed member has proved beneficial; and in *residential care*, where all the relationships of individual patients with one another and with staff are used in treatment.

The term 'therapeutic milieu' implies that the whole of the treatment environment is used to help patients get better. The patients are encouraged to take part in domestic activities and other types of work, and the difficulties and conflicts that occur are explored, usually in group discussion, in order to help each individual patient better understand the current causes of their difficulties and thereby make improvement. Such ways of working make considerable demands upon staff, but it can be extremely helpful for patients with neurotic and personality disorders, especially for problems with relationships.

The concept of the therapeutic community describes settings in which patients are encouraged to identify themselves with the life of the ward or unit so that each develops its own group culture. Acting as a group, patients make decisions affecting their own treatment and that of others; medical and nursing staff have a guiding rather than a controlling role. This has proved helpful, especially for patients with personality disorders. Good leadership and careful training of staff is necessary, as this type of treatment can lead to difficult situations involving both patients and staff; there is a danger of anarchy developing unless the leadership, although discreet, is clear and confident. There are three underlying principles:

1 interpersonal difficulties must be immediately aired and resolved;

2 communication must be maintained at all levels;

3 it must be realized that greater freedom of action involves taking a greater degree of responsibility for one's own actions.

These principles apply to staff and patients alike.

Social skills training

Many psychiatric patients suffer from problems in relationships; there are methods of lessening such deficiencies. *Social skills training* has become a component in treatment. Patients are taught how their verbal and non-verbal behaviour influences how other people feel and act, and how to modify this behaviour so to achieve worthwhile goals in social relationships.

Like other forms of *behavioural modification* (see Chapter 21), the first stage is the analysis of behaviour; breaking down the desired social skill into component parts, so that these may be achieved in sequence. It probably helps if the patient can identify with, and then *model* his behaviour upon, another person who copes satisfactorily in a particular social situation. On a psychiatric ward the role model may be provided by the senior psychiatric nurse conducting a social skills group. After learning how the skill is carried out and seeing this performed, the patient practises it under instruction. It is important to give him information about his performance and to reinforce positively his successes. Frequent *rehearsal* of the skill between treatment sessions is also essential.

Social skills training may be applied in various ways with different patients. A very directive form of training may assist in improving the social competence of those with a learning disability or chronic schizophrenia. Depression impairs social competence, and this in its turn causes further loss of self-esteem and lowering of mood; social skills training is an invaluable part of the management of those depressed patients who demonstrate *learned helplessness*. Amongst patients with neurotic disorders there

is virtually always difficulty with relationships, which social skills training may improve and consequently lessen feelings of failure. Those with sensitive, schizoid and asocial personality disorders may be helped by such training; although it is, of course, a prerequisite that the subject wishes to improve his social functioning and cooperates with treatment.

Some skills are especially amenable to treatment. *Assertiveness training* has been used to help the excessively timid and shy; in contrast, it has been attempted in excessively aggressive people to help them achieve a more socially acceptable form of behaviour. Training is also used to improve social relations with the opposite sex, and for those who have difficulties in initiating or establishing such a relationship. It may therefore form a component of both marital therapy and treatment for sexual dysfunction.

Rehabilitation

Rehabilitation is the process of identifying and then preventing or minimizing *social disablement* which has caused those affected to be unable to perform at a level that could reasonably be expected. Such disablement could be due to psychiatric illness, to disadvantages such as poverty, homelessness or unemployment, or to individual reactions to symptoms. Before rehabilitation can be attempted, a thorough *assessment* in order to determine the type and severity of disability that is present must be made. It is also important to discover what aptitudes the patient has, to agree with him what goals should be aimed for, to make a realistic treatment plan, to determine which members of staff and what treatments are most appropriate, and to monitor the progress made. Such assessment also includes an investigation of his social and family circumstances in order to determine whether further support will be required. The presence of any particular problem behaviour is identified, including an assessment of his ability to carry out everyday activities of living and working.

For many patients rehabilitation implies long-term management. Dealing with those who are mute, inaccessible, apathetic, recurrently disturbed or unhygienic makes considerable demands upon staff, so that a well-trained and harmonious multidisciplinary professional team is essential. The specific techniques used in rehabilitation will include various types of behavioural therapy and individual methods such as occupational and industrial therapy, crisis intervention and the use of appropriate drugs.

Disabled persons

The Disabled Persons (Employment) Act (1944) provided for special officers within the local offices of the Department of Employment known as Disablement Resettlement Officers to keep a register of disabled persons and assist in their rehabilitation and re-employment. Often they work with Industrial Rehabiliation Units, Government Training Schemes and certain forms of protected employment. The interest they show in mentally disordered patients and the skill in placement of such people varies, and to some extent depends upon the amount of support and contact they have from and with members of the psychiatric team.

Occupational therapy

The skills of the occupational therapist complement those of the psychiatrist in both hospital and community treatment of the mentally ill. Occupational therapy uses *activity*, prescribed and carefully planned, to treat and maximize recovery from illness. It has been known since the introduction of humane methods of treatment in the late eighteenth century that congenial, absorbing and sociable employment helped the mentally ill to get better. Occupational therapists work with groups of patients as well as individuals and make a considerable contribution in treating various conditions.

In order to enable the individual to cope with the demands of everyday life programmes of activity are designed for the patient to develop skills needed for work, domestic life, leisure and interpersonal relationships. Sometimes this means learning new skills and sometimes unlearning harmful or destructive habits. The patient then needs to practise these skills in everyday life. Creative and artistic activity is also beneficial for improving personal satisfaction, self-expression and communication.

Industrial and recreational therapy

As well as the more general aims of promoting activity, developing interests, self-confidence and pride of achievement, industrial rehabilitation is used to teach fresh skills that will be useful to the patient on discharge from hospital after improvement from his current illness. Much greater emphasis is now placed upon occupations in which patients are encouraged to work together on group projects, thus bringing about greater social interaction, together with the development of social skills.

With shrinking opportunities for unskilled work and a rise in unemployment, the emphasis of industrial therapy has become less on aiming to make the patient a wage-earner and more upon achieving fulfilment and self-esteem and the more general objectives of rehabilitation. The era when industrial rehabilitation took place on a large scale within the psychiatric hospital is now over. The emphasis is much more upon helping the individual to find sheltered or partly sheltered employment in the community rather than carrying out repetitive factory tasks within the hospital environment. Industrial therapy units that were in the past sited within the psychiatric hospital are increasingly now placed in local authority or other premises closer to where people without mental illnesses work and live. However, it is important to retain the principles that enabled the best hospital units to function effectively, including the careful grading of work in stages towards a greater degree of activity and responsibility, so fitting a patient towards working outside the hospital.

Not all patients, particularly those suffering from chronic mental illness or from severe learning disability, can reach a high level of activity. It is therefore important to select carefully grading of activities and choice of goals with each individual patient in mind, using a variety of different working conditions including industrial therapy units, sheltered workshops, secure occupation outside hospital, and the resources and contacts of voluntary organizations. It is important also, of course, not to damage a patient's fragile feeling of security and self-esteem by clumsy recommendations in this area. A depressed university lecturer will not feel that relief of symptoms is being reinforced by being asked to take part in repetitive manual work. Ingenuity and drive are required of those engaged in organizing programmes so as to make them therapeutic.

The role of the social worker

Most social workers come into regular contact with sufferers from mental disorders, and it is important therefore that they have knowledge of mental illnesses and their treatment. In addition, some social workers have further training and experience with the mentally ill and make a considerable contribution to treatment, rehabilitation and maintenance in the community. Trained social workers have a statutory role in the compulsory admission of the mentally ill under the terms of the Mental Health Act (1983) (see Chapter 24). They also have a significant role in the after-care of discharged hospital inpatients, and, following the implementation of the National Health Service and Community Care Act (1991), the relationship with hospital authorities should be considerably strengthened.

Social workers have an important role in assisting mentally ill people living in the community, both with their relationships and in dealing with the social care system. They form a particularly useful link between the family and the community from which patients come, and hospital-based staff. They are also an important part of the multidisciplinary team for those with learning disability. Probation officers, who have a different type of social work background from those employed by the local authority, are much involved in the rehabilitation of mentally ill offenders and they therefore require knowledge about mental illness.

Some social workers have had further training in family therapy and may form part of the team dealing with disturbed children and adolescents, and their families. In the past, there were many social workers involved in dynamic psychotherapy but this has diminished in recent years. Unfortunately through the 1970s and 80s in Britain there was to some extent a lessening of expertise in the area of mental health amongst the generality of social workers. This was partly caused by shortage of staff because of greatly increased demands of statutory work with children, and partly that within the mental health field itself implementing the Mental Health Act involved an undue proportion of the time that social workers had available. It appears that the balance is now being redressed and that at least some social workers are developing greater expertise in the treatment of the mentally ill.

A social worker can play a useful part within the mental health multidisciplinary team by providing a different slant from the health service professions. Social workers are able to take a discriminating social history thus providing much additional information about and insight into the patient's cultural and family background. To do this properly the social worker requires time and also training which is both practical and theoretical, with understanding of psychiatric concepts and a knowledge of what is likely to be significant in the relatives' account.

The social worker is also in a unique position to help with the emotional needs of the family which may – for instance, in the situation of high expressed emotion in the families of patients with schizophrenia – be an important determinant of the efficacy of treatment. The social worker is able to assess the emotional climate of the patient's home and ascertain serious needs which may call for relief. It is often valuable for the family to have a knowledgeable and sympathetic outsider to talk to, someone who is neither a member of the family nor has the perceived authority of the doctor. There is often a need to interpret the meaning of a patient's mental disorder to anxious or incredulous relatives who may have totally misinterpreted what they were told in the hospital or at the general practitioner's surgery.

Social workers are often called upon to marshal the existing community social services in aid of the patient under treatment; thus children may need to be provided with alternative accommodation, a home help may be required for a patient with schizophrenia or for a widowed mother with a young family. The problems of debt and threatened homelessness may involve negotiations with various helping services. A social worker knows in some detail what is available in the social care system and how to use this for the benefit of each client. Social workers have a particularly important role in after-care when the patient has left hospital; the patient should be seen as having many different needs and also individual resources, rather than being pigeon-holed into any one type of 'problem'. Many treatment plans fail because of difficulties arising from the nature of the disorder itself. For example, the deluded patient who believes that his neighbours are trying to blow poison gas through his letter box will prove difficult to integrate in normal society. Much patience, capacity to listen – particularly to the undertones – and the refusal to be exasperated by failure, are all requisites for those who wish to do social work in the field of mental health.

Apart from this, a social worker with specialized training is a safeguard both to the patient and to his relatives while carrying out statutory work with the Mental Health Act. Social workers are on call day and night to meet emergencies caused by disturbed and excited people in the community. They are involved in the process of compulsory admission (Chapter 24). The way in which these difficult situations are handled may do much to reduce the fear which keeps alive in many people's minds the dread of any form of psychiatric illness and its treatment.

The psychiatric nurse

In hospital the patient has more contact with psychiatric nurses than any other profession.

Nurses are responsible for carrying out treatment – this having been planned jointly by a team of mental health professionals under the clinical direction of the consultant psychiatrist. With so much of psychiatric care now taking place in the community, only the most severely ill and often most disturbed of patients are treated as inpatients. This makes even greater demands than previously on ward nurses, and maintaining their clinical skills, high morale and adequate staffing levels is essential.

Follow-up care at home is increasingly being provided by *community psychiatric nurses*. Psychiatric nursing has changed its role from an emphasis upon custodial care in institutions to more active treatment, greater involvement in rehabilitation, and work in the community. The range of patients with whom the psychiatric nurse now comes into contact has also been considerably expanded, with more types of treatment available.

This has made a considerable impact upon the training of nurses as they now need to know much more about the social management of patients outside hospital, and about individual and group methods of psychological treatment for inpatients and day patients. With better and more intensive training, more nurses are taking on the role of *nurse therapist* in behavioural or dynamic psychotherapy.

The traditional skills and attitudes of nursing, with considerate care and judicious kindness, are very important for dealing with elderly psychiatric patients, especially those with dementia. A good nurse in this situation will put an emphasis upon retaining human dignity and helping the patient to remain a distinct individual with his own ideas and property. The hospital environment is so organized that as far as possible the patient is kept in touch with reality, independence is encouraged, and normal coping is maintained for as long as possible.

Voluntary associations

Social concern for mental disorder expresses itself through voluntary as well as statutory organizations. Thus, national and international councils of mental health have been formed, directed towards the prevention and improved treatment of psychiatric disorders and towards ensuring adequate professional training and standards for those working in the field. In Britain the voluntary organization concerned with the management of all mental disorders is the National Association for Mental Health (MIND).

The range of psychiatric care for mental disorder has greatly widened in the last fifty years and the voluntary bodies have played a large part in ensuring this; there are now about 200 such organizations active in the United Kingdom. Collaboration continues, and voluntary bodies often spearhead progress – for example, with group homes, day hospitals and various other projects to help the mentally ill. The growth of local associations for mental health has often resulted in the extension of good practice from centres of excellence to more remote places.

Voluntary organizations also give an opportunity for patients and their relatives to express their views on the statutory facilities, and to make known their needs. For example, the National Schizophrenia Fellowship and the Manic-Depression Fellowship each play a valuable role in demanding better services for the treatment of the mentally ill, and they are particularly effective when campaigning alongside mental health professionals to gain support from government and local authorities. Age Concern and Help the Aged have a specific remit for the elderly, including both physical and mental disability, and they convey the important message that old age itself is neither illness nor disability but a healthy state of normality. Mencap has a distinguished record in helping people with learning disability and their families in many practical ways.

There has recently been a development of self-help and 'user' organizations. The first of these was Alcoholics Anonymous, but subsequently other organizations have developed to deal with specific conditions, including eating disorders, phobic states and many others. User organizations have developed to give patients and previous patients more control over the resources and methods used for treatment. It is an extension of the consumer movement into health provision, and it can encourage treatment services to be more humane and better directed to the needs and wishes of individual patients.

It is a challenge for modern psychiatry, dedicated to working in the community, to cooperate with voluntary organizations, providing professional advice and information and giving appropriate support and access to health care. Some voluntary organizations provide patients' advocates, volunteers with some knowledge of the law and health and Social Services who help patients obtain their right to adequate treatment; this is particularly useful for those with complex and intertwined problems involving both mental health services and social work agencies. The best provision of care comes when the professionals and volunteers cooperate closely with the needs of individual sufferers uppermost in their minds.

Further reading

Department of Health and Social Security (1975) 'Better services for the mentally ill', London: HMSO.
Goldberg, D. and Huxley, P. (1980) *Mental Illness in the Community: The Patterns to Psychiatric Care*, London: Tavistock Publications.
Huxley, P. (1985) *Social Work Practice in Mental Health*, Aldershot: Gower.
Wing, J.K. and Morris, B. (1981) *Handbook of Psychiatric Rehabilitation Practice*, London: Oxford University Press.

23

Treatment (3): Physical

Modern physical treatments have done much to reduce morbidity, particularly from the psychoses, and have led to patients remaining in hospital for shorter periods than before. However, their action is still poorly understood, and so, like psychological treatments, physical treatments must still be regarded as empirical procedures.

Physical and psychological treatments cannot be entirely dissociated. Every physical procedure exerts a psychological effect, in part derived from the nature of the treatment, from the way it is administered, and from the prestige of the therapist. Of all physical treatments, this is most obvious in drug therapy. About one-third of patients are placebo reactors who respond favourably, perhaps only temporarily, to almost any physical or psychological procedure. Similarly, the way drugs are prescribed and the belief of both patient and doctor in their efficacy may have an effect almost as profound as that of the drug itself. Although inconvenient in research, the placebo effect can be used to maximize the benefits of treatment. It also accounts for side effects in many cases.

For many treatment interventions the best results may be achieved by combining psychosocial with physical methods. It is therefore very important for doctors to know about the indications, precise treatment regime and disadvantages of both types of therapy, and be prepared to use both in combination when appropriate.

General medical care

The need for careful physical examination and such physical investigations as are necessary has already been stressed. Attention should be paid to the general state of physical health of those psychiatric patients who are debilitated by loss of appetite and weight, sleeplessness, and the abuse of alcohol or drugs, as well as to physical illnesses which may be only indirectly associated with the presenting psychiatric disorder but may affect its course. Thus, where anaemia, infection, electrolyte imbalance or other treatable disorder is present, this must be corrected. In alcoholism and in elderly patients where there is poor nutrition, the possibility of avitaminosis should be considered and special attention paid to diet and to replacement.

Many psychiatric patients are under-weight, particularly those who are depressed, tense or anxious. In these a satisfactory gain in weight during treatment may be a sign of recovery. Conversely, in depressed patients who appear to improve but who fail to gain weight, relapse is likely. Weighing should, therefore, be carried out for inpatients at weekly intervals, and the results carefully charted.

Drug treatment

Until the action of drugs upon the central nervous system is better understood, only a working classification, in part based on their general clinical effects and, in part, chemical or pharmacological, is feasible. Although some relationships between chemical structure and clinical effects may be apparent, this is variable. In some cases the effect produced is uncertain, occasionally paradoxical; and it may also vary according to dose and the current condition of the patient. The same is true of side effects.

The following classification includes psychotropic drugs – that is, drugs that have an effect on the mental state and symptoms – and anti-Parkinsonian and anti-epileptic drugs. (Note: as there are so many different preparations available, any attempt at a comprehensive catalogue is out of the question. Nor is it realistic; the position has now been reached where the wisest course of action is for prescribers to acquaint themselves as thoroughly as possible with the action, toxicity and other side effects of relatively few well-tried drugs. Some drugs will be available at the time of publication which were not obtainable at the time of writing, and others may have been withdrawn. Proprietary names are not used here and should be avoided; first, because they vary from one country to another, and, second, because, even in the same country, a drug manufactured by different pharmaceutical companies may be given a different proprietary name.)

1 Anxiolytics
    Benzodiazepines
    Other drugs used for anxiety
2 Hypnotics
3 Antipsychotic drugs
4 Antidepressants
    Tricyclic and related antidepressants
    Monoamine oxidase inhibitors
    5-Hydroxytryptamine reuptake inhibitors (serotonin-specific reuptake inhibitors, SSRIs)

    Lithium
5 Stimulants
6 Anti-Parkinsonian drugs
7 Other drugs
    Anti-epileptics
    Psychotomimetics
    Deterrent drugs
    Cyproterone acetate

Anxiolytics

Anxiolytic drugs are the most commonly used of all the psychotropics in primary care. However, it should be borne in mind from Chapter 21 that, for preference, anxiety should be treated psychologically and not pharmacologically. There are also life circumstances – for example, before examinations – when a certain degree of anxiety is beneficial, and eliminating it, especially with drugs that cause drowsiness, is in fact harmful. In general, psychiatrists more often try to help patients stop taking anxiolytic drugs than prescribe them. Tolerance usually develops within six weeks or less, and therefore if they are used to treat acute anxiety through a specific occasion or episode in life, then short-term prescription is the favoured method.

Benzodiazepines

The pharmacological properties of benzodiazepines are anxiolytic, sedative, hypnotic, muscle relaxant and anticonvulsant. They act through specific receptor sites to enhance GABA neurotransmission and hence to block Noradrenaline and 5-HT systems. Short-acting benzodiazepines, which include temazepam and lorazepam, seem to cause dependency even more rapidly than longer-acting benzodiazepines. Long-acting drugs include diazepam, chlordiazepoxide and nitrazepam. All these drugs are absorbed quickly and, bound to plasma proteins, are rapidly taken up in the brain.

The commonest unwanted actions of benzodiazepines when used to treat anxiety are drowsiness, ataxia and difficulties with concentration and cognition. Impaired coordination affects driving and using dangerous machinery. These effects are potentiated by alcohol and are more severe in elderly patients and in those with renal or hepatic impairment. A paradoxical effect of benzodiazepines has been observed in which, rather than reducing agitation, by diminishing censoring they actually result in an increase in aggressive behaviour. Benzodiazepines are relatively safe even with large over-dosage, but less safe when alcohol or other drugs are also ingested.

Habituation to benzodiazepines occurs quite rapidly, and they should only be used as anxiolytics or hypnotics for a short time, if at all. Withdrawing patients from these drugs can be extremely difficult as there is both physical and emotional dependence in a substantial minority of patients. Withdrawal symptoms of insomnia, apprehensiveness, nausea, tremor and even fits are experienced by patients. Some of these experiences are similar to the original anxiety symptoms for which the drug was prescribed, and this increases the difficulty in withdrawal. Symptoms start within a few days of stopping the drug, and it is recommended therefore that withdrawal after prolonged treatment should take place very gradually over weeks or even months.

Benzodiazepines also have anti-epileptic properties and may be used in disturbed epileptic patients together with anticonvulsants. This property also affects EEG findings so that, where this investigation is contemplated, they should be withdrawn at least two weeks before. Diazepam may also be given intravenously to control status epilepticus, or to control withdrawal symptoms in drug dependence; benzodiazepines have had a useful role in the treatment of delirium tremens. It should be noted, however, that the benzodiazepines are themselves inclined to produce dependence and that epileptic fits can occur on withdrawal. Confusion states due to chronic over-dosage have also been observed.

Hypnotics

Most of the anxiolytic drugs described above are sedative and may also therefore be used as hypnotics. Insomnia is a very frequent complaint

made to a general practitioner. It is probably the most frequent symptom presented in all neurotic disorders and is also a prominent feature of depressive illness. It is a more common complaint in women and amongst the elderly. The most commonly used hypnotics are benzodiazepine drugs, of which a longer-acting example is nitrazepam, and shorter-acting, temazepam. Once again, it is recommended that such drugs, if used at all, should not be used long-term, as after about six weeks' use they tend to become ineffective, tolerance develops, and the patient may become habituated so that withdrawal is difficult. Hypnotics alter the normal pattern of the sleep EEG with reduction of the proportion of rapid eye movement (REM) sleep. On stopping the drug, disturbed sleep may occur with dreams associated with an increase in REM sleep. The longer-acting benzodiazepines are likely to produce some drowsiness the following day. Hypnotic drugs are potentiated by alcohol, which is another reason for always taking a careful history of alcohol intake.

Other hypnotic (and anxiolytic) drugs include the *barbiturates*, which would not now be recommended for this purpose as there are better alternatives and they carry considerable risk of dependency. *Chloral hydrate* and its less irritant derivatives such as dichloralphenazone are useful for children and old people.

Chlormethiazole is occasionally used in psychiatry for the treatment of anxiety; it is markedly anticonvulsant and also hypnotic. It is absorbed extremely rapidly and, like short-acting benzodiazepines, produces pharmacological dependence. It is particularly useful in states of acute excitement and restlessness such as delirium tremens, when it may be administered intravenously.

In general, on request for hypnotic medication the doctor should, as in all other situations, take a careful history and give appropriate advice based on psychological principles. The need for duration of sleep is generally reduced in middle and old age; some people who lead inactive lives tend to have short periods of sleep during the day which will necessarily inhibit sleep at night. Caffeine, taken as tea or coffee in the evening, is likely to promote sleeplessness, as are physical symptoms such as pain, cough or pruritis.

Antipsychotic drugs

The antipsychotic drugs, variously known as *major tranquillizers* or *neuroleptics*, are used to treat psycho-motor excitement and control other symptoms of schizophrenia, mania and organic psychosyndromes. These drugs may also be effective in the prevention of relapse in schizophrenia. The *phenothiazine* group of drugs has been used for longest, and for the largest number of patients. *Butyrophenone* drugs have also proved effective, and more recently other groups of antipsychotic drugs have been added.

Phenothiazines

Chlorpromazine, which remains a widely used major tranquillizer, was introduced to psychiatry in 1952 following the experience of Laborit and Huguenard who used it in the Indo-Chinese War to produce 'artificial hibernation' as a prophylactic agent against severe surgical shock. Chlorpromazine is hypothermic, hypotensive, anti-emetic and weakly antihistaminic. It has a fairly strong sedative action and potentiates the effects of other cerebral depressants, such as anaesthetics, barbiturates and alcohol. There is evidence that it acts by blocking dopamine receptors, and this may contribute to its antipsychotic activity.

The main indications for the use of chlorpromazine are as follows:

1 *To control states of severe excitement and tension* Chlorpromazine appears to be effective without regard to the basis of such states; that is, whether delirium, mania, acute agitated depression or schizophrenic excitement. In severe cases, parenteral administration may be required initially. Care should be taken, as this is liable to produce a fall in blood pressure. It should also be noted that intramuscular injections of chlorpromazine are painful.

2 *As a neuroleptic or psychotropic agent* Apart from controlling excitement, chlorpromazine has a striking effect upon certain schizophrenic symptoms such as hallucinations. Its use in doses ranging from 200 to 1,500 mg daily may improve the mental state in schizophrenia so as to enable resocialization and rehabilitation. Where a satisfactory effect is obtained, long-term maintenance therapy may be required, although today this is probably better done in most cases by the use of depot injections.

3 *As a sedative* Given at night, 50–100 mg will produce sleep in many patients.

4 *As a minor tranquillizer* Small doses – for example, 10–25 mg – one to three times daily, may be effective. However, although controlling anxiety, chlorpromazine depresses some patients. One advantage, however, is that it does not appear to be habit-forming.

Side-effects of chlorpromazine

These are of three main kinds: (1) those which are inherent in the drug's action and include dryness of mouth, constipation, increase of appetite, gain in weight, galactorrhoea, extrapyramidal symptoms; (2) idiosyncratic effects, notably cholestatic jaundice and agranulocytosis – the latter is extremely rare though occasional fatalities have been recorded; and (3) convulsions. Chlorpromazine occasionally induces epileptic fits, particularly in brain-damaged patients.

In larger doses – that is, over 400–500 mg daily – extrapyramidal symptoms are more likely to occur. While Parkinsonism is the commonest variety, other forms, for example *torsion spasm*, *akathisia* (restless treading of the feet) and *tasikinesia* (forced walking-about), can occur, though these are seen more commonly with certain other neuroleptic drugs – for example, trifluoperazine or haloperidol. Parkinsonian symptoms usually disappear when the drug is withdrawn or the dose reduced. Parkinsonian symptoms may usually be adequately controlled by anticholinergic drugs such as procyclidine, benztropine or orphenadrine.

Another side effect, troublesome in subtropical or tropical climates, is that of photosensitive skin reactions. Patients should be told to avoid direct exposure to sunlight and wear long sleeves and a hat. In elderly patients, chlorpromazine needs to be used cautiously owing to its tendency to produce hypotension and hypothermia.

Trifluoperazine is much more potent than chlorpromazine. Its effects are similar, but it is usually much less sedative. Extrapyramidal symptoms are also commoner.

Trifluoperazine may be used in two ways: as a minor, non-dependency-forming tranquillizer (1–2 mg thrice daily); or as a major tranquillizer (10–30 mg daily), either alone or in combination with chlorpromazine primarily in the treatment of more chronic schizophrenic illnesses – especially those of later life and in patients with fairly well-preserved personalities (paraphrenia, see Chapter 18), where it is often of value. Having a more stimulating effect, trifluoperazine may also be useful in younger, withdrawn and anergic schizophrenic patients.

Thioridazine is somewhat similar in action to chlorpromazine in calming agitation and restlessness. It is the least likely of the phenothiazines to cause Parkinsonian symptoms. Retinal pigmentation has been reported with prolonged high doses.

Long-acting phenothiazines, such as *fluphenazine decanoate* in depot injection, are used widely. Whereas the action of these drugs differs little from other phenothiazines, they are prepared in a sesame-oil vehicle and when injected are absorbed only gradually over a period of time. A single injection of 25 mg of fluphenazine decanoate may, therefore, be effective from two to four weeks, or more. It is, however, wise to begin treatment with a small dose to test the effect.

Patients with schizophrenia are often non-compliant with oral medication when this is prescribed. Long-acting phenothiazines, therefore, appear to have considerable value in the maintenance treatment of chronic schizophrenia, and depot injections are now a regular feature in psychiatric outpatient departments, where patients attend for periodic injections. Alternatively, an injection may be given by a community psychiatric nurse who, acting under medical instructions, visits the patient at home or carries out injection clinics in general practice health centres.

Butyrophenones and other antipsychotic drugs

Haloperidol is one of the most widely used neuroleptic agents. It is very likely to produce extrapyramidal symptoms, which are usually readily controlled by anti-Parkinsonian drugs; however, these symptoms may develop very rapidly at any time during treatment. Haloperidol is indicated in the treatment of severe over-activity and excitement. As it does not have the hypothermic and hypotensive effects of chlorpromazine, it may be useful in small doses in elderly agitated patients. It may be used in the treatment of mania, schizophrenic excitement and in delirious states. It also controls aggression and, on this account, may be effective in certain patients with learning disability given to violence. It has been used in the treatment of Gilles de la Tourette Syndrome in adults and children. It can also occasionally be remarkably effective in certain paranoid states. Haloperidol may be given orally or parenterally; twice, or even once-daily administration is often satisfactory. Haloperidol may also be administered in depot formulation and is effective in the prevention of relapse in many chronic schizophrenic patients.

Benperidol, a butyrophenone drug, has been used to reduce sexual activity in some patients involved in repetitive criminal sexual behaviour (page 131).

Pimozide is sometimes used in once-daily dosage for the control of schizophrenic symptoms, and is therefore an alternative to depot injections for maintenance. Its use has been advocated for the treatment of monosymptomatic somatic delusions such as those of infestation (Ekbom's Syndrome, see Chapter 2).

Flupenthixol, which is also available as a long-acting preparation, is chemically related to the phenothiazines. While its action is similar to that of fluphenazine, it is also claimed to have an antidepressant effect, and for this reason to be of value in schizophrenic patients who suffer from depressive symptoms which may sometimes be worsened by fluphenazine.

Clozapine, an azepine drug, has been used for prevention of recurrent schizophrenic episodes. It has been effective in treating some previously resistant patients, but as there is a risk of agranulocytosis, regular monitoring of white blood cells is necessary. *Sulpiride* has also been introduced more recently and may be helpful in reducing the risk of relapse.

The *neuroleptic malignant syndrome* has been reported as an extremely rare complication of almost all of the neuroleptic drugs. The condition develops rapidly, with severe stiffness and generalized muscular rigidity which may affect the throat and chest, causing dysphagia. The patient may show stupor, with impaired consciousness, and hyperpyrexia develops with fluctuating blood pressure, tachycardia, sweating and sometimes excess salivation and urinary incontinence. The creatinine phosphokinase level is usually raised and there is an increased white cell count. Treatment involves stopping neuroleptic drugs, cooling the patient, maintaining fluid balance and treating chest or other infections; dantrolene has been used, as for other causes of malignant hyperthermia.

Antidepressant drugs

There is considerable debate over the range of usefulness of antidepressant drugs, but in selected cases of moderate to severe depressive illness they are generally effective. The two main classes of drugs are the *tricyclics* and related drugs (see British National Formulary), and the *monoamine oxidase inhibitors*. *L tryptophan*, which was used in the past, has now been withdrawn. The *serotonin-specific reuptake inhibitors* (SSRIs) are increasingly used and *lithium* is also used for affective disorders.

Tricyclic and related antidepressants

Tricyclic antidepressants are still the most frequently prescribed. Any difference between the effects of imipramine and amitriptyline appear marginal, although some consider that the latter has more of a tranquillizing effect and is therefore indicated in agitated patients, while imipramine, on the other hand, is more stimulating and may achieve better results in those who are retarded. The same can probably be said of their apparently ever-growing number of derivatives.

Although some appear to suit some patients better than others, properly controlled studies usually demonstrate no significant differences. Imipramine has been extensively studied since its introduction in 1957. There are many reports of its use in depression. Antidepressant drugs alone are often effective in treating mild or moderate states of depression. However, because their action does not become apparent for fourteen to twenty-one days, or even longer in some cases, electroconvulsive therapy is still indicated in severe depressive illnesses, especially those accompanied by delusions and in which the suicidal risk is high. Combined treatment with antidepressant drugs and ECT seems to produce results no faster than ECT alone, although the combination may reduce relapse.

The considerations in choosing which antidepressant drugs are:

1 efficacy;
2 duration;
3 side effects, both uncomfortable and dangerous;
4 toxicity in overdose.

Recently, more attention has been paid to dosage and blood concentration levels but their clinical usefulness is not widely accepted. Once-daily administration of tricyclic antidepressant drugs is sufficient. For preference, the drugs should be administered at bedtime, at least initially, owing to their tendency to produce drowsiness. This may have the double advantage of promoting sleep and reducing drowsiness by day.

Side effects

Unlike the therapeutic action, these occur within a few days of administration. Drowsiness, dry mouth, visual disturbances, postural hypotension, sweating and constipation are common in the initial stages but usually soon wear off. As with the phenothiazines, excessive weight gain may occur. Jaundice can also rarely occur. Night sweats, constipation, urinary retention (usually in males with enlarged prostates, rarely in females), blurring of vision and the precipitation of glaucoma are side effects largely due to the anticholinergic action of tricyclics. More important are cardiac arrhythmias, heart block, and even ventricular fibrillation in those with pre-existing heart disease. It is wise, therefore, to avoid tricyclics when there is a recent history of myocardial infarction. Indeed, in some cases, there are grounds for believing ECT to be safer.

Tricyclic drugs interfere with the control of blood pressure with adrenergic blocking drugs, and they potentiate the action of adrenalin in local anaesthetics. They may precipitate fits in epileptic patients. Withdrawal symptoms such as insomnia, nausea and vomiting, and sweating have been described when they are rapidly withdrawn.

Tricyclic antidepressants seem to have a variable effect on potency. They may sometimes assist those with premature ejaculation by causing some slowness in ejaculation. In other instances they seem to impair potency, although how much of this is due to depression itself and how much due to treatment is often impossible to determine.

Tetracyclic antidepressants and certain other drugs structurally resembling tricyclic antidepressants are used, and claims have been made for fewer side effects, especially cardiac arrhythmia and serious anticholinergic actions.

Monoamine oxidase inhibitors (MAOIs)

These are so-called because they inhibit the action of the enzyme monoamine oxidase and thus prevent the destruction of serotonin (5-HT), noradrenaline (NA) and dopamine (DA). The therapeutic effect was observed first in the treatment of tuberculosis by iproniazid, leading to that drug being taken over into psychiatric practice, initially with encouraging results. But because of its tendency to produce liver necrosis, sometimes fatal, iproniazid and some similar drugs were soon dropped.

MAOIs, although potentially toxic, do have definite antidepressant properties. It would appear that the most effective, although also potentially dangerous, is *tranylcypramine*. Compared with tricyclic antidepressants, tranylcypramine has a much more rapid antidepressant action, having some amphetamine-like properties, leading, for instance, to wakefulness.

Phenelzine is also used, the indications being atypical depressive states, depression unresponsive to tricyclic drugs and phobic anxiety states.

Side-effects arise chiefly out of the action of MAOIs in inactivating the enzymes which oxidize biogenic amines found in some food or ingredients of medicines. Combination of MAOIs with such substances may produce hypertensive crisis or other serious reaction. Because the MAOI drugs will potentiate morphine and other narcotic analgesics, anaesthetists and dentists need to know if a patient is taking them. Because fatalities have been recorded, the patient should carry with him a card stating that he is currently being treated with an MAOI and informing the patient what foodstuffs and drugs are prohibited.

Another potentially fatal side effect is cerebral haemorrhage due to sudden severe hypertension. This is the so-called cheese reaction. If a patient taking an MAOI eats foods containing tyramine, most cheeses (Cheddar cheese in particular), Marmite, yeast-containing substances, broad bean pods, red wine (Chianti notably), or takes some pressor substance such as amphetamine or ephedrine, as may be contained in a nasal decongestant, this may result in a *hypertensive crisis* resembling that produced by a phaeochromocytoma.

Serotonin-specific reuptake inhibitors

Some drugs have a relatively specific action on the serotonin system rather than on other monoamines. 5-HT reuptake blockers include clomipramine and the more recently introduced drugs fluoxetine, fluvoxamine, paroxetine and sertraline. Studies would suggest that these new drugs are effective antidepressants. It is not known, however, how their efficacy compares with longer-established drugs and whether there are patients with a specific 5-HT deficiency whom they could benefit more especially.

Lithium salts

Lithium carbonate was first used by Cade in

Australia to treat schizophrenic and manic excitement. A growing number of investigations by Schou and others have since shown that lithium is effective not only in controlling mania but also, by long-term administration, in preventing the recurrence of manic attacks. It has also been claimed that long-term administration will prevent the occurrence or recurrence of depressive attacks. Although lithium certainly seems to control, at least in part and sometimes completely, the depressive phases of bipolar affective disorder, its effect on recurrent depression appears less certain.

The major therapeutic use of lithium is, therefore, prophylactic, against further episodes of depression or mania. Because of its toxicity and the fact that once started it may need to be taken lifelong, the decision to prescribe should not be undertaken lightly. Three episodes of mania or depression requiring hospitalization within five years would reasonably lead to the use of lithium, but only special circumstances would indicate its prophylactic use with fewer episodes or longer intervals between attacks.

Side effects of lithium toxicity can be serious; gastro-intestinal, cardiac and renal symptoms may occur. Coarse tremor is a sign of toxicity, although fine tremor may occur at therapeutic dose levels. It is important, therefore, and especially so in the early stages, to check serum lithium levels at relatively frequent intervals; these are best kept as low as possible, in the therapeutic range between 0.5 and 1.2 m/mol, to minimize side effects. The daily amount of lithium required to attain this level must be found by careful titration, but usually varies between 600 and 1,600 mg. Once- or twice-daily administration is generally satisfactory.

In an acute condition, the use of lithium for treatment rather than prophylaxis is recommended, although lithium works slowly, and it may, therefore, be necessary to bring manic excitement under control as soon as possible by giving chlorpromazine or haloperidol during the first week or ten days of treatment. Other side effects which may occur at therapeutic dose level include tiredness, thirst and polyuria. In the long term, lithium also depresses thyroid function, particularly in women, so that this should be checked at intervals. If pregnancy occurs, lithium should be stopped as it may be teratogenic; it is certainly contra-indicated during lactation. Women of child-bearing age should consider supervised cessation of lithium before trying to conceive.

If the patient has poor renal function, or if he requires a low-salt diet, lithium should not be used. Decreased dosage and more frequent checks of blood level will be required in the elderly.

Stimulants

Caffeine is a mild stimulant, and amphetamine and cocaine more powerfully so. Although caffeine in moderate dose will maintain vigilance at least for a time, it has no therapeutic use in psychiatry, and an anxiety state occurring in heavy coffee- or tea-drinkers may sometimes be effectively treated by ceasing caffeine ingestion. *Amphetamine* has no role in the treatment of depression. It is not appropriate for appetite suppression in obesity, as dependence readily develops. It is occasionally used for narcolepsy in adults and the hyperkinetic syndrome in children. *Cocaine* has no therapeutic use in psychiatry.

Anti-Parkinsonian drugs

Extrapyramidal symptoms frequently occur as side effects of neuroleptic drugs. These include acute dystonic reactions, opisthotonus, oculogyric crises and akathisia. Tardive dyskinesia, which may take years to develop, is often irreversible; there is pouting and smacking of lips, protrusion of the tongue, other grimacing movements of the mouth and sometimes grunting and fidgeting.

Severe, acute dystonic reactions may be treated by intramuscular or intravenous anticholinergic drugs such as *benztropine* or *procyclidine*. Less acute symptoms may be controlled orally with procyclidine, benztropine, *benzhexol* or *orphenadrine*. Akathisia may be diminished by a benzodiazepine. Anti-Parkinsonian drugs should only be used in conjunction with a neuroleptic if really necessary;

often dosage can be adjusted to provide good control of psychotic symptoms without side effects.

There is no satisfactory treatment for tardive dyskinesia at present, although there is considerable research into the effectiveness of selective dopamine blockers. Prevention is the primary aim, and the use of neuroleptic drugs should be reviewed regularly to see if they are still needed, and, if so, whether the dose may be reduced. In some patients, withdrawal dyskinesia will follow discontinuation of neuroleptic drugs; this may respond to diazepam as a muscle relaxant and minor tranquillizer.

Anti-Parkinsonian drugs such as those listed may, in larger dose, and especially in the elderly, cause an acute brain syndrome with confusion, delirium and hallucinations; this is similar to the atropine psychosis which occurred in the past. Anticholinergic effects may exacerbate glaucoma or provoke acute retention of urine in men. Drowsiness, nausea, dry mouth and constipation may also occur.

Other drugs

Anti-epileptic drugs are used to treat and prevent seizures. For partial or focal seizures *carbamazepine* is the drug of choice and *phenytoin* or *sodium valproate* may also be effective. For generalized seizures of the tonic–clonic type, again, these drugs should be considered first. In myoclonic and absence seizures sodium valproate is usually the drug of first choice. Diazepam, given intravenously, has a use in status epilepticus.

Disulfiram and *citrated calcium carbimide* have been prescribed to deter alcohol abusers from impulsive drinking. They act by blocking oxidation so that acetaldehyde accumulates, causing flushing of the face, headache, choking sensation, anxiety, tachycardia and hypotension. These drugs are prescribed with the patient's full cooperation, and he knows that these symptoms will only occur after the ingestion of alcohol. Some patients find beneficial the deterrent effect of having taken the tablet at a time of day when temptation is at its lowest. The reaction with alcohol is highly unpleasant and potentially dangerous.

Cyproterone acetate is an anti-androgen and, although not acting directly on the central nervous system, affects behaviour by reducing sexual desire in males. It has been used voluntarily for those whose sexually deviant behaviour has resulted in criminal acts and who wish to prevent recurrence.

Special procedures

Electroconvulsive therapy (electroplexy)

Electroconvulsive therapy (ECT) is carried out by the discharge of an electric current of a few milliamps at 100–200 RMS volts from 0.5 to 2 seconds. The charge delivered is often about 200 millicoulombs and sine wave delivery is usual. The two standard placements of electrodes are unilateral, usually parieto-temporal, and bilateral, which is virtually always bitemporal. The passage of current produces a typical grand mal seizure of slow onset over a few seconds. If the latter does not occur, this event is regarded as a sub-convulsive stimulus and should be followed by a second application at a higher voltage.

Atropine is often given before the passing of current to dry up secretions and lessen the risk of arrhythmia. Owing to the risk of fractures, treatment is now always carried out under light anaesthesia delivered by an anaesthetist, together with a short-acting muscle relaxant. This should limit convulsive movements to light twitching of the face and limbs sufficient to show that a seizure has actually occurred. A period of apnoea then follows, during which an airway is inserted and oxygen administered under pressure via a face mask and breathing bag, until normal respiration is restored. The patient can then be safely removed to the recovery room and kept under observation until he regains consciousness, five to ten minutes later. All apparatus necessary for anaesthetic resuscitation, including suction apparatus, cardiac defibrillation and emergency drugs, should be available, though they will very rarely be required. ECT may be given daily for a few days to the very depressed, agitated or restless patient, but is more customarily given two or three times per week. There is no such thing as a standard 'course' of treatment; the number of applications must be tailored to suit individual requirements. Most depressed patients respond adequately to six to eight treatments. These should be followed by an interval of seven to ten days during which, if relapse appears imminent, two or three further applications may be given as necessary. A satisfactory response may often be anticipated during a series of treatments when transient improvement follows the third or fourth application.

Preparation of the patient for ECT is very important. A full physical and psychiatric history and examination will always precede the decision to prescribe treatment. If dental treatment is necessary it should be given before proceeding with ECT to avoid inhaling tooth debris. The procedure, its benefits and dangers must always be explained to the patient and his written consent and cooperation obtained. Compulsorily detained patients who are prescribed ECT should also be asked to sign a form of consent for treatment. If a patient is unwilling to have treatment and ECT is considered essential, the Responsible Medical Officer (the consultant in charge) should invoke the Treatment Section of the Mental Health Act and seek the second opinion of an independently appointed consultant (see page 225). This procedure should also be used if the patient requires ECT and is unable to comprehend what he is being told.

On the morning of treatment no food or drink is given; and immediately prior to treatment the patient should empty his bladder. Dentures, hair-grips and tight clothing should be removed. Calming and encouraging words from the staff administering treatment, together with a humane and caring atmosphere in the treatment room, usually suffice to reassure all but the most agitated patients.

Although it is not known exactly how ECT works, there is some experimental evidence that it mobilizes neurotransmitter substances and possibly prevents the depletion of 5-Hydroxytryptamine in the mid-brain. As this has yet to be confirmed, ECT must continue, for the time being, to be regarded as an empirical procedure. However, the convulsion is a necessary element for the therapeutic effect. Because it is liable to stimulate somewhat frightening fantasies in the minds of lay people, ECT has tended in recent years to receive rather a bad press. This is a pity, for, when properly indicated, it may be remarkably effective and in many cases of depression safer and surer than drugs. Indeed, in some severe cases of depression ECT can be life-saving. The evidence for its effectiveness is amongst the strongest for any medical procedure.

Indications

The most important indication for ECT is severe depressive illness, especially if delusions are present, if there is marked agitation, if the patient is suicidal, or if there has been a failure to respond to antidepressant drugs.

While depressed patients respond best to ECT, certain patients acutely ill with schizophrenia may also receive considerable benefit, though a greater number of treatments may be required. ECT is particularly effective in catatonic states and may also help those who are paranoid, particularly in the presence of affective admixture. Manic states are, on the whole, less responsive and may need more treatment; however, there is some evidence that patients receiving ECT for mania spend less time in hospital, are better on discharge and make a better social recovery than those not treated with ECT. Electroconvulsive therapy may also be used for the relief of depression occurring in organic states such as in syphilitic general paralysis and Parkinsonism, and very occasionally in other physical conditions producing depression. Although not usually advocated for patients with epilepsy, it has been employed to terminate prolonged psycho-motor seizures (epileptic twilight states).

Contra-indications

There are virtually no absolute contra-indications to electroconvulsive therapy, and risks are largely confined to the anaesthetic procedure.

Age is no bar. Treatment may safely be given to both old and young; to pregnant women, without fear of abortion; even to some suffering from quite severe physical illnesses including cardiovascular diseases, though in this instance it is imperative to seek the services of an experienced anaesthetist. With recent experiences of myocardial infarction or cerebrovascular accident, ECT should be withheld for the time being unless there is risk of death from suicide, dehydration or starvation.

Side effects

Except for depersonalization, which may be made worse and may be regarded, therefore, as a contra-indication, the only really inconvenient side effect of modified ECT is its effect upon memory. In younger patients this is of little importance and, in the long run, rarely extends outside the period over which the treatment is given. In those who are older with, perhaps, some degree of cerebral degeneration, the effect of ECT on memory may be more profound and, in some instances, leads to a state of confusion. There is some evidence that unilateral ECT, in which the electrodes are applied only to the side of the head containing the non-dominant cerebral hemisphere, causes less memory disturbance than the more conventional practice of bitemporal placement. The non-dominant hemisphere is on the right side in nearly all right-handed and 70 per cent of left-handed people. There is also some evidence that unilateral is less effective than bilateral application.

ECT is an effective treatment for depression, but occasionally it can convert the illness of a patient with bipolar affective illness from depression into manic phase. A Welsh farmer had been successfully treated for depression with ECT and, after discharge from inpatient care, attended the outpatient clinic flamboyantly wearing morning dress and carrying a cane. Elated and talkative, he told the inexperienced trainee psychiatrist that he had never felt better and wanted to be discharged from outpatient care, with which the psychiatrist acceded. Three hours later the doctor received a telephone call

from the hospital telephonist informing him that there was a gift of six cows from this farmer at reception, and they were wondering what should be done with them!

ECT is compatible with drug treatment, though it is liable to produce confusional states in those who are receiving large doses of phenothiazines. There is also some risk of a fall in blood pressure in those given ECT in conjunction with chlorpromazine. ECT can safely be given together with antidepressant drugs such as imipramine or amitriptyline. Though this does not speed recovery from depression, the combination of antidepressant drugs and ECT may help to prevent relapse.

Light therapy

In so-called *seasonal affective disorder* most episodes of depression are clearly linked to the season of the year. Light therapy has proved effective in some patients and may be prophylactic. It involves the patient in sitting in very bright artificial light for 2 hours every day for one to two weeks. Such treatment is still regarded as experimental.

Psychosurgery

Prefrontal leucotomy, which was first introduced by Moniz in 1935, has largely fallen into disuse. The original technique has been abandoned since the operation was often followed by adverse personality changes. Many modifications have since been introduced, of which the technique of *stereotactic subcaudate tractotomy* probably produces the best results in terms of relief of symptoms and freedom from side effects. Such psychosurgical techniques are now only very rarely used in the United Kingdom.

Indications

The prime indication for surgical intervention is prolonged and persistent tension and anxiety, particularly when this, as it does rarely, occurs almost in pure form. Probably, however, such operations are of greater use in patients in late middle age with chronic agitated depression who have become resistant to other forms of treatment. Although some may later relapse, they may, however, then be found to be responsive once again to other forms of treatment such as ECT. Others who may respond are patients crippled by severe obsessions in whom all other methods of treatment may have been found to be useless. Even so, psychosurgery is by no means always effective.

It is generally agreed that surgery should only be considered after all other treatments – physical, pharmacological and psychological – have been given a thorough trial. The best results, as in all forms of therapy, are obtained in those of good pre-morbid personality characterized by drive, activity and warm affect. Those who are inert, inadequate or of unduly rigid outlook do not do well; neither do those with antisocial traits.

Contra-indications

Psychosurgery is contra-indicated in dementia and particularly in those with cerebral arteriosclerosis who are liable to postoperative cerebral haemorrhage. It is also useless in vegetative and anergic states, as in simple schizophrenia and chronic hebephrenia. It is likely to be harmful in antisocial and inadequate individuals, in whom the operation may aggravate an existing behaviour disorder, leading to aggression and irresponsible actions.

Complications

The operative mortality is very low indeed. Epileptic fits used to occur after the now obsolete leucotomy operations but rarely with modern techniques. Similarly, temporary confusion and enuresis used to be common, but do not usually occur with more up-to-date procedures. Some changes in personality are inevitable, though once again with modern techniques and in the presence of a good pre-morbid personality, these are usually minimal. Some gain in weight is usual. This is occasionally excessive owing to the development of a ravenous appetite (hyperphagia).

Further reading

Crammer, J.L. and Heine, B. (1991) *The Use of Drugs in Psychiatry*, 3rd edn, London: Gaskell.
Fraser, M. (1982) *ECT, A Clinical Guide*, Chichester: Wiley.
Lader, M. and Herrington R. (1990) *Biological Treatments in Psychiatry*, Oxford: Oxford University Press.
Palmer, R. (1981) *Electroconvulsive Therapy: An Appraisal*, Oxford: Oxford University Press.
Royal College of Psychiatrists (1989) *The Practical Administration of Electroconvulsive Therapy*, London: Gaskell.
Trimble, M. (1988) *Biological Psychiatry*, Chichester: Wiley.

24

Psychiatry and the law

In order to begin to understand the relationship between psychiatry and the law, some historical background is essential. In 1700 there were in the United Kingdom very few hospitals receiving mentally ill patients. Throughout the eighteenth century a few more hospitals were founded, many of them associated with religious foundations (for example, The Retreat, established in York in 1792 by the Quaker Tuke family). However, much of the care of the mentally ill – 'lunatics' or 'the insane', in the terminology of the time – was carried out in 'private madhouses'. These establishments were small-scale institutions whose proprietors were paid by relatives of the inmate to accommodate the insane person in a secure setting. Where there was no money, fees of 'pauper lunatics' were sometimes paid for by parish funds. Some have likened the situation to that in the 1980s which saw a boom in entrepreneurial small-scale developments in accommodation for the mentally ill (particularly elderly patients) outside the public sector, but with fees for some drawn from the public purse.

A particular problem with the eighteenth-century private madhouses was a lack of safeguards for inmates. The law offered no protection against wrongful detention of persons who were not insane, nor against ill-treatment; private madhouses became notorious for the appalling conditions in which a great many inmates were held.

As is so often the case, public disquiet,

publicity and official enquiry led to legislative change. A series of Acts of Parliament spanning more than 200 years was begun in 1774, the most recent in 1983. During the first of these two centuries of legislation, two themes were pursued. Various *Lunacy Acts* dealt with procedures for lawful detention of lunatics, while two *Asylums Acts* enabled and later forced county authorities to establish public hospitals for the accommodation of pauper lunatics. By 1850 there were many such county asylums and effective laws governing the care of patients.

Although, during the second half of the last century and the early years of this century, there was gradual yet marked improvement in their care and conditions, there was little public acceptance of the mentally ill. Victorian hospital building had done something *for* the mentally ill but had also done something *about* them: arranged for their care in large institutions standing in even larger grounds, often on the outskirts of towns and cities, if not out in the countryside. It is in the last half-century or so that it has been the focus of law and social policy to bridge the gap between provision for the mentally ill and the population from which the patients have come.

A landmark in this bridging process was the 1930 Mental Treatment Act which permitted voluntary admissions to mental hospitals for the very first time. Arthur Greenwood, introducing the Act as Minister of Health in the 1929–31 Labour government, said that it 'means we have ceased to think of mental disorder as something that is so indecent that it has to be kept in a category of its own'.

Although voluntary admissions were permitted, the situation after 1930 was not as we know it today. There was a three-tier system of voluntary, temporary and certified patients. Voluntary patients were required to sign a written application at the time of admission and, although not subject to detention, they were required to give 72 hours' notice of intention to leave, during which time arrangements could be made for certification if the doctor in charge felt it appropriate. Temporary patients were admitted compulsorily on the application of a relative or a local authority officer supported by two recommendations. Certified patients, except for the initial period in an emergency, were admitted on the basis of an order made by a Justice of the Peace or other judicial authority. Thus, despite a growing proportion of voluntary patients and a gradual development of outpatient clinical activity, the judicial system was involved in a large proportion of admissions even when there was no criminal aspect to the case. In addition, a great many hospital wards remained locked.

Following World War II, with the formation of a National Health Service which included provision for mental illness, a number of changes were set to occur in the 1950s. First, the inertia of the old asylum hierarchy was changing and the effective control of day-to-day policy passed, in many hospitals, to younger and more idealistic medical superintendents who ushered in many changes. They were responsible for the unlocking of doors so that wards in psychiatric hospitals began to become open in the way they are today. Second, there was gradual reduction in hospital size due to a substantial rise in discharge rate, together with the institution of hostels, day hospitals and community-based staff. Dingleton Hospital at Melrose in the Scottish Borders, under the charge of Dr George McDonald Bell, became the first completely open (no locked wards) psychiatric hospital in the English-speaking world. Mapperley Hospital, Nottingham, was, in 1953, the first fully open hospital in England; its superintendent, Dr Duncan MacMillan, was also responsible for an

enormous reduction in the hospital's size. Numbers of psychiatric inpatients in the United Kingdom have been decreasing since 1954. Fewer beds, shorter admissions and increasing community care was in progress long before the government policy of the 1980s made it a contentious issue.

For the changing service, developing beyond the old hospital walls, the legal restrictions were increasingly outmoded. In 1954 a Royal Commission, under the chairmanship of Baron Percy of Newcastle, was set up to examine the law relating to mental illness, and a new law, the Mental Health Act, became statute in 1959. It was a radical accompaniment to the changes in social management of psychiatric patients. It repealed all existing mental health legislation and made it clear that voluntary admission would become the most usual procedure. In practice, enactment of the new legislation was taken as a signal for a huge increase in the proportion of patients admitted informally. David Clark, one of the reforming medical superintendents of the 1950s, related that whilst there were a few voluntary patients on the admission wards, 90 per cent of patients at Fulbourn Hospital, Cambridge, in the middle 1950s were certified; when the appointed day for enactment of the new law arrived in 1959, certification was removed from all the patients. After a brief period of adjustment they settled down to about 12 per cent of admissions and only 8 per cent of the resident hospital population as detained patients.

Throughout the whole country, the 1959 Mental Health Act was well received amongst professional staff working with mental illness and in the wider community. The present Mental Health Act, a revision of the 1959 Act, introduced a number of important changes, but its general spirit is very close to that of its immediate predecessor.

The Mental Health Act (1983)

Although the Act is most evident in relation to patients' admission to and detention in hospital on a compulsory ('formal') basis, one of its most important features is an explicit indication that the great majority of admissions to hospital will be voluntary ('informal'). Except in the designated secure units and special hospitals, about 90 per cent of admissions to psychiatric units and hospitals in the United Kingdom are informal. The proportion of compulsory admissions may reach 20 per cent or even more in some units serving inner-city and metropolitan areas.

The Act deals with many matters other than those concerning compulsory admissions. For example, it states that for informal patients, certain designated treatments which are irreversible or hazardous (for example, psychosurgery) may not be undertaken even with the patient's full and informed consent until a senior psychiatrist from another health district, appointed independently, has carried out certain procedures and is satisfied that the treatment is indicated. It contains regulations about treatment. For compulsorily detained patients, the Act stipulates under which section patients should be detained before certain treatments may be given and the urgent measures that may be taken in an emergency. A large part of the Act refers to the relation between psychiatry and the criminal law, the courts and the prisons.

The parts of the Act of most general relevance deal with compulsory admission to hospital. The general principles guiding its use, rather than the various sections and their numbers, are described here. These principles will be outlined by describing first the application of the most widely used procedure for compulsory admission – that for admission for *assessment* for up to 28 days.

Compulsory admission for assessment

The procedure for admission has three components: medical recommendation, application for admission, and acceptance or receipt of a patient by the hospital managers.

Medical recommendation

A medical recommendation must be made in writing by a *registered* medical practitioner (not a pre-registration house officer) on the appropriate form. An example is shown as Figure 24.1. First, the doctor must be of the opinion that the patient is suffering from *mental disorder*. The phrase 'mental disorder' is a technical term defined in the Act as 'mental illness, arrested or incomplete development of mind, psychopathic disorder and any other disorder or disability of mind'.

Arrested or incomplete development of mind is sub-divided into two categories: severe mental impairment and mental impairment, which are given brief descriptions. A brief comment on psychopathic disorder is also provided in the Act, and these brief descriptions are reproduced in Table 24.1, together with a further note about several situations which are excluded from the category of mental illness. It will be evident that the scanty information conveys little by way of diagnostic guidance. Indeed, the term 'mental illness' is not provided with even the briefest of definitions; it is left entirely to the professional judgement of the medical practitioner to judge whether the patient is suffering from mental illness

Next, mental disorder being present, the doctor must decide whether it is of a nature or degree which warrants detention of the patient in hospital for assessment. No specific guidance is available in the Act upon this issue of severity. However, it is necessary for the practitioner making the recommendation to assert that hospital detention ought to take place in the interests of the patient's own health or safety or with a view to protection of others, or both.

Finally a brief statement must be recorded to support the assertion that, having judged admission to be necessary, it may not be voluntary. For example, the doctor might record that a patient who has recently stopped receiving depot neuroleptic injections has delusions and hallucinations, has threatened violence to his father, and refuses to agree to treatment or admission.

For the patient to be admitted for assessment for a period of up to 28 days, *two medical recommendations* are required. One of these must be completed by a doctor who has, in the terms of

Medical recommendation for admission for assessment

Mental Health Act 1983
Section 2

(full name and
address of medical
practitioner)

I

a registered medical practitioner, recommend that

(full name and address
of patient)

be admitted to a hospital for assessment in accordance with Part II of the Mental Health Act 1983.

I last examined this patient on

(date)

*Delete if not
applicable

*I had previous acquaintance with the patient before I conducted that examination.

* I have been approved by the Secretary of State under section 12 of the Act as having special experience in the diagnosis or treatment of mental disorder.

I am of the opinion

(a) that the patient is suffering from mental disorder of a nature or degree which warrants detention of the patient in a hospital for assessment

AND

Delete (i) or (ii)
unless both apply.

(b) that this patient ought to be so detained
(i) in the interests of the patient's own health or safety
(ii) with a view to the protection of other persons

AND

(c) that informal admission is not appropriate in the circumstances of this case for the following reasons:-

(Reasons should state why informal admission is not appropriate)

Signed _____ Date _____

Figure 24.1 Example of form for medical recommendation for admission for assessment

Table 24.1   *Application of Mental Health Act: 'mental disorder'*

In this Act –

- *'Mental disorder'* means mental illness, arrested or incomplete development of mind, psychopathic disorder and any other disorder or disability of mind and 'mentally disordered' shall be construed accordingly.
- *'Severe mental impairment'* means a state of arrested or incomplete development of mind which includes severe impairment of intelligence and social functioning and is associated with abnormally aggressive or seriously irresponsible conduct on the part of the person concerned.
- *'Mental impairment'* means a state of arrested or incomplete development of mind (not amounting to severe mental impairment) which includes significant impairment of intelligence and social functioning and is associated with abnormally aggressive or seriously irresponsible conduct on the part of the person concerned.
- *'Psychopathic disorder'* means a persistent disorder or disability of mind (whether or not including significant impairment of intelligence) which results in abnormally aggressive or seriously irresponsible conduct on the part of the person concerned.

Nothing in this section shall be construed as implying that a person may be dealt with under this Act as suffering from mental disorder or from any form of mental disorder described in this section, by reason only of promiscuity or other immoral conduct, sexual deviancy or dependence on alcohol or drugs.

the Act, been approved by the Secretary of State for Health as having special experience in the diagnosis or treatment of mental disorder. In practice, this will most often be an experienced psychiatrist, preferably a consultant or senior registrar. Regional Health Authorities each authorize such recognition of doctors on behalf of the Secretary of State, so the policy on who is placed on the list varies between regions.

By preference, the other recommendation is completed by a doctor who already knows the patient – ideally, the general practitioner. However, there are many reasons why it is not always possible to locate such a person and this objective is not mandatory. Any other registered practitioner may make a recommendation, but one of the two must be approved as having special psychiatric experience.

Application for admission

Doctors may 'recommend' a compulsory admission, but it cannot be effected until an *application* is made to the hospital. An application may be made by either an approved social worker or the patient's nearest relative. The nearest relative may, for instance, be a spouse or a parent; the Act contains a list in order of precedence. In practice, however, approved social workers are much more often signatories than are relatives. Indeed, in many areas applications by relatives are all but unknown. Many feel that asking or allowing a nearest relative to make a formal application for compulsory admission is unfortunate and to be avoided if at all possible.

In order to be 'approved' social workers must undergo specific training in the use of the Mental Health Act. Sometimes, for social workers who generally work in areas other than mental health, this training may consist only of a secondment to a relatively short course. Often, though, Approved Social Workers work in the mental health field and are well used to compulsory admission assessments.

Admission of the patient to the hospital

When the necessary forms have been completed the patient may be taken to an appropriate hospital ward. The nursing staff in charge of the ward will receive the patient and the papers on behalf of the hospital managers. A hospital is not obliged to accept a patient, and those making recommendations and applications will have ensured, prior to the patient's arrival, that a bed will be available. It is usual – indeed, good policy – for the Approved Social Worker to accompany the patient to hospital.

Admission as an emergency

It will be evident from the above accounts that compulsory admission may be delayed by failure to locate appropriate professional staff. Such delay may be clinically inappropriate, and use is occasionally made of powers under the Act to admit a patient for assessment as an emergency. Following only *one* medical recommendation and an application, a patient may be admitted for up to 72 hours. When, during that time, the second recommendation is made, the full 28-day order comes into force.

From the point of view of patient protection, this arrangement is clearly less satisfactory and is avoided where possible. Many health districts have policies agreed between medical and social-work staff which confine use of such emergency orders to a very small proportion of compulsory admissions. Urgent assessments may be requested by: general practitioners in patient's homes (or homes of friends or relatives); hospital doctors, usually in accident and emergency departments; or police surgeons dealing with persons in police custody. An effective duty rota of senior psychiatric staff available and willing, when emergencies arise, to assess patients (wherever necessary and at all hours) helps to minimize admissions on an emergency order. It should be possible to effect compulsory admission, even in florid emergency situations, under the full powers of the 28-day assessment order.

Admission for treatment

On occasions, arrangements are made for *admission for treatment* instead of for assessment. The order lasts for up to 6 months instead of for 28 days. Most of the usual drug treatments may be given on an assessment order, but for some patients, often those well-known to psychiatric services, it is clear to those arranging the compulsory admission that treatment, probably for longer than 28 days, will be required. Admission for treatment requires the same kind of application and medical recommendations as does admission for assessment. A treatment order of this kind may also be invoked after admission, when a patient refuses treatment but is deemed likely to benefit from it.

Further detention in hospital

When a 28-day assessment order expires, the patient's status becomes informal; the order may not be renewed. Some patients require further detention in hospital, and a 6-month treatment order is the usual procedure, even if it seems likely that only a week or so will be required before informal care becomes appropriate. The procedure for so detaining patients already in hospital is identical with that for admission for treatment; the two medical recommendations should not, however, both be made by doctors working at the same hospital. Such long-term orders are frequently rescinded by consultants in charge of cases as soon as they feel that informal care has become appropriate.

From time to time informal patients too may require detention on a compulsory basis. When this becomes evident, arrangements are usually made to institute an assessment order or a treatment order, as described above. Where an informal patient *suddenly* wishes to discharge himself without staff agreement, further powers are allowed for under the Act. For example, a depressed patient admitted voluntarily may, before treatment has been effective, worsen and become deluded; when, late at night, he wishes to leave, telling others of self-destructive intent arising from delusional thinking, he may be legally detained. Where there is deemed to be risk to self or others should the patient leave, detention for up to 72 hours may be instituted by the written instruction of the responsible medical officer or his nominated deputy. There is no requirement for a second medical recommendation or an application. Before the doctor attends, a suitably qualified psychiatric nurse may detain the patient for up to 6 hours. As this action has few safeguards against brief confinement in the hospital, its use is usually limited to small numbers of patients. Great efforts are made to move on to the more satisfactory detention procedures as soon as possible after the temporary holding power has been applied.

Duties of local authorities

For many years local authorities have had a responsibility to provide care for those with mental health problems. As well as employing social workers, care includes the provision of residential accommodation and centres for training, occupation and education. The 1983 Mental Health Act also places a specific duty on local authorities to provide after-care for discharged detained patients for so long as it may be necessary.

The 1990s should see this role increasing under the provisions outlined in the government White Paper 'Caring for people' and enacted by the National Health Service and Community Care Act (1991). Local authority Social Services Departments are to have an increased and more central coordinating role in the care of those mentally ill patients who need continuing social help.

Mental Health Act Commission

The Mental Health Act Commission was set up under the legislation changes of 1983. The Commission has members drawn from the ranks of doctors, nurses, social workers, psychologists and others and has various responsibilities. It appoints doctors to provide second opinions about compulsory treatment and the Commission members are required to visit annually each hospital which admits patients compulsorily to interview patients, investigate complaints and undertake a general protective function for detained patients. The Commission is required to publish reports which must be laid before Parliament.

Consent to treatment

Certain psychiatric treatments have legal restrictions upon their use. Even for voluntary patients, psychosurgery cannot be carried out without consent from the patient *and* the statement, in writing, by an independently appointed psychiatrist and two other non-medical persons that the patient's consent is fully informed. For compulsory patients detained on a treatment order, drug treatment may be administered for the first three months. Thereafter, the patient must consent or an independently appointed doctor must see the patient and agree. These stipulations also apply to ECT at any stage during detention for treatment. *Urgent treatment* may, in certain circumstances, be given despite some of these restrictions.

Forensic psychiatry

Forensic psychiatry is a large subject, and one of growing importance, but no more than a brief introduction can be given here. Although there is clearly some overlap, it must be emphasized that crime and mental illness are by no means synonymous. Although there are mental illnesses which may occasionally give rise to criminal behaviour – for example, delusional states may lead to homicide, depression to shoplifting and early dementia to sexual indecency – most offenders, however deviant their behaviour, cannot be considered as mentally abnormal. Likewise, most of those who suffer from mental illness are law abiding. Bearing this in mind, it has to be said that there remains a 'grey area', in which a decision has to be made as to just how much a person who has committed some offence can be held responsible at law on account of their mental condition. Such a decision is clearly necessary not only so that justice can be done but also in order that the person concerned may be dealt with by the court as appropriately as possible.

There are three aspects to be considered. First, the subject may be suffering from a mental disorder at the time of committing an offence, and when brought to trial the issue of criminal responsibility may, therefore, be raised. Second, he may be found to be mentally disordered when called to account for his actions, whereupon the issue may be his fitness to plead. Third, he may be found to be mentally disordered at the time of sentencing, in which case transfer to hospital may be considered.

Criminal responsibility

There has been much discussion of criminal responsibility without arriving at a completely satisfactory compromise between the medical and legal points of view. Interest was first aroused in 1843 when a certain Daniel McNaghton was acquitted of murder on account of suffering from delusions of persecution. After his trial the judges of the country were asked to confer and to express their opinion. This, in summary, was as follows:

> In order to plead insanity in defence of a criminal act, it must be proved that at the time of committing the act, the party accused was labouring under such defect of reason from the disease of the mind as not to know the nature and quality of the act he was doing, or, if he did know it, that he did not know he was doing what was (legally) wrong and punishable.

This is the legal test. The onus rests on the defence to raise the evidence and prove to a 'balance of probabilities' that the insanity of the defendant (usually some form of delusion) was the direct cause of the crime he committed. The defendant is not to be held responsible if he acts in a way which would be permissible if his delusions were true. The McNaghton Rules are now relatively rarely applied; the doctrine of *diminished responsibility*, operative in Scotland for some considerable time, became embodied in English criminal law under Section 2 (1) of the Homicide Act (1957):

> where a person kills or is a party to killing another, he shall not be convicted of murder if he was suffering from such abnormality of mind (whether arising from a condition of arrested or retarded development of mind or any inherent causes or induced by disease or injury) as substantially impaired his mental responsibility for his acts.

Where a defence is successful under the McNaghton Rules, the verdict will be 'not guilty by reason of insanity' leading to mandatory hospital admission with restrictions and without limit of time. In contrast, a plea of diminished responsibility is a plea which, if successful, reduces a charge of murder to one of manslaughter, thus avoiding a mandatory life sentence and allowing the court a greater range of disposal. A defence of diminished responsibility may only be raised in homicide cases.

Automatism

Automatism, such as may occur in association with temporal lobe epileptic seizures, can form a defence if it can be shown that, at the time of committing an offence, the accused was unconscious or his actions were purely automatic. Two types of automatism have been formulated: *insane* and *non-insane*. In the former instance, there will be evidence of mental disease leading to the case being dealt with under the McNaghton Rules. In the case of non-insane automatism (for example, somnambulism), this, if proved, and there being no evidence of insanity, will lead to acquittal.

Infanticide

The charge of infanticide is brought in lieu of murder in the case of a mother who due to a 'disturbance of mind' kills her child within a year and a day of its birth. The charge is, once again, an alternative to one of murder and allows for a wider range of sentence; in the case of infanticide, sentence is often more lenient than for some other forms of homicide.

There are a large number of crimes less serious than murder in which the mental state of the defendant may be considered in terms of *mitigation of sentence*.

Shoplifting

Shoplifting is occasionally associated with a variety of mental disorders, particularly in the young, the elderly and in middle-aged women. These disorders are taken into account when sentencing. The defendant is often placed on probation with or without a requirement of psychiatric treatment.

Sexual offences

Certain sexual offences result from loss of control such as may occur in epilepsy or dementia; sometimes even depressive illness may lead to sexual misdemeanours or crimes. Middle-aged depressed male patients suffering from waning potency sometimes commit acts of indecent exposure, although the large majority of those who do so are younger and are not usually suffering from depressive illness (see Chapter 14).

Fitness to plead

A defendant should be mentally capable of instructing counsel, appreciating the nature of the charge and the significance of pleading 'Guilty' or 'Not guilty', challenging a juror, examining a witness and understanding and following the evidence and court procedure.

The question of his inability to do so on account of 'insanity' may be raised when called upon to account for his actions by the defence, the prosecution or by the judge himself, or in the course of the hearing. When a prisoner is found to be unfit to plead, an order is made out for his detention in a hospital named by the Home Secretary where he is detained under conditions similar to those which pertain to other mentally abnormal offenders admitted to hospital (see below). If his mental condition subsequently improves, the Home Secretary, after consultation with the responsible medical officer, has powers to remit him for trial. This power, however, is used sparingly owing to complications which may arise in the prosecution of a person who has been in hospital a long time.

Admission of mentally abnormal offenders to hospital

Where a person is found guilty of an offence punishable by imprisonment but the court is satisfied on the evidence of two medical practitioners (one approved under the Act as having special psychiatric experience and one a doctor from the receiving hospital) that he is suffering from mental disorder, the court may make an order authorizing his admission to a specified hospital. The mental disorder may be mental illness, psychopathic disorder, mental impairment or severe mental impairment (see Table 24.1). The medical recommendation must state the grounds justifying admission; they are similar to those pertaining to the standard admission for up to 6 months for treatment. The order may be renewed after 6 months, a further 6 months and then at annual intervals, and the responsible medical officer may discharge the patient at any time that he considers appropriate. In the case of a magistrates' court, such an order can be made without recording a conviction. Such an order cannot be made in this way in a Crown court.

In the Crown court, the judge may, additionally, impose restrictions preventing the patient either from being discharged or having leave of absence without the agreement of the Home Secretary. These restriction orders may be applied for a period of time or indeterminately. The judge must hear oral evidence and may only make an order restricting discharge if he is satisfied that it is necessary to protect the public from serious harm.

The court may require a health authority or its representative to give evidence about appropriate facilities for treatment if there is difficulty in finding a hospital place. Regular reports on restricted patients must be sent to the Home Secretary. The patient may be recalled or taken into custody if necessary while conditionally discharged or on leave of absence.

An offender who becomes mentally ill while on remand and awaiting trial or while serving a term of imprisonment may, by order of the Home Secretary, be transferred to a special or ordinary mental hospital after certain specified medical recommendations have been made.

The requirements for consent to treatment apply to patients under all the above detention orders.

Remands to hospital

The Mental Health Act (1983) allows a court to remand an accused person in hospital *for a report* to be prepared on his mental condition (an alternative to remand in custody), or *for treatment* if certain specified medical recommendations are made. There are a number of other powers and orders in this complex part of the Mental Health Act which are not described here but may be read about in the references at the end of this chapter.

Probation with a condition of treatment

Where a court is satisfied, on the evidence of a medical practitioner approved under the Mental Health Act as having special psychiatric experience, that the mental condition of an offender requires and would be susceptible to treatment, it may, instead of ordering compulsory admission to hospital, make a particular kind of probation order. This order, under the Powers of Criminal Courts Act (1973), requires that the offender shall submit, during either a part or all of his probationary period, to psychiatric treatment with a view to bringing about an improvement in his mental condition. Various circumstances may be specified, including treatment as a patient in hospital or as an outpatient. According to changing circumstances, some variation in these provisions can be made on the advice of the medical officer.

Juvenile courts

Juvenile offenders come before special courts in which there is considerable modification of usual law-court procedure. As far as possible, each juvenile offence is dealt with as an individual problem. In some cases the magistrate will call for a medical and psychiatric report.

Civil issues

Contracts

A contract made before the onset of mental dis-
order is binding. A person of unsound mind may make contracts for the necessaries of life, and such contracts are also binding. However, judge and jury may decide what shall be included under the term 'necessaries'.

A person of unsound mind may also make contracts for articles other than necessaries, but such contracts are not binding if they are such as would not have been made but for 'insanity' at the time of making the contract.

Marriage and 'insanity'

A marriage is not valid if at the time of marriage either party was so mentally disordered as not to appreciate the nature of the contract. If such a degree of mental disorder can be proved, the marriage may be decreed null and void after application to the divorce court.

Torts

Torts are offences for which a person is liable in civil as opposed to criminal law. These include libel, slander, trespass and nuisance. A person so wronged by a person of unsound mind would probably be awarded only nominal damages in a court of law.

Receivership

The Court of Protection is an office of the Supreme Court. Its function is to manage and administer the property and affairs of those who, because of mental disorders, cannot do so themselves. The court consists of a Master, 'nominated' judges and a number of Assistant Masters. The court requires an application, usually from a relative or close friend, supported by medical evidence that the individual concerned is incapable, because of mental disorder, of managing his affairs. If the court accepts this evidence, it appoints a Receiver (in Scotland *Curator bonis*), preferably a near relative or friend willing and able to act as such, but failing this, another responsible person, most often the Official Solicitor to the Supreme Court. The powers of the Receiver are strictly defined and limited in such a way as to safeguard absolutely the patient's estate, the administration of which is vested entirely in the court. The court has no control over the patient's person, only his property. Thus the court cannot direct where a patient shall live or that he shall enter or leave a hospital, although it is able to exercise considerable influence over matters of this kind through control of his property. The degree of mental disorder required to give the court jurisdiction is quite distinct from, and much less severe than, that which is required for compulsory detention in hospital under the Mental Health Act.

The court relies greatly on the goodwill and cooperation of doctors. If it becomes apparent to a general practitioner or a hospital doctor that a patient is becoming incapable of managing his affairs, it is the duty of the doctor to advise a patient's relatives of the risks of the situation and, if they refuse to make the necessary application to the court, to do so himself. While a doctor may be reluctant to take such a step, he or she must fully appreciate that the responsibility of any action taken or not taken on medical evidence is entirely that of the court. Some disastrous cases, in which dissipation of a person's entire assets occurs, would be avoided if doctors fully realized their responsibility in this matter.

Testamentary capacity

Only a person with a 'sound disposing mind' can make a valid will. Compulsory detention in itself is no bar, nor is mental disorder necessarily in itself. The following points should be noted when examining a patient with regard to his testamentary capacity:

1 His ability to realize the nature of a will and its consequences.

2 His ability to recall the nature and extent of his property, but not necessarily his ability to recall details of a large estate.
3 His ability to recall the names of all near relatives and to weigh the claims of these and possibly others on his estate.
4 Absence of a morbid state of mind which might pervert the natural feelings of the testator and influence him in his decisions. It is, however, possible for a testator to be deluded and yet to retain a sound disposing mind provided that his delusions are not of such a nature that they are likely to influence his testamentary disposition.
5 A testator may, of course, take the advice of others and have regard to their wishes about the disposition of his property, but must not be influenced by them through fear or by the threat of force. It must be said, however, that such influences are often of a subtler and more intangible kind and not always easy to assess.
6 In case of doubt, the testator should be re-examined after a period of time.

Patients under the jurisdiction of the Court of Protection are discouraged from making wills unless there is medical evidence of testamentary capacity.

Further reading

Bluglass, R. (1983) *A Guide to the Mental Health Act 1983*, Edinburgh: Churchill Livingstone.
Bluglass, R. and Bowden, P. (eds) (1990) *Principles and Practice of Forensic Psychiatry*, Edinburgh: Churchill Livingstone.
Faulk, M. (1988) *Basic Forensic Psychiatry*, Oxford: Blackwell Scientific Publications.
Gostin, L. (1983) *A Practical Guide to Mental Health Law*, London: National Association for Mental Health.

Index

Figures in *italic*, Tables in **bold**.